METHODS IN PHARMACOLOGY AND TOXICOLOGY

Series Editor
Y. James Kang

For further volumes:
http://www.springer.com/series/7653

Ocular Pharmacology and Toxicology

Edited by

Brian C. Gilger

Department of Clinical Sciences, College of Veterinary Medicine, North Carolina State University, Raleigh, NC, USA

Humana Press

Editor
Brian C. Gilger
Department of Clinical Sciences
College of Veterinary Medicine
North Carolina State University
Raleigh, NC, USA

ISSN 1557-2153 ISSN 1940-6053 (electronic)
ISBN 978-1-4939-6069-9 ISBN 978-1-62703-745-7 (eBook)
DOI 10.1007/978-1-62703-745-7
Springer New York Heidelberg Dordrecht London

Softcover reprint of the hardcover 1st edition 2014

Printed on acid-free paper

Humana Press is a brand of Springer
Springer is part of Springer Science+Business Media (www.springer.com)

Preface

This book's subject is ocular pharmacokinetics, pharmacodynamics, and toxicology. There are detailed chapters on study design, analysis, and routes to regulatory approval for various types and routes of ophthalmic drugs.

The vision for this handbook is to provide ophthalmologists, toxicologists, and pharmacologists with both an introduction to the proper methods for ocular pharmacology and toxicology and providing practical methodologies for conducting ocular studies. Proper design and conduct of these studies are essential to accurately determine pharmacokinetics and ocular toxicity from the systemic, topical, periocular, or intraocular administration of drugs or compounds, from the use of ocular medical devices and from ocular surgical procedures. Not only do the studies need to be appropriately designed, the personnel conducting these studies need to be adequately trained in drug administration, examination techniques, and the processing of ocular tissues. The chapters in this book can be a basis of such training.

Ocular toxicology is a special subspecialty of toxicology that not only evaluates the effects of drugs on ocular tissue administered by the traditional routes of drug delivery to the eye, namely topically, periocularly, and intravitreally, but also is a study of the effect on ocular tissue from nonspecific systemic exposure of drugs (general toxicology) and the toxicologic effect of ocular devices and surgical materials in the eye.

The goal of this book is to review the development of ocular therapeutics from preclinical study design to regulatory approval. Ocular anatomy of common animal models will be reviewed in Chapter 2 and techniques in the bioanalysis of ocular tissues and fluids in Chapter 3. Chemistry, manufacturing, and control (CMC) for ocular drugs are reviewed in Chapter 4, while absorption, distribution, metabolism, and excretion (ADME) of drugs in ocular tissue will be discussed in Chapter 5. Formulations, pharmacokinetics, and toxicity of topical and intravitreal ocular drugs will be reviewed in Chapter 6, while Chapter 7 will focus on the development of sustained-release ocular drug delivery systems.

The role of the ophthalmic examination and toxicity in the realm of general toxicology will be reviewed in Chapter 8, while design and methodologies for the study of glaucoma drugs and ocular medical devices will be discussed in Chapters 9 and 10, respectively. Chapter 11 will focus on the techniques and methodologies for microscopic evaluation of ocular toxicity, while Chapter 12 will review the use of nanoparticles for drug and gene therapy of the eye.

I learned a tremendous amount by reviewing these excellent chapters, and together they provide a basis for the pharmacologic and toxicological assessment of ocular drugs and devices, study design, and routes to regulatory approval.

I thank the authors for their dedication and expertise and Springer Protocols for making this book a reality.

Raleigh, NC, USA *Brian C. Gilger*

Contents

Contributors

EVA ABARCA • *Department of Clinical Sciences, North Carolina State University, Raleigh, NC, USA*
IMRAN AHMED • *Alcon Laboratories, A Novartis Company, Fort Worth, TX, USA*
MICHAEL H. BUONARATI • *Intertek Pharmaceutical Services LCMS, El Dorado Hills, CA, USA*
JOSEPH W. CARRAWAY • *NAMSA, Northwood, OH, USA*
KISHORE CHOLKAR • *Division of Pharmaceutical Sciences, School of Pharmacy, University of Missouri-Kansas City, Kansas City, MO, USA*
CHRISTINE CRISH • *Department of Pharmaceutical Sciences, College of Pharmacy, Northeast Ohio Medical University, Rootstown, OH, USA*
SAMUEL D. CRISH • *Department of Pharmaceutical Sciences, College of Pharmacy, Northeast Ohio Medical University, Rootstown, OH, USA*
ELAINE M. DANIEL • *NAMSA, Northwood, OH, USA*
WERNER J. GELDENHUYS • *Department of Pharmaceutical Sciences, College of Pharmacy, Northeast Ohio Medical University, Rootstown, OH, USA*
MALAY GHOSH • *Alcon Laboratories, A Novartis Company, Fort Worth, TX, USA*
BRIAN C. GILGER • *Department of Clinical Sciences, College of Veterinary Medicine, North Carolina State University, Raleigh, NC, USA*
DENISE INMAN • *Department of Pharmaceutical Sciences, College of Pharmacy, Northeast Ohio Medical University, Rootstown, OH, USA*
UDAY B. KOMPELLA • *Nanomedicine and Drug Delivery Laboratory, Department of Pharmaceutical Sciences, Department of Ophthalmology, and Department of Bioengineering, University of Colorado, Aurora, CO, USA*
SHREYA S. KULKARNI • *Nanomedicine and Drug Delivery Laboratory, Department of Pharmaceutical Sciences, University of Colorado, Aurora, CO, USA*
SUSAN S. LEE • *Allergan, Inc., Irvine, CA, USA*
PAUL E. MILLER • *Comparative Ophthalmology, Department of Surgical Sciences, School of Veterinary Medicine, University of Wisconsin-Madison, Madison, WI, USA*
ASHIM K. MITRA • *Division of Pharmaceutical Sciences, School of Pharmacy, University of Missouri-Kansas City, Kansas City, MO, USA*
JAMES A. RENDER • *NAMSA, Northwood, OH, USA*
MICHAEL R. ROBINSON • *Allergan, Inc., Irvine, CA, USA*
JACKLYN H. SALMON • *Department of Clinical Sciences, North Carolina State University, Raleigh, NC, USA*
LEANDRO B.C. TEIXEIRA • *NAMSA, Northwood, OH, USA*
HOANG M. TRINH • *Division of Pharmaceutical Sciences, School of Pharmacy, University of Missouri-Kansas City, Kansas City, MO, USA*
ASWANI DUTT VADLAPUDI • *Division of Pharmaceutical Sciences, School of Pharmacy, University of Missouri-Kansas City, Kansas City, MO, USA*

Cornelis J. Van der Schyf • *Department of Pharmaceutical Sciences, College of Pharmacy, Northeast Ohio Medical University, Rootstown, OH, USA; Department of Biomedical and Pharmaceutical Sciences, College of Pharmacy, Graduate School of Biomedical and Pharmaceutical Sciences, Idaho State University, Pocatello, ID, USA*
Poonam R. Velagaleti • *I-Novion, Inc., Randolph, NJ, USA*
Scott M. Whitcup • *Allergan, Inc., Irvine, CA, USA*
David A. Wilkie • *Comparative Ophthalmology, Department of Veterinary Clinical Sciences, Veterinary Hospital, The Ohio State University, Columbus, OH, USA*

Methods in Pharmacology and Toxicology (2014): 1–6
DOI 10.1007/7653_2013_1

Published online: 29 August 2013

Challenges in Ocular Pharmacokinetics, Pharmacodynamics, and Toxicology

Brian C. Gilger

Abstract

Study of ocular pharmacology, pharmacodynamics, and toxicology is challenging due to the inherent ocular barriers to drug penetration, small ocular tissue sizes and volumes, and sensitive ocular structures. Additionally, wide variation of ocular sizes and physiology among animal models complicates simple translation of results from one species of animal to another. This chapter, and those to follow, will describe the challenges researchers face regarding ocular pharmacology and toxicology as well as providing them with practical methodologies for conducting studies, including study design and specialized methodology, to overcome these challenges and thus improve treatment of ocular disease.

Key words Ocular pharmacokinetics, Pharmacodynamics, Toxicology, Challenges

1 Introduction

This book's subject is ocular pharmacokinetics, pharmacodynamics, and toxicology. There are detailed chapters on study design, analysis, and routes to regulatory approval for various types and routes of ophthalmic drugs, implants, and devices. The practice of ophthalmology can be reduced to the simple goal of getting the right drug at the appropriate therapeutic dose to the target ocular tissue by a method that does not damage healthy tissue [1]. In treatment of ocular disease, however, this simple goal becomes more challenging because of the highly sensitive ocular tissues (e.g., the lens, uveal tract, and retina) and the presence of tissue barriers to drug penetration, namely the lipophilic corneal epithelium, the hydrophilic corneal and scleral stroma, the conjunctival lymphatics, choroidal vasculature, and the blood-ocular barriers [2–8]. Clearly, pharmacokinetics, pharmacodynamics, and toxicology are closely interrelated for all organ systems and drugs, but for the reasons discussed above, the eye poses significantly more challenges than most other tissues.

By definition, *ocular pharmacokinetics* is the study of the mechanisms of drug absorption, distribution, metabolism, and excretion; onset of action; duration of effect; biotransformation;

and effects and routes of excretion of the metabolites of a drug in the eye. *Ocular pharmacodynamics*, on the other hand, is the study of the biochemical and physiological effects of a drug in the eye, including mechanisms of action. *Ocular toxicology* is the study of effects, including adverse effects, of drugs on ocular tissue.

2 Challenges in Ocular Pharmacokinetics and Pharmacodynamics

Traditionally, medication is delivered to the eye by three main mechanisms: topical ocular administration, systemic administration, and intraocular or periocular injection [7]. Each of these methods has significant disadvantages. Topical ocular solutions or ointments have minimal penetration, rapid dilution, and tear washout and rely substantially on patient compliance to administer the medication. Systemically administered medications, in general, have limited ocular penetration and may require high peripheral drug levels with the potential of toxicity. Ocular or periocular injection of medication is traumatic and invasive, is rapidly diluted, and may require repeat procedures for adequate drug levels. Because of these limitations, other mechanisms for delivery of medications to the eye have been, and are being, developed.

When considering drug delivery in ocular therapeutics, there are three important aspects: duration of drug delivery desired, intended tissue target, and patient compliance [1]. Duration of drug delivery varies from minutes, in the case of topical eye drops, to years, in the case of some ocular implants. The route of drug delivery may determine whether or not the drug can reach the targeted tissue. For example, topical ocular medications are likely to reach the cornea and conjunctiva in therapeutic concentrations, but are unlikely to reach the retina and choroid. Finally, the issue of compliance must be considered in ocular drug delivery. If a drug must be given every hour, for example, to reach therapeutic tissue concentrations when treating a chronic disease, it is very unlikely to be given consistently, if at all, by the patient or caregiver. Therefore, the method of ocular drug delivery must correlate to the intended disease in terms of site of drug target and duration of effect to ensure appropriate compliance by the patient [1].

Depending on site of the target tissue, the main problems to address when ocular drug delivery is attempted are how to localize drug action at this site and maintain therapeutic drug levels while minimizing systemic effects. The main route of topical drug entry to the anterior chamber is penetration through the cornea. The time it takes for most drugs to penetrate into the aqueous humor in peak concentration is 20–60 min. The amount of drug penetrating the cornea is linearly related to its concentration in the tear film, unless the drug has other physiochemical properties that alter its penetration (i.e., interaction with other molecules, adherence to proteins, limited solubility of the drug, metabolism by enzymes in tears). Only 1–10 % of a topical dose of medication ever reaches the anterior chamber while the remainder exits with the tear film through the nasolacrimal system, is deposited on the eyelids, or metabolized by enzymes in the tears and surface tissue. Systemic absorption of some drugs can be significant.

The main ocular barriers to intraocular penetration of drugs delivered periocularly or systemically are the cornea, sclera, and the blood-ocular barriers. The cornea is essentially a fat (epithelium)–water (stroma)–fat (endothelium) multilayered sandwich. The epithelium is the major barrier to absorption, especially for hydrophilic medications. The corneal stroma is a major barrier for lipophilic drugs. Therefore, the drug with the optimum ratio of hydrophilocity and lipophilocity provides best corneal transfer. The strong, fibrous ocular scleral layer is a substantial barrier to the penetration of medication into the eye. The ability of a drug to diffuse across the sclera is directly related to the thickness of the sclera and its total surface area and permeability of a drug across the human sclera decreases as scleral thickness increases [9, 10]. Differences in ocular anatomy and physiology related to ocular pharmacology among commonly used animal models are reviewed in Chapter 2.

Delivery of therapeutics to the posterior segment of the eye, especially the vitreous body and retina, poses a significant challenge. Topical ocular medications may not reach therapeutic drug levels in the posterior segment of the eye and traditional medical therapy methods have their disadvantages when targeting the retina. Ocular injections, both intravitreal and retrobulbar, are invasive and require repeated injections to achieve therapeutic drug levels for chronic diseases. Multiple ocular injections may be associated with complications such as inflammation, retinal detachment, and hemorrhage [1]. Recently, transscleral, intrascleral, suprachoroidal, and intravitreal routes of delivery of therapeutics have been suggested for treatment of retinal disease [1, 7, 11–15]. Intravitreal or suprachoroidal reservoir-type diffusion drug delivery devices have also been developed for long-term therapy of posterior segment diseases [1, 12, 16]. Dr. Mitra and colleagues will go into further detail regarding compositions, formulation, pharmacology, pharmacokinetics, and toxicity of topical, periocular, and intravitreal ophthalmic drugs in Chapter 6. Dr. Uday Kompella and colleagues will provide further detail regarding study design and methodologies for drugs targeting ocular posterior segment diseases in Chapter 12.

3 Challenging Features of Ocular Toxicology

Ocular toxicology is a subspecialty of toxicology that not only studies the effects of drugs on ocular tissue administered by the traditional routes of drug delivery to the eye, namely topically, periocularly, and intravitreally, but also is a study of the effect on ocular tissue from nonspecific systemic exposure of drugs (general toxicology) and the toxicologic effect of ocular devices and surgical materials in the eye. The specialized field of the study of glaucoma therapies and devices will be reviewed by Dr. Paul Miller in Chapter 9, while Dr. David Wilkie, in Chapter 8, will be reviewing the general ophthalmic examination as it pertains to general ocular toxicology including species associated findings. Drs. Joseph Carraway and Elaine Daniel will provide details on study design and methodologies for study of ocular medical devices in Chapter 10. Drs. Mike Robinson and Susan Lee will review the federal regulatory process regarding ocular pharmacology, pharmacokinetics, pharmacodynamics, and toxicity of sustained-release ocular drug delivery systems in Chapter 7 and Dr. Imran Ahmed will review the chemistry, manufacturing, and control (CMC) for ocular medications in Chapter 4.

Also important in the study of ocular pharmacology, pharmacokinetics, and toxicology is the bioanalysis of ocular tissues and fluids, which will be reviewed in Chapter 3 by Drs. Poonam Velagaleti and Michael Buonarati, and the absorption, distribution, metabolism, and excretion of drugs in ocular tissue, which will be reviewed in Chapter 5 by Dr. Neels J. Van der Schyf and colleagues. Histopathologic effects of ocular drugs, devices, and therapies will be reviewed by Drs. Leandro Teixeira and James Render in Chapter 11.

4 Summary

The vision for this handbook is to provide ophthalmologists, toxicologists, and pharmacologists with both an introduction to the proper methods for ocular pharmacology and toxicology as well as providing them with practical methodologies for conducting studies, including study design and specialized methodology for ocular tissue. Proper design and conduct of these studies are important because they evaluate the potential for ocular toxicity or other adverse effects arising from the systemic, topical, or other administration of drugs or compounds, the use of medical devices, or certain surgical procedures. While in some cases the studies are designed to provide proof of concept as regards therapeutic efficacy, in the majority of cases studies are being conducted specifically to enable an adequate assessment of safety of test materials and devices in consideration of meeting FDA (or other similar regulating agencies) approval for initiation of human clinical trials (supporting an investigational new drug [IND] and/or investigational device [IDE] application). Therefore, it is important that those conducting these studies be appropriately and adequately trained. This text can be a valuable resource for this training, but it is not a replacement for formal training obtained in residency and/or graduate programs. For example, veterinary ophthalmologists (i.e., Diplomates of the American College of Veterinary Ophthalmologists; see www.acvo.org) are recognized to have the unique training and experience to appropriately conduct ophthalmic examination and surgical procedures as part of preclinical evaluations of ophthalmic drugs, devices, or techniques.

References

1. Weiner AL, Gilger BC (2010) Advancements in ocular drug delivery. Vet Ophthalmol 13 (6):395–406
2. Kim SH, Lutz RJ, Wang NS, Robinson MR (2007) Transport barriers in transscleral drug delivery for retinal diseases. Ophthalmic Res 39 (5):244–254
3. Kim SH, Galban CJ, Lutz RJ, Dedrick RL, Csaky KG, Lizak MJ, Wang NS, Tansey G, Robinson MR (2007) Assessment of subconjunctival and intrascleral drug delivery to the posterior segment using dynamic contrast-enhanced magnetic resonance imaging. Invest Ophthalmol Vis Sci 48(2):808–814
4. Robinson MR, Lee SS, Kim H, Kim S, Lutz RJ, Galban C, Bungay PM, Yuan P, Wang NS, Kim J, Csaky KG (2006) A rabbit model for assessing the ocular barriers to the transscleral delivery of triamcinolone acetonide. Exp Eye Res 82 (3):479–487
5. Kim H, Lizak MJ, Tansey G, Csaky KG, Robinson MR, Yuan P, Wang NS, Lutz RJ (2005) Study of ocular transport of drugs released from an intravitreal implant using magnetic resonance imaging. Ann Biomed Eng 33 (2):150–164
6. Kim H, Robinson MR, Lizak MJ, Tansey G, Lutz RJ, Yuan P, Wang NS, Csaky KG (2004) Controlled drug release from an ocular implant: an evaluation using dynamic three-dimensional magnetic resonance imaging. Invest Ophthalmol Vis Sci 45(8):2722–2731
7. Davis JL, Gilger BC, Robinson MR (2004) Novel approaches to ocular drug delivery. Curr Opin Mol Ther 6(2):195–205
8. Lee TW, Robinson JR (2001) Drug delivery to the posterior segment of the eye: some insights on the penetration pathways after subconjunctival injection. J Ocul Pharmacol Ther 17 (6):565–572
9. Cruysberg LP, Nuijts RM, Gilbert JA, Geroski DH, Hendrikse F, Edelhauser HF (2005) In vitro sustained human transscleral drug delivery of fluorescein-labeled dexamethasone and methotrexate with fibrin sealant. Curr Eye Res 30(8):653–660
10. Lee SB, Geroski DH, Prausnitz MR, Edelhauser HF (2004) Drug delivery through the sclera: effects of thickness, hydration, and sustained release systems. Exp Eye Res 78 (3):599–607
11. Patel SR, Lin AS, Edelhauser HF, Prausnitz MR (2011) Suprachoroidal drug delivery to the back of the eye using hollow microneedles. Pharm Res 28(1):166–176
12. Robinson MR, Whitcup SM (2012) Pharmacologic and clinical profile of dexamethasone intravitreal implant. Exp Rev Clin Pharmacol 5(6):629–647
13. Simpson AE, Gilbert JA, Rudnick DE, Geroski DH, Aaberg TM Jr, Edelhauser HF (2002) Transscleral diffusion of carboplatin: an in vitro and in vivo study. Arch Ophthalmol 120(8):1069–1074
14. Lee SS, Kim H, Wang NS, Bungay PM, Gilger BC, Yuan P, Kim J, Csaky KG, Robinson MR (2007) A pharmacokinetic and safety evaluation of an episcleral cyclosporine implant for potential use in high-risk keratoplasty rejection. Invest Ophthalmol Vis Sci 48(5):2023–2029

15. Gilger BC, Salmon JH, Wilkie DA, Cruysberg LP, Kim J, Hayat M, Kim H, Kim S, Yuan P, Lee SS, Harrington SM, Murray PR, Edelhauser HF, Csaky KG, Robinson MR (2006) A novel bioerodible deep scleral lamellar cyclosporine implant for uveitis. Invest Ophthalmol Vis Sci 47(6):2596–2605

16. Gilger BC, Wilkie DA, Clode AB, McMullen RJ Jr, Utter ME, Komaromy AM, Brooks DE, Salmon JH (2010) Long-term outcome after implantation of a suprachoroidal cyclosporine drug delivery device in horses with recurrent uveitis. Vet Ophthalmol 13(5):294–300

Methods in Pharmacology and Toxicology (2014): 7–32
DOI 10.1007/7653_2013_2

Published online: 29 August 2013

Selection of Appropriate Animal Models in Ocular Research: Ocular Anatomy and Physiology of Common Animal Models

Brian C. Gilger, Eva Abarca, and Jacklyn H. Salmon

Abstract

Selection of appropriate animal models for ocular research is essential to enhance validity of results and to minimize number of animals used. Knowledge of differences in ocular anatomy and physiology of the various animal models is one of the most important parameters in study design. In addition, the researcher must understand the disease process in the animal model and understand how this differs from the primary target animal (human or animal). Finally, the selection of the correct animal model is extremely important when considering route of therapy to translate therapeutic or pharmacokinetic results to larger animals such as humans. The purpose of this chapter is to review the ocular anatomy and physiology differences among common animal models of ocular disease to help researchers select appropriate animal models in experimental designs.

Key words Animal models, Eye, Ocular, Anatomy, Physiology

1 Introduction

Study of animal models of disease has advanced medicine and improved quality of life for both humans and animals. Animals have been studied to understand disease processes, to develop new therapies, and to ensure safety of drugs and potential environmental hazards. However, it is critical that as few animals are used in research as possible, and if used, only done so to understand the structure and function of complex and intricately connected biological systems such as the eye. It is essential, however, that any use of animals in biomedical research is done such that the three Rs are followed, as originally described by Russell and Burch in 1959 [1]. The three Rs include *Replacement*, which usually refers to the use of in vitro or computer models to conduct research instead of animals; *Reduction*, which refers a decrease in the number of animals used by reducing the variables through good experimental design; and *Refinement*, which refers to a change in the study design that leads to a reduction or replacement of animals and minimizes or eliminates pain or distress. Selection of appropriate animal models will greatly enhance the study design and assist, in many cases, the investigator to reduce the use of animals by reducing variability and increasing the validity of results obtained. To select the most appropriate models, the researcher must understand the differences in anatomy and physiology among the different animals. Furthermore, the researcher must understand the disease process in the animal model and understand how this differs from the primary target animal (human or animal). Also, selection of the correct animal model is extremely important when considering route of therapy if one wishes to translate therapeutic or pharmacokinetic results to larger animals such as humans.

The purpose of this chapter is to review the ocular anatomy and physiology differences among common animal models of ocular disease to help researchers select appropriate animal models in experimental designs.

2 Materials

The most common animals used in ocular research include mice, rats, rabbits, guinea pigs, dogs, cats, pigs, and primates (Table 1). In this chapter, we will review the literature to describe the differences in ocular anatomy and physiology in animal models of ocular disease. In these species, effect of drugs (or procedure or device) on induced ocular disease, effect of an induced disease or administered drugs on genetically modified animals, and distribution and

Table 1
Common animal models (and their common genus names) used in ophthalmic research

Mice/mouse (*Mus musculus*)
Rat (*Rattus rattus*)
Rabbits (*Oryctolagus cuniculus*)
Guinea pigs (*Cavia porcellus*)
Dogs (*Canis lupus familiaris*)
Cats (*Felis catus*)
Pigs (*Sus scrofa domesticus*)
Primates
Cynomolgus macaque monkey (*Macaca fascicularis*)
Rhesus macaque (*Macaca mulatta*)

effect of drugs (e.g., pharmacokinetics, pharmacodynamics, and toxicology) on normal ocular tissue are commonly studied. In many species, naturally occurring ocular diseases can also be studied, the results of which may provide a high level of information on a disease and results of therapy, frequently with more valid results than in induced models of disease. An example of the value of study of treatment in naturally occurring disease is the study of the retinal degeneration of RPE 65 −/− deficient dogs, a model of Leber congenital amaurosis (LCA), and their gene therapy treatment studies [2].

Other animal models have been described and also can be very useful for specific purposes. These include the chick eye, salamander retina, etc. [3, 4], but these less common models will not be reviewed in this chapter.

3 Methods

3.1 Ocular Dimensions

One of the most important aspects of selecting appropriate animal models for ocular studies is to understand the ocular anatomic differences among these models. An important determination in these models, especially when use of these models is for pharmacokinetic study, is the ocular dimensions. In Table 2, the relative ocular dimensions of the commonly used ocular animal models are listed.

3.2 Specific Ocular Anatomy and Physiology

Another important aspect of selecting appropriate animal models for ocular studies is to understand the differences in specific ocular anatomy and physiology among common animal models. We will review some important aspects of ocular anatomy and physiology starting from the front of the eye and moving to the back.

3.2.1 Orbit/Lacrimal Gland

Orbital structure among the common animal models is quite varied. Some animals, such as rodents, have minimal orbital protection and very prominent eyes, while other animals, such as dogs, pigs, and primates have deep orbits, which provide much ocular protection (Table 3). Furthermore, the location, number, and type of lacrimal glands vary considerably (Table 3). Three sets of lacrimal glands can be distinguished in mammals: (1) the orbital lacrimal gland (glandula lacrimales superior) located superior temporal to the eye with multiple secretory ducts that open into the lateral half of the superior conjunctival sac; (2) the gland of the nictitating membrane, located inferior nasal associated with the nictitating membrane; and (3) the inferior lacrimal gland (glandula lacrimales inferior) located ventrally, usually far posterior to the eye, with a single secretory duct that opens into the lateral edge of the conjunctival sac. The orbital lacrimal gland is present in man, dogs, pigs, and rabbits. The inferior lacrimal gland includes the

Table 2
Ocular size and dimensions of adult animals commonly used in ophthalmic research

	Animal							
	Mice	Rat	Guinea pig	Rabbit	Cat	Dog	Pig	Non-human primates
Ocular axial length (mm)	3.3 [62–64]	5.6 [65]–6.29 [66]	8.69 [67]	13.75 [68] 17.1 ± 0.41 [69]	20.9 ± 0.5 [70]	20 ± 0.1 [71]	23.9 ± 0.08 [72] Göttingen minipigs <19 mm [73]	Cynomolgus monkey 17.16 ± 0.69 [74]
Corneal thickness (μM)	90.8 [62, 63, 75]	159 ± 14.99 [75]	227.85 ± 14.09 [76]	356.11 ± 14.34 [75]	578 ± 64 [13]	562 ± 6.2 [12]	666[a] [77]	[b]543 [78]
Anterior chamber depth (mm)	0.71 ± 0.02 [68] #14	4.57 [66]	1.31 ± 0.01 [67]	2.8 [68]	5.07 ± 0.3 [70]	3.8 ± 0.1 [71]	2.13 ± 0.22 [79]	Cynomolgus monkey 2.79 ± 0.27 [74] Macaque 3.35 [80]
AH volume (μl)	4.4–5.9 [64, 81]	13.6 [66]	–	287	810 [82]	770 ± 24 [83]	–	Cynomolgus monkey 90–110 [84]

Lens thickness A-P (mm)	1.56 [62, 63]	3.3 [65] #89	3.59 ± 0.15 [67]	3.55 [68]	7.77 ± 0.2 [70]	6.7 ± 1 [71]	7.5–8.14 [5]	Cynomolgus monkey 3.18 ± 0.15 [74]
Vitreal thickness A-P (mm)	0.59–0.71 [62–64]	1.4 [66]–1.5 [65]	3.76 ± 0.15 [67]	7.1 ± 0.45 [69]	7.8	8.54 ± 0.599	–	Cynomolgus monkey 11.25 ± 0.51 [74]
Vitreous volume (μl)	5.3	13.4–13.6 [66, 85]	–	1,060 [86]	2,500 [87]	1,700 ± 86 [83]	Göttingen minipigs 2,000–2,700 [88]	Cynomolgus monkey 1,800–2,000 [74]
Retinal thickness (Central) (μM)	186.9 ± 15.1[c] [62, 63]	192.7[c] [89]–220[d] [17]	140[d] [17]	194.3 ± 7.7[c] [90]	182 ± 11[c] [91]	198.7 ± 9.6[e] [92]	293 ± 13[c] [93]	270–290[e] [94]

[a]Ultrasound pachymetry
[b]Light microscopy
[c]Optical coherence tomography (OCT)
[d]Direct measurement on retinal whole mount
[e]SD-OCT

Table 3
Orbital structures, lacrimal gland, and third eyelid

	Animal							
	Mice	**Rat**	**Guinea pig**	**Rabbit**	**Cat**	**Dog**	**Pig**	**Non-human primate**
Orbit type	Shallow, incomplete	Shallow, incomplete	Shallow, incomplete	Shallow, complete	Deep, incomplete	Deep, incomplete	Deep, incomplete	Deep, complete
Lacrimal gland	Infraorbtial (extraorbital)	Infraorbital (extraorbital)	Infraorbital (extraorbital)	Lacrimal gland, infraorbital (intraorbital)	Lacrimal gland, gland of the nictitating membrane	Lacrimal gland, gland of the nictitating membrane	Lacrimal gland, gland of the nictitating membrane	Lacrimal gland (superior-temporal)
Harderian gland	Intraorbital	Intraorbital	Intraorbital	Intraorbital	None	None	None	None
Third eyelid	Yes	Yes	Yes	Yes	Yes	Yes	Yes	No

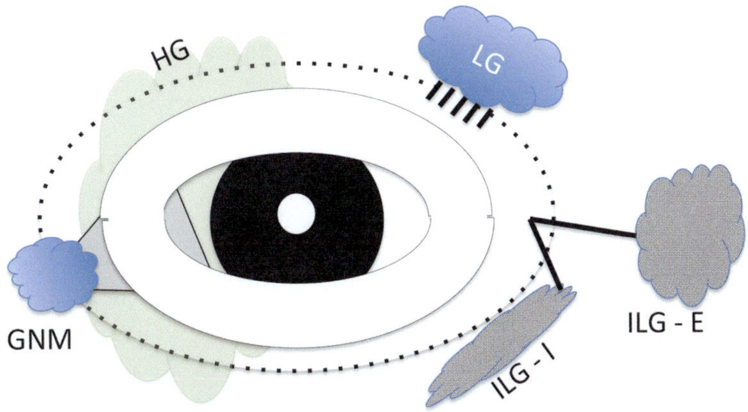

Fig. 1 Illustration showing relative positioning of major orbital glands in mammals. The harderian gland (HG) is located medially and behind the globe, in many species filling a large portion of the orbit. The gland of the nictitans (GNM) is a lacrimal gland that is located medially and a component of the base of the nictitating membrane. The lacrimal gland (LG) is located superior-temporal and has 5–6 ducts that empty onto the conjunctival surface. In contrast, the infraorbital lacrimal gland (ILG) is located ventrally in the orbit (ILG-I) or ventral laterally extraorbitally (ILG-E)

infraorbital gland of rodents (Fig. 1; Table 3). Some mammals also have the Harder's or harderian gland, which is different from the gland of the nictitating membrane (Table 3). It is extraglandular tissue that extends into the orbit from the nictitans gland [5]. The Harder's gland is considerably larger than the gland of the third eyelid and is deeply seated in the orbit. The Harder's or harderian gland contributes lipids and phospholipids to the ocular surface [6–8]. Lipid secretions from the Harder's gland contribute to the tear film and may have a profound effect on the pharmacokinetics of topically applied ocular drugs. See more information on tear film components later in this chapter.

3.2.2 Eyelids/Third Eyelid: Blink Rate

The major structural differences between the animals regarding eyelid anatomy and function generally revolves around the presence or absence of a third eyelid (palpebra tertia, plica semilunaris, or third eyelid) (Table 3). In most animals with a third eyelid, the action of the eyelid is generally passive and elevated only with retraction of the globe (via retractor bulbi muscles) or when there is decreased sympathetic tone. The presence of a third eyelid can make examination of animals more difficult and depending on the drug or device being evaluated, may make application of the product more difficult. For example, the third eyelid can make placement of a corneal contact lens on the ocular surface quite challenging and may reduce retention time.

Table 4
Average blink rates of normal eyes (modified from Venzina) (9)

	Animal							
	Mice	Rat	Guinea pig (95)	Rabbit	Cat	Dog	Pig	Non-human primate
Blink rates	1 per 5 min	1 per 5 min	1 per 10 to 1 per 4 min	1 per 6 min	1 per 18 s	1 per 10–20 s	1 per 20–30 s	1 per 6 s

The normal blink rate of animals varies tremendously also (Table 4) [9]. Knowledge of the normal blink rate is important when accessing ocular irritation of drugs where an increased blink rate, especially if prolonged, is a parameter suggesting increased irritation.

3.2.3 Tear Film

Components of tear film are quite varied and depend on whether or not the eye is inflamed and if the animal has a harderian gland. In general, the tear film is composed of lipids (usually secreted by eyelid meibomian glands), mucins (usually secreted by conjunctival goblet cells and in some animals the orbital lacrimal gland), and an aqueous component (secreted mostly by the lacrimal gland and accessory glands in the conjunctiva). Table 5 lists the common tear film components in the normal eye of the various animal models. In a recent study evaluating the meibomian gland lipids of rabbits, dogs, and mice, it was determined that mouse and dog meibomian gland lipids were closer biochemically to humans than the rabbit [8].

3.2.4 Cornea

The cornea of most laboratory animals consists of the corneal epithelium externally, the corneal stroma, Descemet's membrane, and corneal endothelial cells [10, 11]. Descemet's membrane is the basement membrane for the endothelial cells and becomes thicker with age as it is continuously produced. The corneal stroma consists primarily of collagen fibrils, keratocytes, nerves, and glycosaminoglycans. Corneal collagen fibrils exist in broad belts called lamellae that run approximately parallel to the corneal surface. Corneal thickness, as measured by ultrasonic pachymetry, confocal microscopy, or OCT, and endothelial cell counts are listed in Table 6. The peripheral cornea is thicker on average than the central cornea and corneal thickness increases gradually with age [12, 13].

3.2.5 Anterior Chamber/Aqueous Humor

The components of aqueous humor also vary among animal species and differ greatly if there is active inflation. Table 7 lists the common tear film components in the normal eye of the various animal models.

Table 5
Components of normal tear film

Tear component	Animal							
	Mice	Rat	Guinea pig	Rabbit	Cat	Dog	Pig	Non-human primates
Lactoferrin	Present (96)	Present (96)	600 ng/ml (97)	Present (96)	Present (96)	Present (96)	–	Rhesus monkey: Present (98)
Epidermal growth factor	79.3 ± 7 (99)	Present (100)	–	Present (101)			–	
Lipocalin (Von von Ebner's gland protein; VEGP)	Not present (102)	Present (102)	Not present (102)	*Sexual dimorphism*[a] (103) Intact male 159.75 ± 7.81 Intact female 127.66 ± 8.54	Not detected (102)	Present (102)	Present (102)	Rhesus monkey: Present (98)
Lysozyme	–	–	–	0.003 ± 0.0007 mg/ml (104)		Present (low concentration) (105)	–	Present (high concentrations) (105)
Secretory IgA	20 μg/ml (106)	200 μg/ml (107)	–	Present (108)	Present (109)	25.28 ± 1.9 mg/dl (110)	–	Cynomolgus monkey: 9.5 mg/dl (111)
Mucins (MUC5AC)	Present (112) (Muc5AC)	Present (112) (rMuc5AC)		Present (113)		Present (114)		

(continued)

Table 5
(continued)

Tear component	Animal							
	Mice	Rat	Guinea pig	Rabbit	Cat	Dog	Pig	Non-human primates
Meibomian lipid	Major composition: WE CE (115) OAHFA major amphiphiles (115)	–	–	Major composition: DiHL-esters DiAD (115) OAHFA major amphiphiles (115)	–	179 ± 60 MU[b] (116) Major composition: WE CE (115) OAHFA major amphiphiles (115)	–	–

Major lipid components: *CE* cholesteryl esters, *WE* wax esters, *OAHFA* (O-acyl)-omega-hydroxy fatty acids, *CE-OAHFA* esters of OAHFA, *DiHL-esters* 24,25-dihydro-Δ8-lanostero, *DiAD* diacylated diols

[a]Units: densitometry analysis of Western blots

[b]Meibometer units

Table 6
Parameters of the cornea of common animal models used in ocular research

	Animal							
	Mice	Rat	Guinea pig	Rabbit	Cat	Dog	Pig	Non-human primates
Corneal thickness (Central) μm	[a]120 ± 6 (117) [c]122–137[f] (118)	[a]170 ± 5 (117)	[b]227.85 (76)	[a]354 ± 6 (117) [b]407 ± 20 (119) [g]385 (120)	[b]578 ± 64 (13) [a]545 (117) [a]592 (121) [h]600 (122)	[a]550 (117) [a]585 (121) [b]562 ± 6.2 (12) [h]535 (122)	[b]666 (123)	[c]543 (78)[d] *Western lowland gorilla* [a]580 (124)
Epithelial thickness (Central) (μm)	[c]44.6 ± 1.7 (125) [e]37.1–46.8[f] (118)	–	[b]45.54 (76)	[i]45.8 ± 2.2 (126)	[c]38 (127) [h]60 (122)	[h]55 (122)	–	[c]26 (78)[d] *Western lowland gorilla* [c]33 (124)
Stromal thickness (Central) (μm)	[c]115.9 ± 5.4 (125) [e]80.5–90.8[f] (118)	[e]88 (128)	[b]163.69 (76) [e]270 (128)	[e]250 (128)	[h]540 (122)	[h]480 (122)	–	–
Descemet's membrane thickness (Central) (μm)	[c]2.17 ± 0.3 (118)	[e]3.5 (128)	[b]3.96 (76) [e]13 (128)	[e]5.6 (128)	–	10–15 (129)	–	*Western lowland gorilla* [c]7.5 (124)
Endothelial cell count (cells/m^2)	[a]2,875 (117) [c]2,282–3,060 (130)	[a]2,242 (117)	[a]2,352 (76)	[a]3,233 (117) [j]6,098 (131)	[a]2,731 (117) [a]2,846 (121) [k]2,530 (132)	[a]2,818 (117) [a]3,175 (121) [j]7,190 (133)	–	*Rhesus M* [k]2,959–3,128 (134)

[a]In vivo confocal microscopy
[b]Ultrasound pachymetry
[c]Light microscopy (for endothelium count cells: Flatmounts stained with alizarin red)
[d]Primates studied: *L. mustelinus*, *C. torquatus*, *C. aethiops*, *C. cephus*, *E. patas*, Mirus, *P. troglodytes*, *G. gorilla*, *C. jacchus*, *A. caraya*, *A. paniscus*, *L. lagotricha*
[e]TEM
[f]Mice strains studied: 129/SVJ; C_{57}BL/6; BALB/C
[g]AS-OCT
[h]SD-OCT
[i]Ultrahigh resolution OCT
[j]SEM
[k]Specular microscopy

Table 7
Components of the aqueous humor of common animal models used in ocular research

Aqueous humor component	Animal							
	Mice	Rat	Guinea pig	Rabbit	Cat	Dog	Pig	Non-human primates
K^+ (mEq/l)				6 (135)	4.4 (136)	5.0 (137)	3.6 (135)	3.9 ± 0.1 (138)
Na^+ (mEq/L)				136.9 (135)	158.5 (136)	149.4 (137)	131.3 (135)	152.3 ± 4.2 (138)
Cl^- (mEq/L)				103.4 (135)		124.8 (137)	106.8 (135)	124.8 ± 1.0 (138)
HCO_3^- (mEq/l)				33.6 (137)	30.4 (136)			22.5 ± 1.7 (138)
Phosphorus (mg/dl)				0.89 (137)	0.48 (136)	0.53 (137)		1.3 ± 0.1 (138)
Glucose (μmol/ml)				6.9 (136)	4.55 (136)	5.11 (136)		2.9 (138)
Total protein (mg/dl)	22 (81)	100 (139)		25.9 (137)	50 (140)	36.4 (137)	10.6 (141)	33.3 ± 2.6 (138)
pH				7.58 (142)				7.49 (138)
Calcium (μmol/l or mEq/l)				1.7 (μmol/l) (143)	2.7 (mEq/l) (136)	2.9 (mEq/l) (136)		2.5 (μmol/l)(143)
Mg (mg/dl)				0.8 (137)				1.9 ± 0.1 (138)
Ascorbic acid (mM)		0.09 (144) 0 (145)	1.03 (144) 0.75 (145)	1.06 (144) 1.7 (145)	0.1 (136)	0.55 (136)	0.57 (145)	1.18 (138)
Lactate (μmol/l)				9.9 (143)				4.3 (138)
Urea nitrogen (μmol/ml)				6.3 (146)	5.16 (136)	7.45 (136)		6.1 (138)
H_2O_2 (μM)	–	9 (147)	47 (147)	59 (147)	4.9 (147)	9 (147)		27 (147)

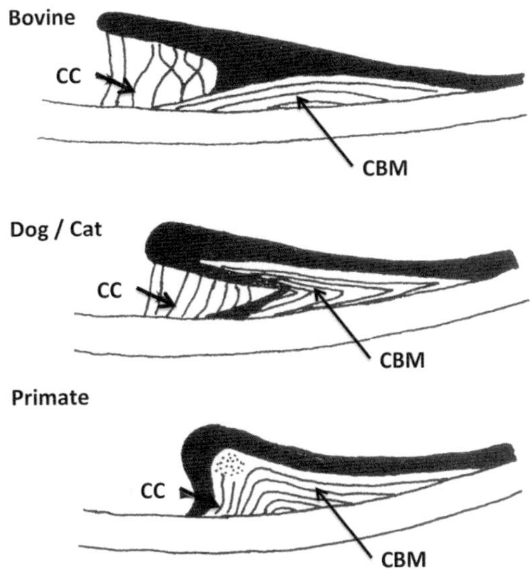

Fig. 2 Comparison of ciliary body musculature (CBM) in mammalian iridocorneal angles of the bovine, carnivore (dog or cat), and the primate. Development of the CBM is most pronounced in primates and least pronounced in ungulates (i.e., bovines). The size of the ciliary cleft (CC) is inversely large and pronounced in the bovine (Modified from Duke-Elder S. System of Ophthalmology, Vol. I. The Eye in Evolution. London: Henry Kimpton, 1958)

3.2.6 Glaucoma/ Iridocorneal Angle

The aqueous humor drainage angle is similar in most species in that there is a trabecular meshwork, ciliary cleft, and aqueous collecting veins. However, of the common species used in ophthalmic research, only rodents (mice) and primates have a Schlemms's canal [14]. Furthermore, the size and significance of the scleral spur and ciliary musculature differs in animal models (Fig. 2). In general, primates tend to have larger ciliary musculature (high amount of accommodative ability) versus rodents and ungulates, which in general have smaller musculature [5]. Certain anti-glaucoma medications, such as miotics which act by opening the iridocorneal angle by constriction of ciliary musculature and the resultant pull on the scleral spur, may have less of an effect on animals with smaller ciliary musculature [15]. See Chapter 10 for details of selection of animal models and design of glaucoma studies.

3.2.7 Lens

The lens of common laboratory animals varies greatly by size and volume of the eye they occupy. The lenses of rodents typically occupy a large portion of eye, thus resulting in a small vitreous body. This relatively large lens and small vitreal body makes intravitreal injections in rodents difficult and subject to lens trauma or toxicity. See Table 1 for dimensions of the lens.

3.2.8 Vitreous Body

The vitreous body mostly varies in size (Table 1) and firmness of structure. Younger animals, which are the age usually studied in most laboratories, have a well-formed vitreal collagen structure. This organized structure may differ substantially from older individuals with vitreal degeneration and syneresis. In young animals, the vitreous is gel-like because of a network of fine collagen fibrils; however, in older animals collagen fibrils progressively aggregate resulting in vitreous liquefaction [16]. These size and age differences should be taken into account in studies evaluating vitreal injections, especially regarding drug distribution and toxicity.

3.2.9 Retina/Optic Nerve

There are several important differences in retinal anatomy among common animal models, including differences in retinal thickness, retinal vascular pattern, rod and cone density, and presence of an area of ganglion cell density, e.g., a macula. Retinal thickness varies from approximately 190 μm in mice to 260 μm in humans (Tables 1 and 8) [17, 18]. In all species, there are fewer ganglion cells in the periphery of the retina than in the center, greatly reducing the visual acuity of the peripheral visual field. The visual streak (superior to optic nerve), area centralis (temporal to optic nerve), or macula (temporal to optic nerve) all have increased density of glanglion cells and cones and therefore, provide the best visual acuity (Table 8) [19].

In dogs, cats, pigs, and primates, the retina contains a plexus of blood vessels that extend throughout the light-sensitive portion of the retina (holangiotic pattern) (Fig. 3). In the rabbit, retinal blood vessels are confined to a broad horizontal band coincident with the area of dispersion of the myelinated nerve fibers of the optic nerve (merangiotic pattern) (Fig. 4). In the guinea pig, the retinal blood vessels are restricted to the peri-papillary portion of the optic disc (paurangiotic pattern) (Fig. 5; Table 8) [20].

4 Notes

4.1 Selection of Appropriate Animal Models

4.1.1 Models for Mechanistic Determination Versus Pharmacology/Pharmacokinetics

Eyes of various laboratory animals can be evaluated for signs of ocular toxicity when evaluating general toxicity. Several chapters in this book review the methods and procedures of selecting appropriate animal models and the methods to determine ocular toxicity. However, when testing effectiveness of drugs on models of ocular disease, there are two separate but important testing questions or goals. First, is the drug effective in the ocular disease state that is being tested? For this goal, usually rats or mice are evaluated and dosed by a routine route, e.g., orally, subcutaneously, or intraperitoneally. These studies also play a role in determining pathogenesis of disease–drug mechanisms, therefore the wide array of reagents and genetically modified mice and rats are a major asset. Determination of the appropriate dose (i.e., dose ranging studies) is usually also performed in these first set of studies.

Table 8
Retinal anatomy of common animal models used in ocular research

Retinal component	Animal							
	Mice	Rat	Guinea pig	Rabbit	Cat	Dog	Pig	Non-human primates
Retinal thickness (μM)	186.9 ± 15.1 (62, 63)	192.7 (89) 220 μm (17)	140 (17)		250[b] (17)		293 ± 13 (93)	
Area of cone density	Visual streak	Visual streak	Visual streak	Visual streak	Area centralis (temporal)	Area centralis (temporal)	Visual streak	Macula/fovea
Retinal vacular pattern	Holangiotic	Holangiotic	Paurangiotic	Meriangiotic	Holangiotic	Holangiotic	Holangiotic	Holangiotic
Vascular supply	Posterior ciliary arteries	Posterior ciliary arteries		Posterior ciliary arteries	Short posterior ciliary arteries	Short posterior ciliary arteries		Central retinal artery

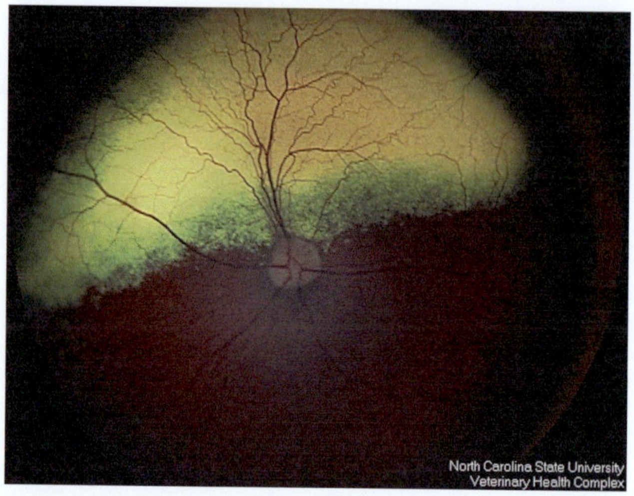

Fig. 3 Ocular fundus photograph of the dog demonstrating a holangiotic pattern of retinal vasculature. This vascular pattern is typical of dogs, cats, pigs, and primates and is characterized by blood vessels that extend throughout the light-sensitive portion of the retina

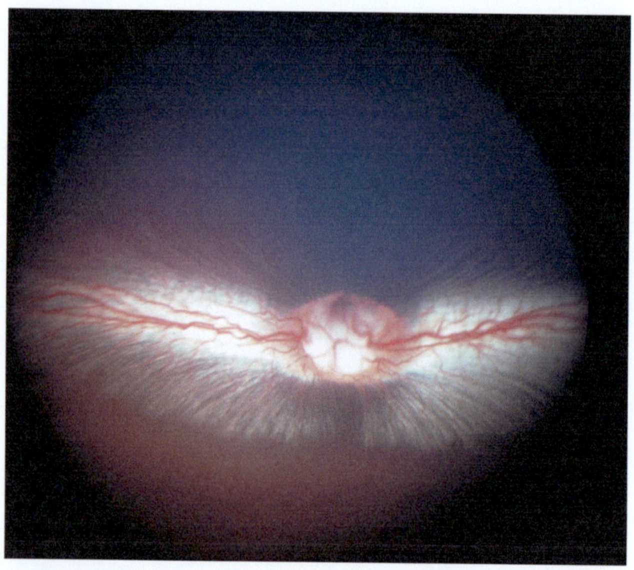

Fig. 4 Ocular fundus photograph of a rabbit demonstrating a merangiotic pattern of retinal vasculature. This vascular pattern is characterized by a broad horizontal band coincident with the area of dispersion of the myelinated nerve fibers of the optic nerve

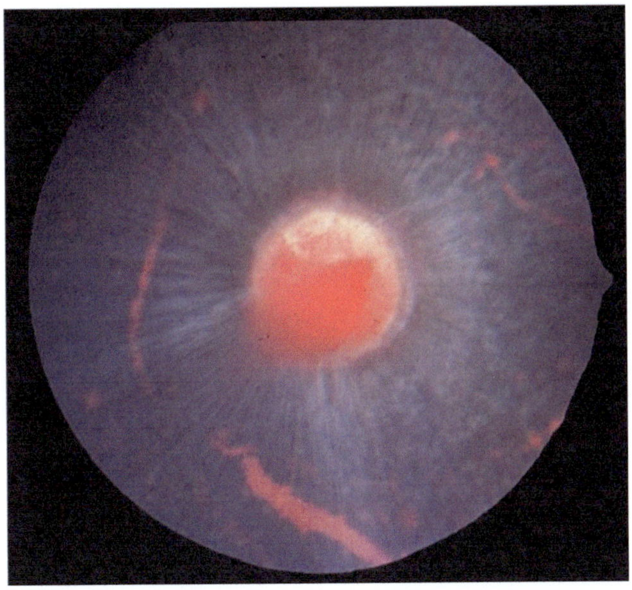

Fig. 5 Ocular fundus photograph of a guinea pig demonstrating a paurangiotic pattern of retinal vasculature. This vascular pattern is typical of guinea pigs, some marsupials, and horses and is characterized by retinal vasculature restricted to the peri-papillary portion of the optic disc

The second goal is to determine if an appropriate dose can reach the ocular target tissue and be effective in the eye using a dosing route and frequency that is clinically feasible. These studies would determine the pharmacokinetics and pharmacodynamics of a specific route of administration of a drug, typically in a normal eye, then repeated using the optimal dosing and routes in eyes of models of the disease state. For this second group of studies to be clinically valid in most instances, the animal models would have to have eyes anatomically similar to the target species and in the case of humans, use of the dog, pig, or primate eye would be most appropriate. Finally, when selecting the appropriate animal model, the target tissue and disease state has to be paired with the most appropriate route of therapy (Fig. 6). This determination is important for pharmacokinetic, toxicologic, and efficacy studies.

4.1.2 Induced Models Versus Naturally Occurring Models of Ocular Disease

When evaluating living ocular tissues for evaluation of ocular pharmacokinetics, pharmacodynamics, and toxicity, normal animals are typically studied, the more uniform to each other the better to minimize biologic variability (and thus increase statistical power of the experiments). These animals are purpose bred for biomedical studies, and in the case of rodents, have similar if not identical genetic background.

To determine the effect of a drug on ocular disease, whether the disease is induced or naturally occurring, animal models of the

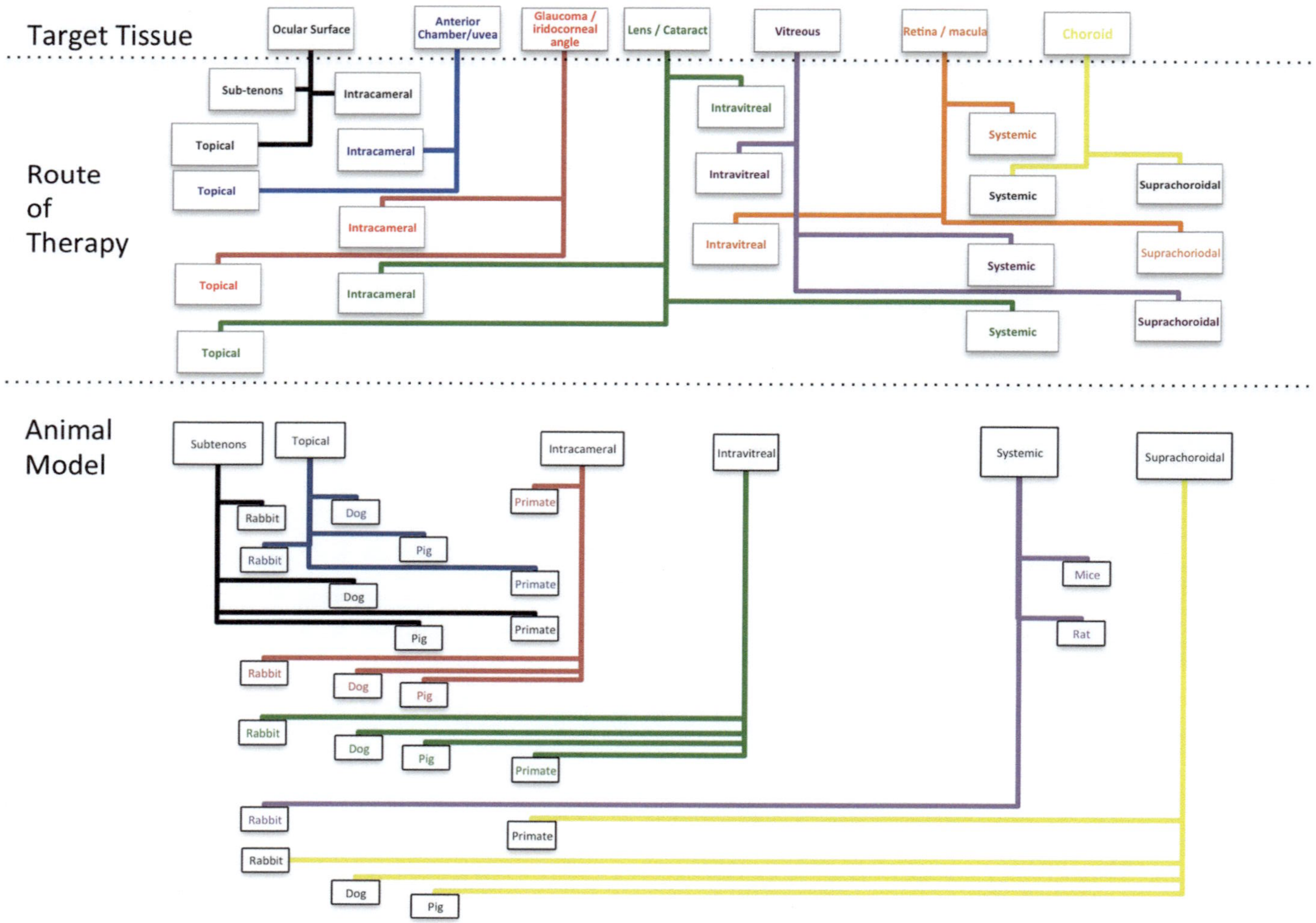

Fig. 6 When selecting the appropriate animal model, the target tissue and disease state has to be paired with the most appropriate route of therapy. Secondly, the route of therapy (i.e., a clinically feasible dosing route and frequency) must be matched to an animal model that would allow clinically valid pharmacokinetic, pharmacodynamic, efficacy, and toxicology studies to be performed

disease are commonly studied. Induced animal models of ocular disease are most valid when they are similar clinically and pathologically to the target ocular disease. Examples of induced ocular disease used to study the effectiveness of therapeutics, and in some cases to study the pathogenesis of disease, include corneal scrape and infectious keratitis models [21–23], endotoxin induced uveitis [24–26], glaucoma models [27–31], and laser induced choroidal neovascularization models [32–34], to name just a few. Genetically modified models of ocular disease are potentially powerful tools to study the pathogenesis of ocular disease and also can be used to determine clinical efficacy of medications. There are numerous examples of these genetically modified models of ocular disease [35–38].

Study of naturally occurring ocular diseases may provide a high level of information regarding a specific ocular disease and results of therapy, frequently with more valid results than in induced models of disease because of the similarity of the ocular disease to that observed in humans. Examples include, but are not limited to, the open-angle glaucoma model in beagles [39–42], retinal disease models in dogs [2, 43–49], recurrent uveitis in horses [50–57], and cataractogenesis in diabetic dogs [58–61].

Additional models of ocular disease, both induced and naturally occurring will be discussed in subsequent chapters of this book.

5 Conclusions

Understanding the differences in ocular anatomy and physiology along with understanding the relationship of the chosen animal model to the target species is essential when planning studies to determine ocular pharmacology, toxicity, and efficacy. For example, determining that a drug applied topically to a mouse eye provides a therapeutic concentration of a drug and/or is effective in treating a disease, has virtually no relation to treatment of the human eye with eye drops. On the other hand, success of treatment of a larger animal, such as a pig or dog, with a similar size and ocular anatomy to the human eye, would provide much more valid results, in most cases. Another example is selecting appropriate animal for treatment of retinal disease should involve use of animals with similar retinal anatomy and retinal vascular supply. Use of appropriate models is essential to decrease variability, minimize the number of animals used in studies, and to increase study validity. It is the responsibility of all researchers that perform biomedical research to actively follow the three Rs (i.e., Replacement, Reduction, and Refinement) [1] when designing studies.

References

1. Russell W, Burch R (1959) The principles of humane experimental technique. Methuen, London
2. Acland GM, Aguirre GD, Bennett J, Aleman TS, Cideciyan AV, Bennicelli J, Dejneka NS, Pearce-Kelling SE, Maguire AM, Palczewski K, Hauswirth WW, Jacobson SG (2005) Long-term restoration of rod and cone vision by single dose rAAV-mediated gene transfer to the retina in a canine model of childhood blindness. Mol Ther 12(6):1072–1082, doi: S1525-0016(05)01561-3 [pii]10.1016/j.ymthe.2005.08.008
3. Beattie JR, Finnegan S, Hamilton RW, Ali M, Inglehearn CF, Stitt AW, McGarvey JJ, Hocking PM, Curry WJ (2012) Profiling retinal biochemistry in the MPDZ mutant retinal dysplasia and degeneration chick: a model of human RP and LCA. Invest Ophthalmol Vis Sci 53(1):413–420, doi:10.1167/iovs.11-8591iovs.11-8591 [pii]
4. Gross RL, Hensley SH, Gao F, Wu SM (1999) Retinal ganglion cell dysfunction induced by hypoxia and glutamate: potential neuroprotective effects of beta-blockers. Surv Ophthalmol 43(Suppl 1):S162–170
5. Samuelson D (2007) Ophthalmic anatomy. In: Gelatt K (ed) Veterinary ophthalmology, vol 1, 4th edn. Blackwell, Ames, IA
6. Barabino S, Chen W, Dana MR (2004) Tear film and ocular surface tests in animal models of dry eye: uses and limitations. Exp Eye Res 79(5):613–621, doi:S0014-4835(04)00196-4 [pii]10.1016/j.exer.2004.07.002
7. Bareggi R, Narducci-Bareggi P, Crescenzi A (1979) Lipids in the Harder's gland of certain rodents. III: Glycolipids. Basic Appl Histochem 23(2):165–169
8. Butovich IA, Lu H, McMahon A, Eule JC (2012) Toward an animal model of the human tear film: biochemical comparison of the mouse, canine, rabbit, and human meibomian lipidomes. Invest Ophthalmol Vis Sci 53 (11):6881–6896, doi:10.1167/iovs.12-10516iovs.12-10516 [pii]
9. Vezina M (2012) Comparative ocular anatomy in commonly used laboratory animals. In: Weir A, Collins M (eds) Assessing ocular toxicology in laboratory animals. Molecular and integrative toxicology. Springer Science & Business Media, Philadelphia, PA, pp 1–21
10. Shively JN, Epling GP (1970) Fine structure of the canine eye: cornea. Am J Vet Res 31 (4):713–722
11. Spreull JS (1966) Symposium: the corneal ulcer I. Anatomy and physiology of the cornea of the dog. J Small Anim Pract 7(3):253–255
12. Gilger BC, Whitley RD, McLaughlin SA, Wright JC, Drane JW (1991) Canine corneal thickness measured by ultrasonic pachymetry. Am J Vet Res 52(10):1570–1572
13. Gilger BC, Wright JC, Whitley RD, McLaughlin SA (1993) Corneal thickness measured by ultrasonic pachymetry in cats. Am J Vet Res 54(2):228–230
14. Lei Y, Overby DR, Boussommier-Calleja A, Stamer WD, Ethier CR (2011) Outflow physiology of the mouse eye: pressure dependence and washout. Invest Ophthalmol Vis Sci 52 (3):1865–1871, doi:10.1167/iovs.10-6019 iovs.10-6019 [pii]
15. van der Woerdt A, Gilger BC, Wilkie DA, Strauch SM, Orczeck SM (1998) Normal variation in, and effect of 2% pilocarpine on, intraocular pressure and pupil size in female horses. Am J Vet Res 59(11):1459–1462
16. Le Goff MM, Bishop PN (2008) Adult vitreous structure and postnatal changes. Eye (Lond) 22(10):1214–1222, doi:10.1038/eye.2008.21eye200821 [pii]
17. Buttery RG, Hinrichsen CF, Weller WL, Haight JR (1991) How thick should a retina be? A comparative study of mammalian species with and without intraretinal vasculature. Vision Res 31(2):169–187
18. Bentaleb-Machkour Z, Jouffroy E, Rabilloud M, Grange JD, Kodjikian L (2012) Comparison of central macular thickness measured by three OCT models and study of interoperator variability. ScientificWorldJournal 2012:84 2795. doi:10.1100/2012/842795
19. Hebel R (1976) Distribution of retinal ganglion cells in five mammalian species (pig, sheep, ox, horse, dog). Anat Embryol (Berl) 150(1):45–51
20. De Schaepdrijver L, Simoens P, Lauwers H, De Geest JP (1989) Retinal vascular patterns in domestic animals. Res Vet Sci 47(1):34–42
21. McCarey B, Edelhauser H, Williams K (2006) Comparison of the effect of moxifloxacin and gatifloxacin on corneal epithelial wound healing in the rabbit model. Cornea 25:S35–S38
22. Tam C, Lewis SE, Li WY, Lee E, Evans DJ, Fleiszig SM (2007) Mutation of the phospholipase catalytic domain of the Pseudomonas aeruginosa cytotoxin ExoU abolishes colonization promoting activity and reduces corneal disease severity. Exp Eye Res 85(6):799–805,

doi:S0014-4835(07)00241-2 [pii]10.1016/j.exer.2007.08.015

23. Wu TG, Wilhelmus KR, Mitchell BM (2003) Experimental keratomycosis in a mouse model. Invest Ophthalmol Vis Sci 44(1):210–216
24. Rosenbaum JT, McDevitt HO, Guss RB, Egbert PR (1980) Endotoxin-induced uveitis in rats as a model for human disease. Nature 286(5773):611–613
25. Chan CC, Ni M, Miele L, Cordella-Miele E, Ferrick M, Mukherjee AB, Nussenblatt RB (1991) Effects of antiflammins on endotoxin-induced uveitis in rats. Arch Ophthalmol 109(2):278–281
26. Allen JB, McGahan MC, Ogawa Y, Sellon DC, Clark BD, Fleisher LN (1996) Intravitreal transforming growth factor-beta 2 decreases cellular infiltration in endotoxin-induced ocular inflammation in rabbits. Curr Eye Res 15(1):95–103
27. Rasmussen CA, Kaufman PL (2005) Primate glaucoma models. J Glaucoma 14 (4):311–314, doi: 00061198-200508000-00015 [pii]
28. Weinreb RN, Lindsey JD (2005) The importance of models in glaucoma research. J Glaucoma 14(4):302–304, doi:00061198-200508000-00012 [pii]
29. Rezaie T, Waitzman DM, Seeman JL, Kaufman PL, Sarfarazi M (2005) Molecular cloning and expression profiling of optineurin in the rhesus monkey. Invest Ophthalmol Vis Sci 46(7):2404–2410, doi:46/7/2404 [pii] 10.1167/iovs.04-1243
30. Ruiz-Ederra J, Garcia M, Hernandez M, Urcola H, Hernandez-Barbachano E, Araiz J, Vecino E (2005) The pig eye as a novel model of glaucoma. Exp Eye Res 81 (5):561–569, doi:S0014-4835(05)00106-5 [pii]10.1016/j.exer.2005.03.014
31. Prasanna G, Hulet C, Desai D, Krishnamoorthy RR, Narayan S, Brun AM, Suburo AM, Yorio T (2005) Effect of elevated intraocular pressure on endothelin-1 in a rat model of glaucoma. Pharmacol Res 51(1):41–50, doi:S1043661804001057 [pii]10.1016/j.phrs.2004.04.006
32. Semkova I, Peters S, Welsandt G, Janicki H, Jordan J, Schraermeyer U (2003) Investigation of laser-induced choroidal neovascularization in the rat. Invest Ophthalmol Vis Sci 44(12):5349–5354
33. Ciulla TA, Criswell MH, Danis RP, Hill TE (2001) Intravitreal triamcinolone acetonide inhibits choroidal neovascularization in a laser-treated rat model. Arch Ophthalmol 119(3):399–404, doi:els90067 [pii]
34. Ishibashi T, Hata Y, Yoshikawa H, Nakagawa K, Sueishi K, Inomata H (1997) Expression of vascular endothelial growth factor in experimental choroidal neovascularization. Graefes Arch Clin Exp Ophthalmol 235(3):159–167
35. Cotroneo MS, Haag JD, Zan Y, Lopez CC, Thuwajit P, Petukhova GV, Camerini-Otero RD, Gendron-Fitzpatrick A, Griep AE, Murphy CJ, Dubielzig RR, Gould MN (2007) Characterizing a rat Brca2 knockout model. Oncogene 26(11):1626–1635, doi:1209960 [pii]10.1038/sj.onc.1209960
36. Biswas S, Bhattacherjee P, Paterson CA, Tilley SL, Koller BH (2006) Ocular inflammatory responses in the EP2 and EP4 receptor knockout mice. Ocul Immunol Inflamm 14 (3):157–163, doi:R1X0564408P78744 [pii] 10.1080/09273940600665879
37. Song XJ, Li DQ, Farley W, Luo LH, Heuckeroth RO, Milbrandt J, Pflugfelder SC (2003) Neurturin-deficient mice develop dry eye and keratoconjunctivitis sicca. Invest Ophthalmol Vis Sci 44(10):4223–4229
38. Kaifi JT, Hall LR, Diaz C, Sypek J, Diaconu E, Lass JH, Pearlman E (2000) Impaired eosinophil recruitment to the cornea in P-selectin-deficient mice in Onchocerca volvulus keratitis (River blindness). Invest Ophthalmol Vis Sci 41(12):3856–3861
39. Kuchtey J, Olson LM, Rinkoski T, Mackay EO, Iverson TM, Gelatt KN, Haines JL, Kuchtey RW (2011) Mapping of the disease locus and identification of ADAMTS10 as a candidate gene in a canine model of primary open angle glaucoma. PLoS Genet 7(2):e1001306. doi:10.1371/journal.pgen.1001306
40. Hart H, Samuelson DA, Tajwar H, MacKay EO, Lewis PA, Kallberg M, Gelatt KN (2007) Immunolocalization of myocilin protein in the anterior eye of normal and primary open-angle glaucomatous dogs. Vet Ophthalmol 10(Suppl 1):28–37, doi:VOP517 [pii] 10.1111/j.1463-5224.2007.00517.x
41. Ricard CS, Mukherjee A, Silver FL, Wagenknecht PL (2006) Canine myocilin is associated with lipid modified by palmitic acid. Mol Vis 12:1427–1436, doi:v12/a161 [pii]
42. Gelatt KN, Peiffer RL Jr, Gwin RM, Gum GG, Williams LW (1977) Clinical manifestations of inherited glaucoma in the beagle. Invest Ophthalmol Vis Sci 16 (12):1135–1142
43. Kijas JW, Cideciyan AV, Aleman TS, Pianta MJ, Pearce-Kelling SE, Miller BJ, Jacobson SG, Aguirre GD, Acland GM (2002) Naturally occurring rhodopsin mutation in the dog causes retinal dysfunction and degeneration mimicking

human dominant retinitis pigmentosa. Proc Natl Acad Sci U S A 99(9):6328–6333, doi: 10.1073/pnas.0827 14499 082714499 [pii]

44. Wang W, Zhang Q, Acland GM, Mellersh C, Ostrander EA, Ray K, Aguirre GD (1999) Molecular characterization and mapping of canine cGMP-phosphodiesterase delta subunit (PDE6D). Gene 236(2):325–332, doi: S0378111999002462 [pii]
45. Aguirre GD, Baldwin V, Pearce-Kelling S, Narfstrom K, Ray K, Acland GM (1998) Congenital stationary night blindness in the dog: common mutation in the RPE65 gene indicates founder effect. Mol Vis 4:23
46. Acland GM, Aguirre GD (1987) Retinal degenerations in the dog: IV. Early retinal degeneration (erd) in Norwegian elkhounds. Exp Eye Res 44(4):491–521
47. Aguirre G, Farber D, Lolley R, O'Brien P, Alligood J, Fletcher RT, Chader G (1982) Retinal degeneration in the dog III. Abnormal cyclic nucleotide metabolism in rod-cone dysplasia. Exp Eye Res 35(6):625–642
48. Buyukmihci N, Aguirre G, Marshall J (1980) Retinal degenerations in the dog II. Development of the retina in rod-cone dysplasia. Exp Eye Res 30(5):575–591, doi:0014-4835(80) 90041-X [pii]
49. Aguirre G (1978) Retinal degenerations in the dog. I. Rod dysplasia. Exp Eye Res 26 (3):233–253, doi:0014-4835(78)90072-6 [pii]
50. Deeg CA, Hauck SM, Amann B, Pompetzki D, Altmann F, Raith A, Schmalzl T, Stangassinger M, Ueffing M (2008) Equine recurrent uveitis—a spontaneous horse model of uveitis. Ophthal Res 40(3–4):151–153, doi:10.1159/000119867 000119867 [pii]
51. Gilger BC, Salmon JH, Wilkie DA, Cruysberg LP, Kim J, Hayat M, Kim H, Kim S, Yuan P, Lee SS, Harrington SM, Murray PR, Edelhauser HF, Csaky KG, Robinson MR (2006) A novel bioerodible deep scleral lamellar cyclosporine implant for uveitis. Invest Ophthalmol Vis Sci 47(6):2596–2605, doi:47/6/2596 [pii]10.1167/iovs.05-1540
52. Deeg CA, Amann B, Raith AJ, Kaspers B (2006) Inter- and intramolecular epitope spreading in equine recurrent uveitis. Invest Ophthalmol Vis Sci 47(2):652–656, doi:47/ 2/652 [pii] 10.1167/iovs.05-0789
53. Paglia DT, Miller PE, Dubielzig RR (2004) James Wardrop and equine recurrent uveitis. Arch Ophthalmol 122(8):1218–1223, doi:10.1001/archopht.122.8.1218 122/8/ 1218 [pii]
54. Deeg CA, Ehrenhofer M, Thurau SR, Reese S, Wildner G, Kaspers B (2002) Immunopathology of recurrent uveitis in spontaneously diseased horses. Exp Eye Res 75(2):127–133, doi:S0014483502920117 [pii]
55. Gilger BC, Yang P, Salmon JH, Jaffe GJ, Allen JB (2002) Expression of a chemokine by ciliary body epithelium in horses with naturally occurring recurrent uveitis and in cultured ciliary body epithelial cells. Am J Vet Res 63 (7):942–947
56. Deeg CA, Kaspers B, Gerhards H, Thurau SR, Wollanke B, Wildner G (2001) Immune responses to retinal autoantigens and peptides in equine recurrent uveitis. Invest Ophthalmol Vis Sci 42(2):393–398
57. Gilger BC, Malok E, Cutter KV, Stewart T, Horohov DW, Allen JB (1999) Characterization of T-lymphocytes in the anterior uvea of eyes with chronic equine recurrent uveitis. Vet Immunol Immunopathol 71(1):17–28, doi: S0165-2427(99)00082-3 [pii]
58. Abrams KL, Stabila PF, Kauper K, Elliott S (2011) Vascular endothelial growth factor in diabetic and nondiabetic canine cataract patients. Vet Ophthalmol 14(2):93–99. doi:10.1111/j.1463-5224.2010.00846.x
59. Kador PF, Betts D, Wyman M, Blessing K, Randazzo J (2006) Effects of topical administration of an aldose reductase inhibitor on cataract formation in dogs fed a diet high in galactose. Am J Vet Res 67(10):1783–1787. doi:10.2460/ajvr.67.10.1783
60. Wilkie DA, Gemensky-Metzler AJ, Colitz CM, Bras ID, Kuonen VJ, Norris KN, Basham CR (2006) Canine cataracts, diabetes mellitus and spontaneous lens capsule rupture: a retrospective study of 18 dogs. Vet Ophthalmol 9(5):328–334, doi:VOP490 [pii] 10.1111/j.1463-5224.2006.00490.x
61. Basher AW, Roberts SM (1995) Ocular manifestations of diabetes mellitus: diabetic cataracts in dogs. Vet Clin North Am Small Anim Pract 25(3):661–676
62. Zhou X, Xie J, Shen M, Wang J, Jiang L, Qu J, Lu F (2008) Biometric measurement of the mouse eye using optical coherence tomography with focal plane advancement. Vision Res 48 (9):1137–1143, doi:10.1016/j.visres.2008. 01.030 S0042-6989(08)00070-9 [pii]
63. Wang L, Povazay B, Chen YP, Hofer B, Drexler W, Guggenheim JA (2011) Heritability of ocular component dimensions in mice phenotyped using depth-enhanced swept source optical coherence tomography. Exp Eye Res 93 (4):482–490, doi:10.1016/j.exer.2011.06. 008 S0014-4835(11)00198-9 [pii]
64. Remtulla S, Hallett PE (1985) A schematic eye for the mouse, and comparisons with the rat. Vision Res 25(1):21–31, doi:0042-6989 (85)90076-8 [pii]

65. Guggenheim JA, Creer RC, Qin XJ (2004) Postnatal refractive development in the Brown Norway rat: limitations of standard refractive and ocular component dimension measurement techniques. Curr Eye Res 29(4–5):369–376, doi:QU0MJL6N0UU7PTKA [pii] 10.1080/02713680490515991
66. Hughes A (1979) A schematic eye for the rat. Vision Res 19(5):569–588
67. Zhou X, Qu J, Xie R, Wang R, Jiang L, Zhao H, Wen J, Lu F (2006) Normal development of refractive state and ocular dimensions in guinea pigs. Vision Res 46(18):2815–2823, doi:S0042-6989(06)00063-0 [pii] 10.1016/j.visres.2006.01.027
68. Herse P (2005) Effects of hyperglycaemia on ocular development in rabbit: refraction and biometric changes. Ophthalmic Physiol Opt 25(2):97–104, doi:OPO262 [pii] 10.1111/j.1475-1313.2004.00262.x
69. Toni MC, Meirelles AE, Gava FN, Camacho AA, Laus JL, Canola JC (2010) Rabbits' eye globe sonographic biometry. Vet Ophthalmol 13(6):384–386. doi:10.1111/j.1463-5224.2010.00831.x
70. Gilger BC, Davidson MG, Howard PB (1998) Keratometry, ultrasonic biometry, and prediction of intraocular lens power in the feline eye. Am J Vet Res 59(2):131–134
71. Williams DL (2004) Lens morphometry determined by B-mode ultrasonography of the normal and cataractous canine lens. Vet Ophthalmol 7(2):91–95, doi:10.1111/j.1463-5224.2004.04005.x VOP04005 [pii]
72. Sanchez I, Martin R, Ussa F, Fernandez-Bueno I (2011) The parameters of the porcine eyeball. Graefes Arch Clin Exp Ophthalmol 249(4):475–482. doi:10.1007/s00417-011-1617-9
73. Nielsen L, Lind N (2005) Measurements of three ocular parameters in the Göttingen Minipig. Scand J Lab Anim Sci 32:9–16
74. Kaufman PL, Calkins BT, Erickson KA (1981) Ocular biometry of the cynomolgus monkey. Curr Eye Res 1(5):307–309
75. Schulz D, Iliev ME, Frueh BE, Goldblum D (2003) In vivo pachymetry in normal eyes of rats, mice and rabbits with the optical low coherence reflectometer. Vision Res 43 (6):723–728, doi:S0042698903000051 [pii]
76. Cafaro TA, Ortiz SG, Maldonado C, Esposito FA, Croxatto JO, Berra A, Ale OL, Torrealday JI, Urrets-Zavalia EA, Urrets-Zavalia JA, Serra HM (2009) The cornea of Guinea pig: structural and functional studies. Vet Ophthalmol 12(4):234–241, doi:10.1111/j.1463-5224.2009.00708.xVOP708 [pii]
77. Faber C, Scherfig E, Prause J (2008) Corneal thickness in pigs measured by ultrasound pachymetry in vivo. Lab Anim Sci 35(1):39–43
78. Merindano MD, Canals M, Potau JM, Costa J, Ruano D (1997) Morphological and morphometric aspects of primate cornea: a comparative study with human cornea. Eur J Morphol 35(2):95–104
79. Asejczyk-Widlicka M, Schachar RA, Pierscionek BK (2008) Optical coherence tomography measurements of the fresh porcine eye and response of the outer coats of the eye to volume increase. J Biomed Opt 13 (2):024002. doi:10.1117/1.2907453
80. Lapuerta P, Schein SJ (1995) A four-surface schematic eye of macaque monkey obtained by an optical method. Vision Res 35 (16):2245–2254, doi:0042-6989(94)00320-L [pii]
81. Aihara M, Lindsey JD, Weinreb RN (2003) Aqueous humor dynamics in mice. Invest Ophthalmol Vis Sci 44(12):5168–5173
82. Toris CB, Yablonski ME, Wang YL, Hayashi M (1995) Prostaglandin A2 increases uveoscleral outflow and trabecular outflow facility in the cat. Exp Eye Res 61(6):649–657
83. Gilger BC, Reeves KA, Salmon JH (2005) Ocular parameters related to drug delivery in the canine and equine eye: aqueous and vitreous humor volume and scleral surface area and thickness. Vet Ophthalmol 8 (4):265–269, doi:VOP00401 [pii] 10.1111/j.1463-5224.2005.00401.x
84. Toris CB, Zhan GL, Wang YL, Zhao J, McLaughlin MA, Camras CB, Yablonski ME (2000) Aqueous humor dynamics in monkeys with laser-induced glaucoma. J Ocul Pharmacol Ther 16(1):19–27
85. Dureau P, Bonnel S, Menasche M, Dufier JL, Abitbol M (2001) Quantitative analysis of intravitreal injections in the rat. Curr Eye Res 22(1):74–77
86. Iyer MN, He F, Wensel TG, Mieler WF, Benz MS, Holz ER (2005) Intravitreal clearance of moxifloxacin. Trans Am Ophthalmol Soc 103:76–81, discussion 81–73
87. Izumi N, Nagaoka T, Sato E, Sogawa K, Kagokawa H, Takahashi A, Kawahara A, Yoshida A (2008) Role of nitric oxide in regulation of retinal blood flow in response to hyperoxia in cats. Invest Ophthalmol Vis Sci 49(10):4595–4603, doi:10.1167/iovs.07-1667 iovs.07-1667 [pii]
88. Shafiee A, McIntire GL, Sidebotham LC, Ward KW (2008) Experimental determination and allometric prediction of vitreous volume, and retina and lens weights in

Gottingen minipigs. Vet Ophthalmol 11 (3):193–196, doi:10.1111/j.1463-5224.2008.00619.xVOP619 [pii]
89. Lozano DC, Twa MD (2012) Quantitative evaluation of factors influencing the repeatability of SD-OCT thickness measurements in the rat. Invest Ophthalmol Vis Sci 53 (13):8378–8385, doi:10.1167/iovs.12-9940 iovs.12-9940 [pii]
90. Muraoka Y, Ikeda HO, Nakano N, Hangai M, Toda Y, Okamoto-Furuta K, Kohda H, Kondo M, Terasaki H, Kakizuka A, Yoshimura N (2012) Real-time imaging of rabbit retina with retinal degeneration by using spectral-domain optical coherence tomography. PLoS One 7(4):e36135, doi:10.1371/journal.pone.0036135 PONE-D-11-23574 [pii]
91. Gekeler F, Gmeiner H, Volker M, Sachs H, Messias A, Eule C, Bartz-Schmidt KU, Zrenner E, Shinoda K (2007) Assessment of the posterior segment of the cat eye by optical coherence tomography (OCT). Vet Ophthalmol 10(3):173–178, doi:VOP532 [pii] 10.1111/j.1463-5224.2007.00532.x
92. Hernandez-Merino E, Kecova H, Jacobson SJ, Hamouche KN, Nzokwe RN, Grozdanic SD (2011) Spectral domain optical coherence tomography (SD-OCT) assessment of the healthy female canine retina and optic nerve. Vet Ophthalmol 14(6):400–405. doi:10.1111/j.1463-5224.2011.00887.x
93. Gilger B, Abarca E, Salmon J, Patel S (2013) Treatment of acute posterior uveitis in a porcine model by injection of triamcinolone acetonide into the suprachoroidal space using microneedles. Invest Ophthalmol Vis Sci 54(4):2483–2492
94. Rosolen SG, Riviere ML, Lavillegrand S, Gautier B, Picaud S, LeGargasson JF (2012) Use of a combined slit-lamp SD-OCT to obtain anterior and posterior segment images in selected animal species. Vet Ophthalmol 15 (Suppl 2):105–115. doi:10.1111/j.1463-5224.2012.01037.x
95. Trost K, Skalicky M, Nell B (2007) Schirmer tear test, phenol red thread tear test, eye blink frequency and corneal sensitivity in the guinea pig. Vet Ophthalmol 10(3):143–146, doi: VOP521 [pii]10.1111/j.1463-5224.2007.00521.x
96. Hemsley S, Cole N, Canfield P, Willcox M (2000) Protein microanalysis of animal tears. Res Vet Sci 68:207–209
97. Boonstra A, Kijlstra A (1987) Guinea pig tears contain lactoferrin and transferrin. Curr Eye Res 6(9):1115–1123
98. Morimoto-Tochigi A, Walkup R, Nakajima E (2010) Mechanism for Carbachol-induced secretion of lacritin in cultured monkey lacrimal acinar cells. Invest Ophthalmol Vis Sci 51:4395–4406
99. Tsutsumi O, Tsutsumi A, Oka T (1988) Epidermal growth factor-like, corneal wound healing substance in mouse tears. J Clin Invest 81(4):1067–1071
100. van Setten G, Tervo K, Virtanen I (1990) Immunohistochemical demonstration of epidermal growth factor in the lacrimal and submandibular glands of rats. Acta Ophthalmol (Copenh) 68(4):477–80
101. Klenkler B, Sheardown H, Jones L (2007) Growth factors in the tear film: role in tissue maintenance, wound healing, and ocular pathology. Ocul Surf 5(3):228–239
102. Redl B (2000) Human tear lipocalin. Biochim Biophys Acta 1482:241–248
103. Seamon V, Vellala K, Zylberberg C, Ponamareva O, Azzarolo AM (2008) Sex hormone regulation of tear lipocalin in the rabbit lacrimal gland. Exp Eye Res 87(3):184–190, doi:10.1016/j.exer.2008.05.012 S0014-4835(08)00158-9 [pii]
104. Zhou L, Beuerman R, Barathi A, Tan D (2003) Analysis of rabbit tear proteins by high-pressure liquid chromatography/electrospray ionization mass spectrometry. Rapid Commun Mass Spectrom 17(5):401–412
105. Davidson H, Kuonen V (2004) The tear film and ocular mucins. Vet Ophthalmol 7:71–77
106. Masinick S, Montgomery C, Montgomery P (1997) Secretory IgA inhibits Pseudomonas aeruginosa binding to cornea and protects against keratitis. Invest Ophthalmol Vis Sci 38(5):910–918
107. Sullivan D, Allansmith M (1984) Source of IgA in tears of rats. Immunology 53:791–796
108. Schechter J, Warren D, Mircheff A (2010) A Lacrimal gland is a lacrimal gland, but Rodent's and Rabbit's are not human. Ocul Surf 8(3):111–134
109. Schultz R, Scott F, Duncan J (1974) Feline immunoglobulins. Infect Immun 9 (2):391–393
110. Ginel P, Novales M, García M (1993) Immunoglobulins in stimulated tears of dogs. Am J Vet Res 54(7):1060–1063
111. Cole M, Bowen W (1976) Immunoglobulins A, G, and M in serum and in some secretions of monkeys (Macaca fascicularis). Infect Immun 13(5):1354–1359
112. Gipson I, Argüeso P (2003) The role of mucins in the function of the corneal and conjunctival epithelia. Int Rev Cytol 231:1–49
113. Inatomi T, Tisdale A, Zhan Q (1997) Cloning of rat muc5ac mucin gene: comparison of its structure and tissue distribution to that of

human and mouse homologues. Biochem Biophys Res Commun 236:789–797

114. Hicks S, Carrington S, Kaswan R (1997) Demonstration of discrete secreted and membrane-bound ocular mucins in the dog. Exp Eye Res 64:597–607

115. Butovich I, Lu H, McMahon A (2012) Toward an animal model of the human tear film: biochemical comparison of the mouse, canine, rabbit, and human meibomian lipidomes. Invest Ophthalmol Vis Sci 53 (11):6881–6896

116. Ofri R, Keren O, Kass P (2007) Canine meibometry: establishing baseline values for meibomian gland secretions in dogs. Vet Ophthalmol 174(3):536–540

117. Reichard M, Hovakimyan M, Wree A, Meyer-Lindenberg A, Nolte I, Junghans C, Guthoff R, Stachs O (2010) Comparative in vivo confocal microscopical study of the cornea anatomy of different laboratory animals. Curr Eye Res 35(12):1072–1080. doi:10.3109/02713 683.2010.513796

118. Henriksson JT, McDermott AM, Bergmanson JP (2009) Dimensions and morphology of the cornea in three strains of mice. Invest Ophthalmol Vis Sci 50(8):3648–3654, doi:10.1167/iovs.08-2941iovs.08-2941 [pii]

119. Chan T, Payor S, Holden BA (1983) Corneal thickness profiles in rabbits using an ultrasonic pachometer. Invest Ophthalmol Vis Sci 24(10):1408–1410

120. Wang X, Wu Q (2013) Normal corneal thickness measurements in pigmented rabbits using spectral-domain anterior segment optical coherence tomography. Vet Ophthalmol 16(2):130–134. doi:10.1111/j.1463-5224.2012.01041.x

121. Kafarnik C, Fritsche J, Reese S (2007) In vivo confocal microscopy in the normal corneas of cats, dogs and birds. Vet Ophthalmol 10 (4):222–230, doi:VOP543 [pii]10.1111/j.1463-5224.2007.00543.x

122. Famose F (2013) Assessment of the use of spectral domain optical coherence tomography (SD-OCT) for evaluation of the healthy and pathological cornea in dogs and cats. Vet Ophthalmol. doi:10.1111/vop.12028

123. Faber C, Wang M, Scherfig E, Sorensen KE, Prause JU, Ehlers N, Nissen MH (2009) Orthotopic porcine corneal xenotransplantation using a human graft. Acta Ophthalmol 87(8):917–919, doi:10.1111/j.1755-3768.2008.01489.xAOS1489 [pii]

124. Knapp S, McCulley JP, Alvarado TP, Hogan RN (2007) Comparative ocular anatomy of the western lowland gorilla. Vet Ophthalmol 10(6):357–362, doi:VOP568 [pii]10.1111/j.1463-5224.2007.00568.x

125. Henriksson JT, Bron AJ, Bergmanson JP (2012) An explanation for the central to peripheral thickness variation in the mouse cornea. Clin Exp Ophthalmol 40(2):174–181. doi:10.1111/j.1442-9071.2011.02652.x

126. Reiser BJ, Ignacio TS, Wang Y, Taban M, Graff JM, Sweet P, Chen Z, Chuck RS (2005) In vitro measurement of rabbit corneal epithelial thickness using ultrahigh resolution optical coherence tomography. Vet Ophthalmol 8(2):85–88, doi:VOP00345 [pii] 10.1111/j.1463-5224.2005.00345.x

127. Choo J, Caroline P, Harlin D (2008) Morphologic changes in cat epithelium following continuous wear of orthokeratology lenses: a pilot study. Cont Lens Anter Eye 31:29–37

128. Hayashi S, Osawa T, Tohyama K (2002) Comparative observations on corneas, with special reference to Bowman's layer and Descemet's membrane in mammals and amphibians. J Morphol 254(3):247–258. doi:10.1002/jmor.10030

129. Murphy C, Pollock R (1993) The eye. In: HE E (ed) Miller's anatomy of the dog, 3rd edn. WB Saunders, Philadelphia, PA, pp 1009–1055

130. Lively GD, Jiang B, Hedberg-Buenz A, Chang B, Petersen GE, Wang K, Kuehn MH, Anderson MG (2010) Genetic dependence of central corneal thickness among inbred strains of mice. Invest Ophthalmol Vis Sci 51(1):160–171, doi:10.1167/iovs.09-3429 iovs.09-3429 [pii]

131. Doughty MJ (2006) Subjective vs. objective analysis of the corneal endothelial cells in the rabbit cornea by scanning electron microscopy—a comparison of two different methods of corneal fixation. Vet Ophthalmol 9(2):127–135, doi:VOP449 [pii] 10.1111/j.1463-5224.2006.00449.x

132. Peiffer RL Jr, DeVanzo RJ, Cohen KL (1981) Specular microscopic observations of clinically normal feline corneal endothelium. Am J Vet Res 42(5):854–855

133. Rodrigues GN, Laus JL, Santos JM, Rigueiro MP, Smith RL (2006) Corneal endothelial cell morphology of normal dogs in different ages. Vet Ophthalmol 9(2):101–107, doi: VOP427 [pii] 10.1111/j.1463-5224.2006.00427.x

134. Lu ST, D'Andrea J, Chalfin S, Crane C, Marchello D, Garay R, Hatcher D, Ziriax J (2010) Absence of corneal endothelium injury in non-human primates treated with and without ophthalmologic drugs and

exposed to 2.8 GHz pulsed microwaves. Bioelectromagnetics 31(4):324–333. doi:10.1002/bem.20556

135. Gerometta RM, Malgor LA, Vilalta E, Leiva J, Candia OA (2005) Cl- concentrations of bovine, porcine and ovine aqueous humor are higher than in plasma. Exp Eye Res 80 (3):307–312, doi:S0014-4835(04)00282-9 [pii]10.1016/j.exer.2004.10.001
136. Gum G, Gelatt K, Esson D (2007) Physiology of the eye. In: Gelatt K (ed) Veterinary ophthalmology, 4th edn. Blackwell Publishing, Ames, IA, pp 160–170
137. Aubin ML, Gionfriddo JR, Mama KR, Powell CC (2001) Analysis of aqueous humor obtained from normal eyes of llamas and alpacas. Am J Vet Res 62(7):1060–1062
138. Gaasterland DE, Pederson JE, MacLellan HM, Reddy VN (1979) Rhesus monkey aqueous humor composition and a primate ocular perfusate. Invest Ophthalmol Vis Sci 18(11):1139–1150
139. Stjernschantz J, Uusitalo R, Palkama A (1973) The aqueous proteins of the rat in normal eye and after aqueous withdrawal. Exp Eye Res 16(3):215–221, doi:0014-4835(73)90216-9 [pii]
140. Rotatori DS, Kerr NC, Raphael B, McLaughlin BJ, Shimizu R, Stern GA, Schultz GS (1994) Elevation of transforming growth factor alpha in cat aqueous humor after corneal endothelial injury. Invest Ophthalmol Vis Sci 35(1):143–149
141. Abe A, Hiraoka M, Inatomi S, Ohguro I, Ohguro H (2012) Lysosomal phospholipase A2 activity in pig aqueous humor. Invest Ophthalmol Vis Sci 53(1):152–156, doi:10.1167/iovs.11-7891iovs.11-7891 [pii]
142. Schwartz B (1964) The ph-temperature coefficient of rabbit anterior chamber aqueous humor. Invest Ophthalmol 3:96–99
143. Bito LZ (1970) Intraocular fluid dynamics. I. Steady-state concentration gradients of magnesium, potassium and calcium in relation to the sites and mechanisms of ocular cation transport processes. Exp Eye Res 10 (1):102–116
144. Giblin FJ, McCready JP, Kodama T, Reddy VN (1984) A direct correlation between the levels of ascorbic acid and H2O2 in aqueous humor. Exp Eye Res 38(1):87–93, doi:0014-4835(84)90142-8 [pii]
145. Varma SD, Richards RD (1988) Ascorbic acid and the eye lens. Ophthalmic Res 20 (3):164–173
146. Kinsey VE (1953) Comparative chemistry of aqueous humor in posterior and anterior chambers of rabbit eye, its physiologic significance. AMA Arch Ophthalmol 50 (4):401–417
147. Spector A, Ma W, Wang RR (1998) The aqueous humor is capable of generating and degrading H_2O_2. Invest Ophthalmol Vis Sci 39(7):1188–1197

Methods in Pharmacology and Toxicology (2014): 33–52
DOI 10.1007/7653_2013_6

Published online: 17 July 2013

Challenges and Strategies in Drug Residue Measurement (Bioanalysis) of Ocular Tissues

Poonam R. Velagaleti and Michael H. Buonarati

Abstract

Bioanalysis (quantification of drug/metabolite residue in biological fluids and tissues) plays an important role in support of drug efficacy and safety studies during drug development. Bioanalysis can be very challenging when the drug or the metabolites to be measured are unstable or are difficult to extract from biological matrices or when significant matrix interference is experienced during detection of the analytes of interest. Ocular tissue bioanalysis is particularly challenging because of the anatomical complexity of the eye. Furthermore, several heterogeneous tissues of the eye such as conjunctiva, sclera, cornea, and retina may act as barriers to drug absorption and distribution within the eye and therefore each ocular tissue must be collected individually and analyzed to determine drug and metabolite concentrations. Many ophthalmic drugs are administered topically and less than 5 % of the applied drug is likely to penetrate the eye. Most of the topically applied drug may be washed away by tears, cleared by other mechanisms, and/or absorbed into the systemic circulation. Because of the limited bioavailability, the drugs may not always reach targeted therapeutic concentrations in the ocular tissue(s). Without sensitive and accurate bioanalytical methods to measure and demonstrate that drug concentrations within the ocular tissues reach appropriate levels, following drug administration, erroneous conclusions may be drawn regarding efficacy and/or local safety. Pharmacokinetic measurements in blood/plasma for assessing systemic bioavailability, or residence time and drug distribution, are generally not useful in ocular studies since systemic exposure may not be directly related to exposure in the tissues of the eye after local ocular routes of administration. Systemic exposure, nonetheless, is very important in evaluating drug safety. Limited availability of control matrices needed for ocular bioanalysis studies poses additional challenges that may be partially addressed by using surrogate matrices. This chapter discusses the unique challenges and their resolution during eye tissue collection, method development, and the conduct of sample analysis for ocular bioanalytical studies.

Key words Ocular bioanalysis, Ocular tissues, Eye dissection, Tissue homogenization, Drug extraction, Drug analysis, Surrogate matrix

1 Introduction

Drug exposure assessment, systemic and/or at the site of action, in human or animal studies is a vital part of drug development. This allows correlations of drug-mediated biological responses to time of exposure (pharmacokinetics) that relate both to the desirable therapeutic effect and to undesirable adverse responses (toxicity) to the administered drugs. Measurement of drugs and their metabolites in biological matrices in typical bioanalytical studies (blood, serum, plasma, urine, and feces) is rarely straightforward. Ocular tissue bioanalysis, with an additional unique set of associated challenges, is much more complex. Ocular tissue bioanalysis, being invasive in nature, is typically conducted in preclinical studies. The rabbit is the species most commonly utilized for ocular investigations; other species include guinea pig, pig, monkey, and dog.

The eye is among the most complex organs in the body and is composed of several heterogeneous tissues and fluids including the sclera, conjunctiva, cornea, lens, iris, ciliary body, choroid, retina, aqueous humor, and vitreous humor. Classical tissue bioanalytical studies often rely on the preparation and analysis of homogenates of the entire organ or the representative sections of that organ. However, the eye is typically dissected to obtain component tissues and fluids for analysis. This is necessary due to the heterogeneity of the eye and because ocular drug administration often requires the placement of the dosed material relatively far from the site of action within the eye; i.e., the administered drug may have to traverse several tissue barriers and ocular fluids to reach its target tissue. Measurements of drug concentrations from the site of administration through the various tissues and fluids leading to the targeted tissue, along with the targeted tissue itself, provide critical information about the drug and its formulation. These data are critical in guiding lead candidate selection and in the development of appropriate pro-drugs or formulations for ocular administration to ensure that sufficient drug is reaching the targeted site of action.

The eye is constructed of various physical and biological barriers to absorption, which can be a challenge for drug delivery to intended sites of action. Although therapies for ocular disorders can be administered systemically, bioavailability to the eye is limited by the blood–ocular barrier. Localized routes of administration, including topical, periocular, and intravitreal, are usually required to generate greater ocular tissue exposures. It is estimated that approximately 80 % of a topically applied drug is washed away by tears and enters the general circulation via the nasolacrimal canal or is absorbed from the conjunctival sac via local blood capillaries. Typically, less than 5 % of topically applied drug is bioavailable to the eye [1–5]. Drugs can be directly injected into the eye (including sub-conjunctival, sub-tenon, or intra-vitreal injections) or administered by various ocular devices which are frequently implanted in the vitreous cavity, outside the path of vision. The concentration of drug and/or metabolites in systemic circulation following localized ocular administration is usually low, often at or below the level of detection of the analytical method being used. Hence, assessment of systemic exposure may require the development of highly sensitive bioanalytical methods for drug and metabolites in blood, serum, or plasma.

Following intraocular absorption, some drugs distribute rapidly and reach approximately equivalent concentrations in the aqueous humor, iris, and ciliary body with lower concentrations in the lens and vitreous humor [2]. Due to extensive vascularization of the iris and ciliary body, this often results in efficient drug clearance from those tissues [2, 6]. However, the vitreous humor, which occupies approximately 80 % of the eye volume in humans, has very low turnover. If the drug is successful in reaching the vitreous humor, this fluid can act as a reservoir to continuously deliver administered drug over an extended period of time to other eye tissues, especially the retina. Therefore it is necessary to know the drug concentration and the time course in applicable individual eye tissues to assess whether the drug is reaching the assumed site of action and in sufficient quantities to be efficacious. Lack of efficacy of a drug with known biological activity after ocular or systemic administration may simply be due to poor ocular distribution and/or ocular biotransformation of the drug to inactive metabolites.

After entry into eye tissues, the drug may undergo rapid conversion to inactive metabolites, effectively lowering drug-mediated responses [1, 2]. There is ample documentation in the literature that the eye contains "detoxifying enzymes" for protection against continuous exposure to foreign substances [7–14]. Although present in much lower levels than in the liver, cytochrome P-450 [15–21], monoamine oxidase [22, 23], and diamine oxidase [24] activities have been reported in ocular tissues. Aldehyde dehydrogenases are reported to be highly expressed in the cornea [25]. Esterases, including acetylcholinesterase and butyrylcholinesterase, are abundant in eye tissues [26–29] and may even be elevated in inflamed tissue [30]. Additionally, oxidoreductase activities have been reported [31–34]. Phase II (conjugating) enzymes present in ocular tissues include glutathione-S-transferases and UDP-glucuronosyltransferases [35, 36]. A number of drug transporters are also present in ocular tissues. These transporters, some of which are highly expressed, may also play a significant role in ocular drug absorption or lack thereof [37]. While many of the drug-metabolizing enzymes will not have significant activity in collected ex vivo samples, some of the enzymes, such as the esterases, can remain active post sample collection. Such activity can have considerable impact on final drug concentration determinations and must be considered in the development of suitable bioanalytical methods. While metabolic degradation can result in significant losses of drug, these same processes also can be exploited using a pro-drug approach. Pro-drugs, with little or no biological activity, can have superior drug absorption and distribution characteristics over their metabolically or chemically generated active drugs. These characteristics may be exploited to facilitate delivery of the pro-drug to the target sites within the eye where it is converted to the active drug at adequate concentrations leading to a desired biological response. Examples of pro-drugs used successfully in ocular indications include latanoprost and travoprost [38].

In such cases, bioanalytical methods need to be developed keeping in mind that not only the drug but also the pro-drug needs to be stabilized during sample collection and storage to insure accurate measurement of pro-drug and drug concentrations [39]. Regulatory agencies may require both pro-drug (when feasible) and drug concentrations to be measured in blood/plasma in the clinical/nonclinical investigations as well as in ocular tissues in the animal studies.

The tissue sample collection procedure itself will also have impact on bioanalytical results. Since the biological barriers present in viable ocular tissues break down immediately upon euthanasia, concentrations of drugs and other xenobiotics may equilibrate rapidly throughout the eye. Hence, after euthanasia, it is critical that the eyes be enucleated as soon as possible and be frozen instantly by submersion into liquid nitrogen or a dry ice/alcohol bath to prevent drug migration to adjacent tissues. As mentioned earlier, since enzymes present in the ocular tissues can continue to be active after the eye is enucleated, rapid flash freezing also inhibits any remaining enzymatic activity. Likewise, the eyes need to be kept frozen during dissection. In addition in the analysis of pro-drugs, appropriate enzyme inhibitors (such as esterase or protease inhibitors) [39–42] may need to be added to the collection vial/container prior to tissue collection in order to prevent pro-drug conversion to drug. If this is not feasible, the inhibitors should be added immediately upon thawing of the samples prior to tissue homogenization/extraction. However, it is preferred that the inhibitors be added to the collection containers prior to tissue collection.

Ocular bioanalytical studies differ from classical pharmacokinetic studies sampling blood, serum, or plasma in that sample collection typically follows termination of the source animal; hence, control ocular tissue matrices are not readily available. Surrogate matrices (e.g., plasma) are therefore commonly used for assay qualifications, validations, and sample analyses for ocular methods. While the use of a surrogate matrix can alleviate the problem of scarcity of ocular tissues, it can complicate the study design for method qualifications and validations. Furthermore, many of the ocular tissues and fluids collected in bioanalytical studies are present in such low volume or weight that reanalysis may be difficult or impossible, depending on the assay approach utilized.

Ocular tissues must be processed appropriately so that the processed sample is representative of the entire original tissue sample. Ocular tissues such as sclera, cornea, and conjunctiva can be difficult to homogenize because of their structural complexity. Because of the physical and chemical characteristics of biological samples, bioanalytical methods typically have several associated processing steps that yield a sufficiently clean and compatible sample for the analytical system used in quantification of drug concentrations. Interfering endogenous compounds, tissue fragments, and particulates are either removed from the sample or the drug is extracted from the biological sample and a more purified sample generated. For effective tissue extraction, various strategies can be employed that will depend on the type of drug molecule to be extracted. Small organic molecules can be effectively extracted by employing various organic solvents. Macromolecules, such as proteins, need aqueous processing conditions [43, 44] to avoid denaturation and loss of solubility. The reader may want to consult the excellent review article on bioanalytical approaches to analyzing peptides and proteins by LCMS [45]. In addition, endogenous components in ocular tissues, such as melanin, can bind some drugs tightly and require the development of more rigorous extraction techniques than with other biological matrices. Typically, extracted samples are concentrated and the concentrates reconstituted and/or further subjected to additional cleanup procedures. Following extraction, the samples are analyzed using various separation techniques coupled with an appropriate detector, depending on the type of molecule being analyzed. Macromolecules are typically detected by an enzyme-linked immunosorbent assay (ELISA technique) [43–47] while smaller molecules are analyzed by HPLC/UV or HPLC-MS/MS procedures [46].

This chapter does not discuss bioanalytical techniques or a method validation in great detail as these are well documented in the literature [45, 46, 48]. Rather, this chapter focuses on the various challenges encountered with ocular fluid and tissue bioanalysis and attempts to provide some recommendations on how these challenges may be overcome.

2 Types and Collection of Various Ocular Tissues

2.1 Types of Matrices Collected

The following are the matrices that are often collected and analyzed in ocular bioanalytical studies. Figure 1 provides an anatomical sketch of the rabbit eye, identifying the ocular tissues that are generally collected for bioanalysis.

1. Blood (Serum/Plasma)
   Ocular therapies reach their target tissues after direct administration to the eye (e.g., topical, injection, or via an ocular implant device), or from the systemic circulation after intravenous or extravascular administration. Regardless of the route of administration, the determination of blood concentrations is necessary to evaluate potential drug toxicity due to systemic exposure. In human ocular studies, blood may well be the only matrix available for assessing drug exposure. While some drugs are measured in whole blood, the majority of bioanalytical assays for experimental drugs use plasma or serum as the matrix of choice. Because of the typically low concentrations of drug in plasma or serum after

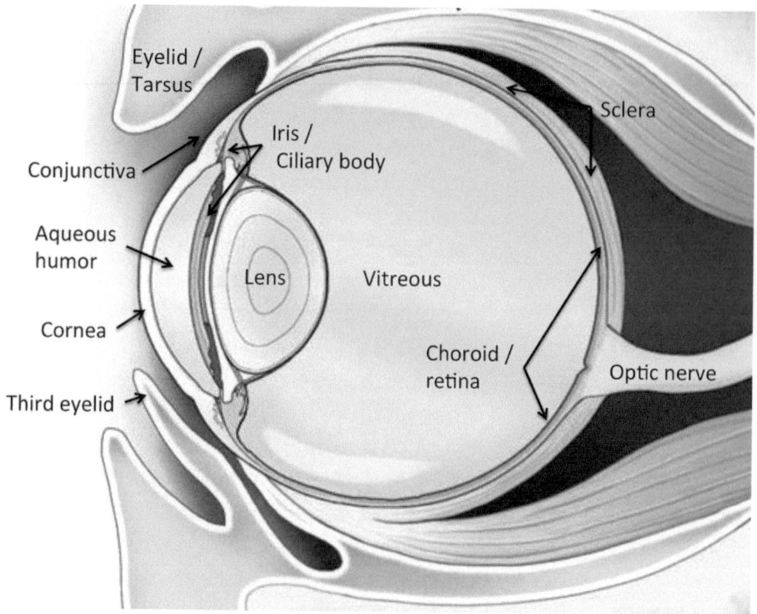

Fig. 1 An anatomical sketch of the rabbit eye

ocular administration, highly sensitive assays are commonly required and pose a major challenge for this matrix. The challenges associated with interferences are well known and must always be taken into account when developing highly sensitive methods. Vacutainers containing appropriate antioxidant and/or enzyme inhibitors may need to be utilized for blood sample collection to prevent potential oxidation and/or hydrolysis of pro-drug/drug/metabolite molecules due to the of action of esterases, proteases, etc. present in blood. The presence of high protein concentrations in plasma and serum can be of some concern as interfering components in assays; however, proteins also serve as protective agents in the prevention of nonspecific binding of certain drugs to sample containers and tubes used during sample processing. When sampling blood, volume and collection times should be appropriate for the assay and the pharmacokinetic evaluation and should minimize negative impact on the study animal. Too large an amount of blood collected at multiple time points (e.g., 8–10 time points for a PK study) within a short time window can cause adverse effects such as hemorrhagic shock and tissue anoxia [49] and can also affect the pharmacokinetics of the drug. Typically 0.5–1.5 mL/time point blood should be sufficient for bioanalytical work, depending on assay sensitivity requirements and aliquot volume used.

2. Tears

   Tear film secreted by the lacrimal glands is composed of proteins, lipids, carbohydrates, and electrolytes [50]. Protein concentration is about 10–15 % that of plasma [50, 51]. Nonspecific binding should be considered when there is poor or erratic recovery of the analyte during assay development. Tears are typically collected using Schirmer Tear Test Strips [52] and drug is extracted from the strips before drug/metabolite analysis. Each strip (contained in a small tube) must be weighed both before and after tear collection in order to calculate the weight of the tear sample collected.

3. Aqueous Humor

   The aqueous humor acts as a surrogate for blood to provide nutrients to the lens, cornea, and trabecular meshwork. It resembles plasma ultrafiltrate in composition, having similar electrolyte concentrations as plasma, but very low protein concentrations [50, 51]. In fact, the protein concentration in aqueous humor is about 0.5 % that of plasma and consists mainly of albumin and low-molecular-weight globulins. As such, it is a relatively clean matrix from a bioanalytical viewpoint, but the low protein concentrations can pose challenges in developing assays for drugs that have nonspecific binding characteristics to storage and extraction vessels. Because of its relative cleanliness as a biological matrix, simple sample processing procedures for aqueous humor can often be developed for drug analysis.

4. Vitreous Humor

   The vitreous humor, which resides within the vitreous chamber in the posterior segment of the eye, comprises approximately 80 % of the volume of the human eye. The vitreous humor is composed mostly of water but contains collagens, hyaluronic acid, and other proteoglycans and glycosaminoglycans that give this matrix gel-like properties [50, 51, 53]. The vitreous humor can differ in its liquid-like or gel-like properties with age, species, and the area of the eye sampled. Any vitreous sample should be considered as nonhomogeneous for sampling purposes and therefore must either be analyzed in whole or must be pretreated to produce a homogenous sample prior to aliquoting.

5. Cornea/Sclera/Lens

   The cornea, sclera, and lens have structural components that can dictate the approach required for sample processing. These tissues contain collagen, glycosaminoglycans, and proteoglycans [51, 54–56]. These tissues are difficult to homogenize and multiple and/or longer homogenization steps may be required during sample processing.

6. Iris/Ciliary Body/Retina/Choroid

   The pigment melanin is found in several tissues of the eye including those of the uveal tract (iris, ciliary body, and choroid) and the retina. Melanin may play a critical role in drug binding and has been associated with long residence times, drug efficacy, and possible ocular toxicity [57]. Melanin binding, however, may not be predictive of ocular toxicity [58]. Melanin is a polymer composed of dihydroxyindolyl and dihydroxyindole-2-carboxyl units and is ultimately derived from tyrosine [59, 60]. As such, melanin has multiple sites containing hydroxyl and carboxylic acid groups, which can interact with drugs, especially basic drugs [58, 59]. Examples of drugs known to bind to melanin in the eye include ephedrine, atropine, chlorpromazine, timolol, chloroquine, and levofloxacin [57, 59, 61]. When developing bioanalytical assays for iris, ciliary body, choroid, or retina, the drug binding characteristics of melanin must be taken into consideration. Drug binding to melanin can sequester the drug, making it unavailable for analysis. This may not be of consequence when melanin-containing tissues are used to generate calibration curves as long as drug binding is comparable across the concentration range of the assay and when sensitivity is sufficient. However, when using a surrogate matrix for the calibration curve (including tissues from non-pigmented animals such as New Zealand White rabbits), recovery from the pigmented tissues and surrogate matrix may be different and this must be accounted for when developing the assay. The use of high concentrations of salts (such as NaCl or $MgCl_2$) or other agents to disrupt the melanin–drug binding may be required for the development of an appropriate assay [60].

2.2 Eye Dissection and Ocular Tissue Collection

Proper sample collection is critical for ocular bioanalytical studies. Improper sample collection procedures can result in cross contamination of tissues or fluids which will compromise the value of even the best bioanalytical techniques. The main challenges encountered during sample collection are the following:

1. The biological ocular barriers that stop foreign substances including drugs from penetrating eyes or traveling across various tissues within the eye are destroyed immediately upon euthanasia of the animal, allowing drugs to equilibrate across tissues within the eye. As mentioned earlier, to prevent this equilibration, eyes need to be enucleated immediately upon euthanasia and flash frozen in liquid nitrogen or in a dry ice/alcohol bath as soon as possible. The eyes must be maintained in a frozen state during dissection to prevent or minimize drug diffusion to adjacent tissues.
2. As mentioned previously, ocular tissues contain several drug-metabolizing enzymes. These may provide a challenge

for the bioanalyst in that they must be prevented from acting on pro-drug or active drug after the sample is collected. Therefore, before undertaking a study, it is important to determine how to stabilize pro-drugs or metabolically unstable drugs and metabolites in collected samples. It may be necessary to add a known amount of modifier (antioxidant, protease inhibitor, or esterase inhibitor as the case may be) to the vials prior to dissection and sample collection.

3. During eye dissection, cross contamination of ocular tissues must be avoided. Taking certain precautions during sample collection will help in this regard. If the samples are being collected after systemic exposure, the animals may need to be perfused with chilled saline solution before necropsy to avoid contamination from blood since some eye tissues (choroid, conjunctiva) are highly vascularized structures. If the samples are being collected after topical administration, the enucleated eyeball can be rinsed in cold buffer such as phosphate-buffered saline (PBS) followed by flash freezing of the eye. If several groups of animals are to be euthanized in a day, the placebo group should always be the first one to be euthanized and/or dissected followed by the low-dose group with the longest time point ahead of shorter time points, followed by the higher dosed groups in a similar fashion. It is also essential to keep instruments clean during dissection to avoid cross contamination of the various eye tissues.

The technique for eye dissection should be practiced using cadaver eyes from rabbit or another model animal before dissecting ocular tissues from actual study samples. The procedure and sequence for ocular tissue collection in rabbits is briefly described in this section. All equipment required during surgery, dry ice/alcohol bath, and pre-labeled/pre-weighed vials need to be arranged prior to euthanasia. Eyes are enucleated as soon as possible following euthanasia and the eyeball should be quickly rinsed in cold buffer, blotted dry, and immediately flash frozen. If needed, eyelids, conjunctiva, and lacrimal glands are then collected and frozen. Dissection of the frozen eye can be performed immediately or on a later day. The frozen eye is placed on a cooled ceramic tile to avoid thawing of the eye during dissection. In order to prevent cross contamination of ocular tissues, instruments should be thoroughly rinsed with PBS followed by methanol followed by PBS and blotted dry (beakers of PBS and methanol need to be placed adjacent to dissection area for rinsing of instruments). The eye globe is separated in half using a long razor blade (a new blade is to be used for each eye), typically into a dorsal and ventral half. The frozen aqueous humor is removed first and is placed into its labeled vial. Depending on technician's preference, the aqueous humor can also be aspirated from the eye with a needle and syringe before the eye is enucleated and flash frozen. The cornea sections are removed next from the frozen eye, followed by lens, and vitreous humor. The iris and ciliary body are usually removed together followed by the retina and choroid. The remaining sclera fragments are then placed in a vial. Since collected ocular tissue samples are very small in weight/volume, the entire sample is usually processed for drug quantification. It is therefore highly recommended that at the in-life facility, samples are collected in pre-weighed, pre-labeled vials and weighed again prior to storage under frozen conditions. The balance used for weighing samples needs to be calibrated prior to its use and must be able to weigh ocular tissues accurately in the mg range. The weight data needs to be provided to the bioanalytical laboratory along with the samples as the analytical laboratory will rely on the information provided by the in-life facility to calculate concentrations (ng/g) in various ocular tissues. All samples are stored frozen until analysis. If the bioanalytical laboratory is at a different location, samples need to be shipped frozen over dry ice using an overnight courier. The shipment should be made only Monday through Wednesday so as to avoid thawing of samples if held over the weekend.

3 Ocular Tissue/Fluid Sample Analysis

The processing of ocular tissues is complicated because of sample size and the nature of the matrix.

Sample processing must result in suitable recovery of the drug and its metabolites (analytes) from a biological matrix using sufficient sample cleanup to remove interfering matrix components to allow for detection and quantification of the drug. The techniques chosen should result in a suitable assay sensitivity as well as acceptable selectivity, precision, and accuracy for the method developed. For liquid biological matrices such as plasma or aqueous humor, sample processing is relatively straightforward and usually involves aliquoting a portion of the sample coupled with one or more cleanup steps prior to detection. For an ocular tissue, the sample must first be converted from a semisolid to a semiliquid matrix or to an assay-compatible solution, either via direct extraction of the drug from the tissue into a solvent or through tissue homogenization.

3.1 Tissue Homogenization

Tissue homogenization techniques have been reviewed in the literature [62, 63] and include mechanical homogenization, sonication, and enzymatic or chemical digestions. Ultimately the choice of the sample processing approach will depend on the amount and type of tissue, and the drug being analyzed. Ocular tissue weights vary with tissue type, species, and collection technique, ranging from as low as 10 mg up to 1 g. Multiple homogenization steps may be required for ocular tissue matrices to achieve acceptable overall drug recovery. The sample tube must be compatible with the drug, matrix, and processing method to be used during sample homogenization and/or extraction, with respect to tube material, volume, and cap seal. Loss of drug due to nonspecific binding via interaction with the walls of sample tubes or with the cap seals can be an issue for some drugs, especially in low-protein matrices like aqueous humor, and must be evaluated (e.g., by container-to-container sample transfer experiments). If nonspecific binding is found to be significant, preventive measures such as addition of detergents to sample tubes must be used to allow for acceptable and consistent recovery of drug.

Mechanical tissue homogenization with more traditional rotating blade homogenizers (handheld or semi-automated devices) or with newer bead beater-type homogenizers is commonly used for analysis of ocular tissue samples as part of sample processing [64–66]. Bead beater-type homogenizers are well suited where very small amounts of tissue are available for analysis. Beads made of steel, zirconium, ceramics, or glass are placed into an enclosed container with the tissue and the sample is mixed at a very high speed to produce the homogenate. Reenforced polypropylene tubes varying in volume from 2 to 7 mL are typically used for this procedure. With bead beating, cross contamination during homogenization is eliminated and multiple samples can be processed at the same time. With the more traditional homogenization techniques, very thorough cleaning of the homogenization apparatus between samples is required to prevent sample-to-sample cross contamination. Regardless of the mechanical homogenization approach used, sample processing at cold temperature is required to avoid drug instability due to heat generated during homogenization. Temperature control is also critical under conditions of tissue disruption by high-energy sonication. Similarly, drug stability must be considered under conditions of chemical or enzymatic tissue digestion processes. While simple centrifugation of the homogenate to remove solid tissue fragments can be used as a final processing step under certain situations, more extensive cleanup of the homogenate is generally required.

3.2 Tissue Extraction and Analyte (Drug/Metabolite) Analysis

Three main sample extraction techniques (or variants thereof) used in the bioanalysis of small molecules are protein precipitation, liquid–liquid extraction, and solid-phase extraction (SPE). All can be applied to ocular fluid and tissue analysis. The analyses are typically coupled with chromatography prior to sample detection. High-pressure liquid chromatography (HPLC) coupled with a triple quadrupole mass spectrometer (LC/MS/MS) is the method of choice for most small-molecule drugs because of the superior selectivity and sensitivity of the technique. Recently, the use of high-resolution mass spectrometry (HRMS) has become available for the quantification of drugs in biological matrices.

Other detection systems coupled to HPLC such as ultraviolet (UV)/visible light or fluorescence detection with their advantage of wider linear ranges have also been used in bioanalytical studies, but these detectors typically have less selectivity and far less sensitivity than MS detection and therefore are becoming obsolete in bioanalysis. Radiolabeling can also be used to aid in the determination of distributional characteristics of drugs, especially when highly sensitive bioanalytical methods cannot be easily developed. The disadvantage of measuring drug distribution using radioactivity however, is that the method cannot distinguish radioactivity originating from the parent drug or its metabolites. If LC/MS/MS detection is to be utilized on radiolabeled samples, it must be remembered that the molecular mass will increase depending on the radiolabeled tag used and knowing the exact mass is critical for MS/MS detection.

For macromolecules or larger size molecules such as high-molecular-weight peptides, immunoassays are most often the quantitative method of choice for bioanalysis. Immunoassays have been used for the analysis of proteins in ocular fluids (aqueous and vitreous humor) [67, 68], and tissues [44, 69]. For macromolecules, sample processing techniques prior to the analysis procedure itself are limited as sample cleanup must not adversely affect the structural integrity of the protein to be analyzed. However, for many matrices, the characteristics of antibodies that selectively bind to protein drugs along with the associated washing steps of immunoassays typically constitute sufficient sample cleanup for quantification. Conversely, small-molecule drugs can be processed through a variety of sample processing techniques, typically without impact on chemical structure, and can be extracted from tissues and ocular fluids with relatively high efficiency.

As with homogenization, the choice of extraction procedure must take into account the chemical characteristics of the drug along with the associated challenges of the matrix. Protein precipitation involves, in addition to proteins, the removal of other macromolecules and cellular debris from the sample matrix using a solvent such as acetonitrile or an acid such as trichloroacetic acid. Solvents should ordinarily be added in a ratio of at least 2:1 (organic solvent:aqueous sample), but this should be assessed during method development activities to provide for high drug recovery and is dependent on the characteristics of the drug to be analyzed. In some cases, homogenates may need to be prepared in an aqueous: organic solvent solution due to aqueous solubility characteristics of the drug. After centrifugation of the precipitated sample, the drug typically remains in the supernatant, which is subsequently analyzed. Protein precipitation can leave many interfering matrix components in the supernatant and highly selective detection systems (LC/MS/MS) are typically required for analysis. However, protein precipitation is a very simple technique and is a suitable sample processing procedure for many ocular bioanalytical studies.

Liquid–liquid and SPE extractions tend to produce much cleaner samples. Liquid–liquid extractions involve the addition of an immiscible organic solvent such as methyl-t-butyl ether (MTBE) or ethyl acetate to an aqueous matrix sample, typically at a ratio of 3:1 (organic solvent:aqueous sample) or higher to achieve suitable recovery in a single extraction step. After mixing, the organic and aqueous layers are allowed to separate. The organic solvent layer containing the extracted drug is evaporated and the sample is reconstituted in a compatible solvent for analysis. For ionizable drugs, the pH can be adjusted to provide for additional cleanup steps. For instance, a sample can be made basic to keep an acidic drug in an ionized state and therefore not extractable. The organic solvent can then be used to remove interfering matrix components with an initial extraction, leaving the drug behind in the aqueous layer. After pH adjustment to an acidic condition, the organic solvent can be added again and the now non-ionized acid drug extracted. Liquid–liquid extraction is suitable for ocular fluids, tissue homogenates, and even intact tissues (liquid–solid extraction using vigorous conditions) and can yield very clean extracts for analysis. When using liquid–liquid extraction for intact ocular tissues and homogenates, very long mixing times or multiple extraction steps may be required for acceptable recovery of drug. Lastly, SPE has been used successfully in assays of plasma and other biological fluids, but it is less suitable for tissue homogenates since homogenates contain solid particles which can clog the SPE columns. For SPE to have utility for ocular tissue matrices, the extraction procedure must be coupled to one or more additional sample cleanup procedures to produce a suitable solution for loading onto the SPE column. For instance, organic supernatant of a precipitated tissue homogenate may be diluted with aqueous buffer and then loaded onto a SPE column for additional sample cleanup. Care must be taken to ensure that a high percentage of drug is released into the homogenization buffer or solvent prior to loading the SPE column and to ensure that drug bound to soluble tissue components does not simply flow through the SPE column to waste.

Regardless of the extraction procedure used, it is important to include an internal standard within the assay. The internal standard is a chemical which is structurally similar to the drug to be analyzed and is added in equal amounts to all samples in an analytical run. The internal standard is used to correct for sample-to-sample inconsistencies in sample processing and chromatographic analysis. An internal standard can be added at one of several steps of the extraction procedure depending on assay design and need for reanalysis of the sample. The internal standard should be added as early as possible in the procedure to compensate for losses through processing. Use of a poor internal standard can result in difficulties in method development, restrictions in sample processing methodology, and an assay, which is subject to high failure rates, especially with complex ocular tissue assays. There are two types of internal standards, structural analogues and stable isotopically labeled molecules. Typically, an analogue internal standard will differ only slightly in chemical structure from the drug and will have similar extractability and chromatographic behavior. Analogue internal standards can be used with LC/MS/MS; however, stable labeled internal standards are superior and are the internal standard of choice. Besides almost identical extractability, a stable labeled internal standard will have nearly identical chromatographic characteristics to the drug and will elute at approximately the same retention time. This is important in controlling ionization effects in LC/MS/MS methods caused by matrix components which can suppress or enhance peak response. Under certain conditions, with highly efficient LC columns, drug and stable labeled internal standard can chromatographically separate, which may not be desirable.

The % recovery of a drug (and internal standard) is an important component of bioanalytical method development. Recovery can be estimated by spiking the drug and the internal standard into control matrix (e.g., quality control samples) and comparing assay response after sample processing to that of a reference sample at theoretical concentrations representing 100 % recovery. Recovery of drug across several concentrations as well as that of the internal standard at the concentration used for extraction should be similar. For LC/MS/MS, the reference sample should be prepared in an extracted blank of the biological matrix of interest to account for any ion suppression or enhancement of mass spectrometer response (matrix effects) by endogenous components of the biological matrix. With tissues, it is difficult to determine the true recovery of a drug [62, 63]. Homogenates can be prepared and spiked with drug, but recovery estimation in homogenates only addresses the extraction component of the assay. Therefore, it is important to have recovery assessments from intact tissues, when feasible, to allow for the measurement of drug loss through the homogenization and extraction procedures. However, it must be recognized that exogenous fortification of a control tissue sample does not necessarily equate with biologically incurred drug present in tissue samples following drug administration. Nonetheless, assessments of recovery from both homogenates and intact tissues can better lead to the development of an acceptable method which can enter into assay qualification or validation studies.

3.3 Method Qualification/Validation

Bioanalytical assays used in studies for submissions to regulatory agencies must meet certain requirements to be acceptable and must be assessed prior to use. Method assessments of assay performance generally fall into two categories, the more rigorous method validation and the abbreviated method qualification. Method qualifications are validation-like studies that assess a subset of components normally required for a validation. For bioanalytical assays developed to assess systemic exposure such as for plasma, the methods must typically undergo rigorous validation procedures as prescribed in various regulatory guidance documents [70, 71]. However, for ocular studies, the scarcity of control matrices may make it difficult, if not impossible, to follow the applicable guidance for validations. When ocular fluid or tissue-specific exposure data is critical for supporting regulated safety studies, a method validation or at least a method qualification study should be performed, before utilizing the method for sample analysis. As with plasma validations, ocular tissue method validations and/or method qualifications should assess the accuracy and precision of the method across multiple analytical runs. The assessment of accuracy and precision is a critical component of a validation or a qualification study as these parameters define the capability of a method to measure the true or the theoretical concentration values of assayed samples and the degree of consistency across replicates. Selectivity, or the ability of an assay to differentiate the drug from other components in the matrix such as endogenous compounds, is another important component of validations. Additional parameters to be assessed include calibration curve performance, short-term matrix stability, long-term matrix freezer stability, extract stability, reinjection performance, recovery, and other applicable assay parameters. When a control matrix is difficult to obtain and not all validation parameters can be tested, a method qualification is run and a justification provided when used for regulatory studies. For bioanalytical assays supporting internal decision making such as for lead drug candidate selection or early formulation studies, a full validation may not be necessary and a method qualification assessing at least 1 day of accuracy and precision, and perhaps some stability, may be sufficient. While method qualification studies are less extensive than method validation studies, sufficient evaluation must be conducted to allow for high confidence in the method used for the samples of interest. For instance, establishment of benchtop stability, a lack of matrix interference, and/or a lack of matrix effects to reduce assay bias in reporting results for the study samples may be deemed critical for a method qualification, but parameters such as percent recovery need not be run as in validations. In addition, method qualifications may be run with a single day of accuracy and precision, while validations should consist of multiple runs over several days. With method qualifications, acceptance criteria are often relaxed from those of validated methods, and for small molecules, ±20 % acceptance criteria are often used. However, criteria may need to be tighter or can sometimes be relaxed further, and should be based on the use and critical nature of the data.

As with any quantitative assay, calibration standards should be prepared in sufficient numbers across the assay range to be used. In the case of regulated bioanalytical methods, a calibration curve range should consist of at least six different concentration levels [70, 71]. During validation, the suitability of the curve range is tested by preparing calibration curves for each analytical run in the study. The suitability of the calibration curve is determined by consistent and acceptable accuracy and precision of the calibration samples, as well as acceptable accuracy of quality control (QC) samples prepared at concentrations within the range of the assay. QC samples are prepared independently of calibration samples at low, mid, and high concentrations within the curve range, and are used to assess both accuracy and precision of the method as well as stability of the drug in matrix and in the prepared extracts.

3.4 Use of a Surrogate Matrix

It is advisable to prepare calibration standards in the same matrix as the study samples to be analyzed. However, this will not always be feasible due to the limited availability of control matrix on ethical grounds for animal welfare. When this occurs, the choice of a surrogate matrix of high similarity to the ocular study sample matrix is recommended to allow for appropriate assay performance. If a closely related surrogate matrix is not available and a less closely related one is utilized (e.g., plasma as a surrogate matrix for ocular tissues), use of a stable labeled internal standard becomes even more important (when using LC/MS/MS). Also critical is a thorough sample cleanup procedure, to ensure comparability of the final extracted samples derived from the surrogate and study sample matrices. This is important because of potential differences in the recovery of drug and/or due to variable amounts of endogenous compounds present in the surrogate and study sample matrices that can affect quantification. A stable labeled internal standard is likely to compensate for the differences. As discussed previously for melanin-containing tissues, surrogate matrix may not yield comparable drug peak response to that of the study sample matrix, but with adequate internal standard correction, an assay can often be developed to appropriately quantify drug in the tissues of interest under these circumstances.

3.5 Sample Analysis

After a method validation or qualification study has been completed and the bioanalytical method has been shown to be acceptable for its purpose, the sample analysis phase can be initiated. Acceptance criteria are set for the calibration curve and for the QC samples used during sample analysis based on the type of study, the performance of the method during validation or qualification, and regulatory requirements. Criteria are often set as per the regulatory guidance documents [70, 71] with calibration curves having at least 75 % of the calibration standards within 15 % of nominal concentration (20 % at the LLOQ) and two-thirds of QC samples within 15 % of nominal concentration. It may be acceptable to widen the acceptance criteria, especially during the early phases of drug development. Although meeting the acceptance criteria is critical in the decision to report study sample drug concentrations from a given analytical run, additional parameters of assay performance should also be assessed. For LC/MS/MS or other chromatographic methods, each analytical run must be inspected to ensure that peak shape and peak response of the study samples are comparable to those of the calibration standards and QC samples. Study samples can be subject to interferences from metabolites or components of formulations not present in spiked samples used for calibration and this can result in a bias in the reported concentrations. Some metabolites such as glucuronides can potentially revert back to the drug within the source of the mass spectrometer and these can interfere when eluting near the retention time of the drug or worse, bias drug concentration when eluting at the same retention time. Trends in peak response anomalies can also occur and these can be checked by comparing the internal standard response in the calibration standards and QC samples with that of the study samples; the responses should be comparable in magnitude. Study samples can even cause the peak response throughout a run to shift, differing substantially from that encountered during validation where only spiked samples are used. Unusual assay responses caused by or associated with the study samples may require post-validation investigations and even method modifications and subsequent revalidations. Atypical responses from ocular tissue study samples are not uncommon and differences between study and calibration samples can be even more substantial when using surrogate matrix curves.

Since it is often necessary to cover a large analytical range for quantification, the calibration range limitations of existing instrumentation can be a challenge for the analysis of ocular tissue samples. Due to the relatively small size of ocular tissue samples, methods often do not allow for re-extraction of over-range samples by dilution such as with plasma or serum assays. For early pilot distribution studies where tissue concentrations are unknown, a broad calibration curve outside the normal linear range of the detector (e.g., three orders of magnitude for mass spectrometers) may be used with a quadratic regression. After the pilot studies, the calibration range can be reduced in magnitude for subsequent studies such that a linear regression can be used. An alternative approach which may be more suitable for validation is to employ multiple calibration ranges for the assay. A low calibration curve range can be prepared for an initial processing of samples and a higher calibration curve range prepared with subsequent dilution of sample extracts to fall within acceptable detection limits. After an initial analysis using the low calibration range, any over-range samples can be analyzed using the high-concentration calibration curve with the more dilute extracts.

Acknowledgments

The authors express their gratitude to Prof. Neal Castagnoli, Peters Professor of Chemistry, Virginia Tech, Blacksburg, VA, for making literature available for ocular metabolism and for critical review of the manuscript. Authors also wish to thank Dr. James E. Patrick of Patrick's Pharmaceutical Consulting, LLC, Mr. Sidney Weiss of I-Novion, Inc, and Mr. Lee Hamm of Intertek Pharmaceutical Services for providing a critical review of this manuscript.

References

1. Bodor N, Buchwald P (2005) Ophthalmic drug design based on the metabolic activity of the eye: soft drugs and chemical delivery systems. AAPS J 7(4):E820–E833
2. Shell J (1982) Pharmacokinetics of topically applied ophthalmic drugs. Surv Ophthalmol 26(4):207–218
3. Urtti A (2006) Challenges and obstacles of ocular pharmacokinetics and drug delivery. Adv Drug Deliv Rev 58:1131–1135
4. Gaudana R, Ananthula HK, Parenky A, Mitra AK (2010) Ocular drug delivery. AAPS J 12 (3):348–360
5. Duvvuri S, Majumdar S, Mitra MK (2004) Role of metabolism in ocular drug delivery. Curr Drug Metab 5:507–515
6. Macoid MC, Sieg JW, Robinson JR (1976) Corneal drug absorption, an illustration of parallel first-order absorption and rapid loss of drug from absorption depot. J Pharm Sci 65:150–152
7. Al-Ghananeem A, Crooks P (2007) Phase I and phase II ocular metabolic activities and the role of metabolism in ophthalmic prodrug and codrug design and delivery. Molecules 12:373–388
8. Chandegara NP, Chorawala MR (2012) Soft and dissociative steroids: a new approach for the treatment of inflammatory airway and eye diseases. Int J Pharmaceut Sci Res 3 (2):311–319
9. Noble S, Goa KL (1998) Loteprednol etabonate: clinical potential in the management of ocular inflammation. BioDrugs 10:329–339
10. Benedetti MS, Whomsley R, Poggesi I et al (2009) Drug metabolism and pharmacokinetics. Drug Metabol Rev 41(3):344–390
11. Attar M, Shen J, Ling KJ, Tang-Liu D (2005) Ophthalmic drug delivery considerations at the cellular level: drug-metabolising enzymes and transporters. Expert Opin Drug Deliv 2 (5):891–908
12. Shichi H (1984) Biotransformation and drug metabolism. Handbook Exp Pharmacol 69 (1):117–148
13. Leinweber FJ (1991) Drug disposition in the mammalian eye and brain: a comparison of mechanisms. Drug Metab Rev 23(1–2):133–246
14. Bergamini MVW (1984) In: Glaucoma: Appl Pharmacol Med Treat [Proc Meet] Drance SM, Neufeld AH (ed) p 151–184
15. Jaanus SD (1992) Ocular side effects of selected systemic drugs. Optom Clin 2:73–96
16. Kishida K, Matsumoto K, Manabe R, Sugiyama T (1986) Cytochrome P450 and related components of the microsomal electron transport system in the bovine ciliary body. Curr Eye Res 5:529–533
17. Schwartzman ML, Abraham NG, Masferrer J et al (1985) Cytochrome P450 dependent metabolism of arachidonic acid in bovine corneal epithelium. Biochem Biophys Res Commun 132:343–351
18. Schwartzman ML, Masferrer J, Dunn MW, Mcgiff JC, Abraham NG (1987) Cytochrome P450, drug metabolizing enzymes and arachidonic acid metabolism in bovine ocular tissues. Curr Eye Res 6:623–630
19. Asakura T, Shishi H (1992) Cytochrome P450-mediated prostaglandin omega/omega-1 hydroxylase activities in porcine ciliary body epithelial cells. Exp Eye Res 55:377–384
20. Shichi H, Atlas SA, Nebert DW (1975) Genetically regulated arylhydrocarbon hydroxylase induction in the eye: possible significance of the drug-metabolising enzyme system for the retinal pigmented epithelium-choriod. Exp Eye Res 21:557–567
21. Schwartzman ML, Pageno PJ, Mcgriff JC, Abraham NG (1987) Immunochemical studies

on the contribution of NADPH cytochrome P450 reductase to the cytochrome P450 dependent metabolism of arachidonic acid. Arch Biochem Biophys 252:635–645

22. Shanthaveerappa TR, Bourne GH (1964) Monoamine oxidase distribution in the rabbit eye. J Histochem Cytochem 12:281–287
23. Sparks DL, Thomas TN, Buckholtz NS (1981) Monoamine oxidase activity in bovine retina: subcellular distribution and drug sensitivities. Neurosci Lett 21:201–206
24. Crabbe MJC (1985) Ocular diamine oxidase activity. Exp Eye Res 41:777–778
25. Muzio G, Maggiora M, Paiuzzi E, Oraldi M, Canuto RA (2012) Aldehyde dehydrogenases and cell proliferation. Free Radic Biol Med 52 (4):735–746
26. Lee VH (1983) Esterase activities in adult rabbit eyes. J Pharm Sci 72(3):239–244
27. Sanchez-Chavez G, Vidal CJ, Salceda R (1995) Acetyl- and butyrylcholinesterase activities in the rat retina and retinal pigment epithelium. J Neurosci Res 41:655–662
28. Coupland SE, Hoffman HH, Penfoldand PL, Billson FA (1993) Increased hydroxylase activities in the human trabecular meshwork of glaucomatous eyes. Ger J Ophthalmol 2:107–112
29. Appleyard ME, McDonald B, Benjamin L (1991) Presence of a soluble form of acetylcholinesterase in human ocular fluids. Br J Ophthalmol 75:276–279
30. Physlactos AC (1991) The lysosomal enzymes of the iris-ciliary body are retained in their organelles and exhibit increased activities during acute uveal inflamation. Acta Ophthalmol (Copenh) 69:33–38
31. Rao PV, Zigler JS Jr (1991) Zeta-crystallin from guinea pig lens is capable of functioning catalytically as an oxidoreductase. Arch Biochem Biophys 284:181–185
32. Gondhowiardojo TD, van Haeringen NJ, Hoekzema R, Pels L, Kijlstra A (1991) Detection of aldehyde dehydrogenase activity in human corneal extracts. Curr Eye Res 10:1001–1007
33. Godbout R (1992) High levels of aldehyde dehydrogenase transcripts in the undifferentiated chick retina. Exp Eye Res 54:297–305
34. Holmes RS, Vandeberg JL (1986) Ocular NAD-dependent alcohol dehydrogenase and aldyhyde dehydrogenase in the baboon. Exp Eye Res 43:383–398
35. Watkins J, Wirthwein DP, Sanders RA (1991) Comparative study of phase II biotransformation in rabbit ocular tissues. Drug Metab Dispos 19:708–713
36. Ahmed H, Singh SV, Medh RD, Ansari GAS, Kurosoku A, Awasthi YC (1988) Differential expression of omega, beta, and pi classes isozymes of glutathione S-transferase in bovine lens, cornea and retina. Arch Biochem Biophys 266:416–426
37. Zhang T, Xiang CD, Gale D, Carreiro S, Zhang EY (2008) Drug transporter and cytochrome P450 mRNA expression in human ocular barriers: implications for ocular drug disposition. Drug Metab Dispos 36:1300–1307
38. Faulkner R, Sharif NA, Orr S, Sall K, Dubiner H, Whitson JT, Moster M, Craven ER, Curtis M, Pailliotet C, Martens K, Dahlin D (2010) Aqueous humor concentrations of bimatoprost free acid, bimatoprost and travoprost free acid in cataract surgical patients administered multiple topical ocular doses of lumigan or travatan. J Ocul Pharmacol Ther 26 (2):147–156
39. Fung NE, Zheng N, Arnold EM, Zeng J (2010) Effective screening approach to select esterase inhibitors used for stabilizing ester-containing prodrugs analyzed by LC-MS/MS. Bioanalysis 2(4):733–743
40. Wolf R, Rosche F, Hoffmann T, Demuth HU (2001) Immunoprecipitation and liquid chromatography–mass spectrometric determination of the peptide glucose-dependent insulinotropic polypeptides GIP1–42 and GIP3–42 from human plasma samples. New sensitive method to analyze physiological concentrations of peptide hormones. J Chromatogr A 926:21–27
41. Fanciulli G, Azara E, Wood TD, Delitala G, Marchetti M (2007) Liquid chromatography-–mass spectrometry assay for quantification of gluten exorphin B5 in cerebrospinal fluid. J Chromatogr B 852:485–490
42. Aoyagi T, Umezawa H (1981) The relationships between enzyme inhibitors and function of mammalian cells. Acta Biol Med Ger 40 (10–11):1523–1529
43. Gaudreault J, Fei D, Rusit J, Suboc P, Shiu V (2005) Preclinical pharmacokinetics of ranibizumab (rhuFabV2) after a single intravitreal administration. Invest Ophthalmol Vis Sci 46 (2):726–733
44. Xu Y, You Y, Du W, Zhao C, Li J, Mao J, Chen H, Cheng L (2012) Ocular pharmacokinetics of bevacizumab in vitrectomized eyes with silicone oil tamponade. Invest Ophthalmol Vis Sci 53(9):5221–5226
45. Ewles M, Goodwin L (2011) Bioanalytical approaches to analyzing peptides and proteins by LC–MS/MS. Bioanalysis 3(12):1379–1397
46. Venn RF (ed) (2000) Principles and practice of bioanalysis. Taylor and Francis, London

47. Deneka N, Wan S, Bond O, Kornburst D, Reich S (2008) Ocular biodistribution of bevasiranib following a single intravitreal injection to rabbit eyes. Mol Vis 14:997–1005
48. Lakshmana Prabu S, Suriyaprakash TNK (2012) Extraction of drug from the biological matrix: a review, applied biological engineering—principles and practice, Naik G R (ed.), ISBN: 978-953-51-0412-4, InTech. http://www.intechopen.com/books/applied-biological-engineering-principlesand-practice/extraction-of-the-drug-from-the-biological-matrix
49. Kwon Y (2001) Handbook of essential pharmacokinetics, pharmacodynamics, and drug metabolism for industrial scientists. Kluwer Academic/Plenum Publishers, New York
50. Grus FH, Joachim SC, Pfeiffer N (2007) Proteomics in ocular fluids. Proteomics Clin Appl 1:876–888
51. Riley MV, Green K (1992) Comparative physiology and biochemistry of the eye. In: Otto H et al (eds) Manual of oculotoxicity testing of drugs. Gustav Fischer Verlag, Stuttgart, Jenna, New York
52. Schirmer O (1903) Studien zur Physiologie und Pathophysiolgie der Tränenabsonderung und Tränenabfuhr. Albrecht Von Graefes Arch Ophthalmol 56:197–291
53. Mains J, Tan LE, Zhang T, Young L, Shi R, Wilson C (2012) Species variations in small molecule components of animal vitreous. Invest Ophthalmol Vis Sci 53 (8):4778–4786
54. Meek KM, Fullwood NJ (2001) Corneal and scleral collagens—a microscopist's perspective. Micron 32(3):261–272
55. Austin BA, Coulon C, Liu CY, Kao WW, Rada JA (2002) Altered collagen fibril formation in the sclera of lumican-deficient mice. Invest Ophthalmol Vis Sci 43(6):1695–1701
56. Kelley PB, Sado Y, Duncan MK (2002) Collagen IV in the developing lens capsule. Matrix Biol 21(5):415–423
57. Salazar-Bookman MM, Wainer I, Patil PN (1994) Relevance of drug-melanin interactions to ocular pharmacology and toxicology. J Ocul Pharmacol 10:217–239
58. Leblanc B, Jezequel S, Davies T, Hanton G, Taradach C (1998) Binding of drugs to melanin is not predictive of ocular toxicity. Regul Toxicol Pharmacol 28:124–132
59. Howells L, Godfrey M, Sauer MJ (1994) Melanin as an adsorbent of drug residues. Analyst 119:2691–2693
60. Fukuda M, Morita Y, Sasaki K (2000) Studies on the binding mechanism of fluoroquinolones to melanin. J Infect Chemother 6:72–76
61. Tanaka M, Takashina H, Tsutsumi S (2004) Comparative assessment of ocular tissue distribution of drug-related radioactivity after chronic oral administration of ^{14}C-levofloxacin and ^{14}C-chloroquine in pigmented rats. J Pharm Pharmacol 56:977–983
62. Xue YJ, Gao H, Ji QC, Lam Z, Fang X, Lin ZJ, Hoffman M, Schulz-Jander D, Weng N (2012) Bioanalysis of drug in tissue: current status and challenges. Bioanalysis 4(21):2637–2653
63. Smith KM, Xu Y (2012) Tissue sample preparation in bioanalytical assays. Bioanalysis 4 (6):741–749
64. Ichhpujani P, Katz LJ, Hollo G, Shields CL, Shields JA, Marr B, Eagle R, Alvim H, Wizov SS, Acheampong A, Chen J, Wheeler LA (2012) Comparison of human ocular distribution of bimatoprost and latanoprost. J Ocul Pharmacol Ther 28(2):134–145
65. Si EC, Bowman LM, Hosseini K (2011) Pharmacokinetic comparisons of bromfenac in duraSite and xibrom. J Ocul Pharmacol Ther 27 (1):61–66
66. Kadam RS, Jadhav G, Ogidigben M, Kompella UB (2011) Ocular pharmacokinetics of dorzolamide and brinzolamide after single and multiple topical dosing: implications for effects on ocular blood flow. Drug Metab Dispos 39 (9):1529–1537
67. Sinapis CI, Routsias JG, Sinapis AI, Sinapis DI, Agrogiannis GD, Pantopoulou A, Theocharis SE, Baltatzis S, Patsouris E, Perrea D (2011) Pharmacokinetics of intravitreal bevacizumab (Avastin®) in rabbits. Clin Ophthalmol 2011 (5):697–704
68. Chen JJ, Ebmeier SE, Sutherland WM, Ghazi NG (2011) Potential penetration of topical ranibizumab (Lucentis) in the rabbit eye. Eye (Lond) 25:1504–1511
69. Nomoto H, Shiraga F, Kuno N, Kimura E, Fujii S, Shinomiya K, Nugent AK, Hirooka K, Baba T (2009) Pharmacokinetics of bevacizumab after topical, subconjunctival, and intravitreal administration in rabbits. Invest Ophthalmol Vis Sci 50(10):4807–4813
70. Guidance for Industry: Bioanalytical Method Validation, U.S. Department of Health and Human Services, Food and Drug Administration, May 2001
71. Guideline on Bioanalytical Method Validation, European Medicines Agency, July 2011

Methods in Pharmacology and Toxicology (2014): 53–79
DOI 10.1007/7653_2013_9

Published online: 17 July 2013

Chemistry, Manufacturing, and Control of Ophthalmic Formulations

Malay Ghosh and Imran Ahmed

Abstract

A road map to develop ophthalmic formulations for topical ocular applications is provided in this chapter. This includes design of appropriate studies, development of formulations matching target product profile, selection of suitable packaging, stability assessment, and critical aspects of manufacturing. Uniqueness and challenges associated with ophthalmic formulation development are also described. The chapter further outlines the regulatory requirements necessary to file IND and NDA.

Key words Preformulation, Drug substance, Drug product, Pharmaceutical development, Dosage form, Impurities, Tests and specifications, Container closure system, Manufacturing, Sterilization, Stability, ICH, FDA, Regulatory submission

1 Introduction

Ophthalmic preparations are sterile products that may be administered topically to the eye or injected into ocular tissue compartments in the anterior or the posterior segments of the eye (Fig. 1) [1, 2]. Dosage forms for the eye include, but are not restricted to, solutions, suspensions, emulsions, gels, ointments, implants, and inserts [3]. Ophthalmic formulations, like dosage forms used for other routes of delivery, must fulfill the essential requirements of safety, stability, manufacturability, and bioavailability. In addition to fulfilling these common requirements ophthalmic dosage forms must be designed with special attention to formulation factors that may affect ocular tolerability and safety, such as the pH, buffer type, buffer capacity, excipient type and levels, osmolarity, sterility, endotoxin content, preservatives, and particulate matter. As such, the chemistry, manufacturing, and controls (CMC) of ophthalmic formulations is especially constrained by issues related to patient safety and tolerability, compendia requirement, and regulatory guidelines [1].

This chapter provides CMC guidance for the design and development of ophthalmic formulations with emphasis on topical ocular drug delivery. The development scientist may utilize the information presented herein to help design and carry out the

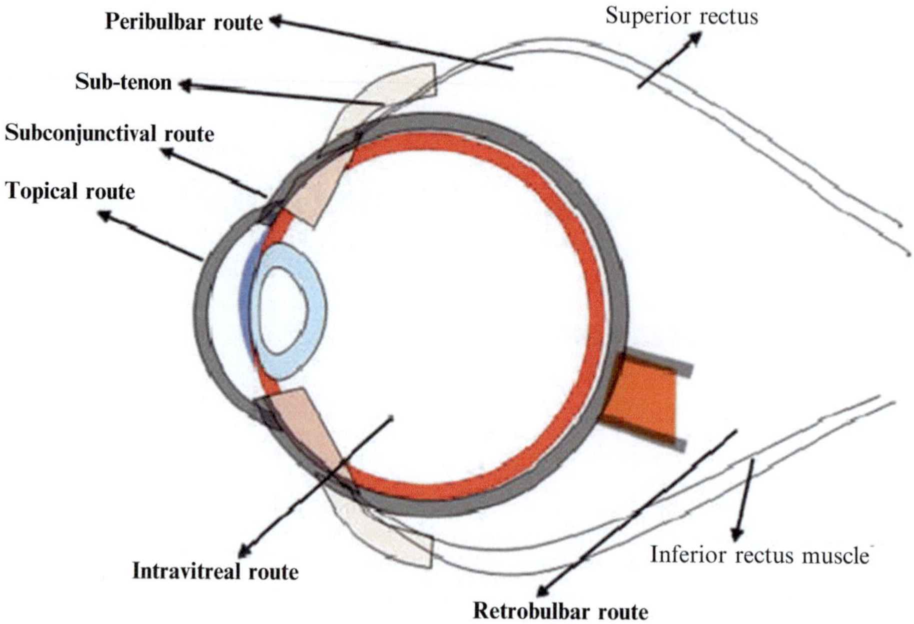

Fig. 1 Routes of administration into the eye. © 2013 U.S. Pharmacopeial Convention, used by permission

activities for selecting the qualitative and quantitative (Q Q) composition, specifications and controls, packaging, and manufacturing process for ophthalmic drug products. It is important to note that this is not a prescriptive document and specific chemical and physical characteristics of the molecule should be considered and need to be addressed as part of the development process. The approach described herein is based upon rational formulation design concepts and quality by design (QbD) approaches for selecting the preferred drug product composition consistent with regulatory guidance.

2 Ophthalmic Formulation Development Planning

The topical ophthalmic product development flow chart shown in Fig. 2 describes critical steps/studies necessary to develop the target formulation with desired attributes meeting pharmaceutical and regulatory requirements.

The essential first step in rational product development is to construct the quality target product profile (QTPP) that identifies quality attributes critical for product performance [4]. Although identification of all the product attributes may not be possible at the onset of development, it is important to identify as many quality attributes as possible in order to understand the formulation and the final targeted product. An example of a QTPP is provided in Table 1.

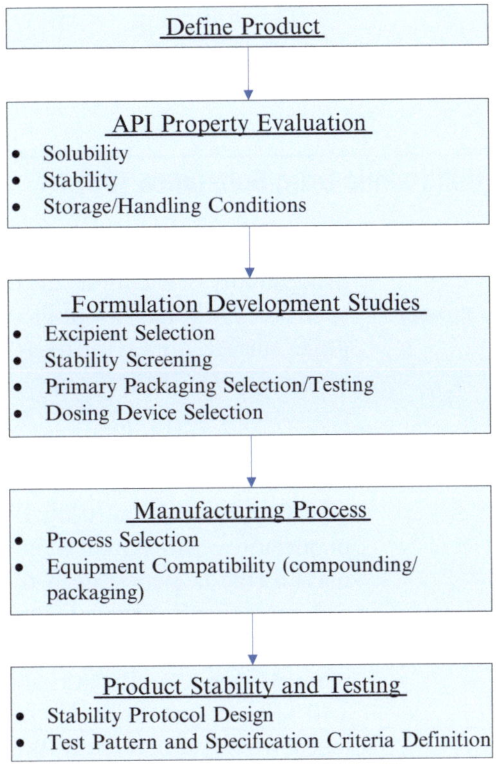

Fig. 2 Topical ophthalmic product development flow chart

Table 1
Representative QTPP of a topical ocular product

	Must	Preferred
Route of administration	Topical ocular	Same
Dosage form	Solution, suspension, emulsion	Solution
Efficacy	Must meet desired criteria	Same
Excipients	Toxicologically acceptable and ICH Q8 justifiable	Same
Target pH	5–7.5	7.4
Safety	No adverse effect	Same
Shelf life	18 months at 15–25 °C	24 months at 2–30 °C
Preservative effectiveness	Meets USP and Ph. Eur B Requirements	Ph. Eur A Requirements
Endotoxin	<0.5 EU/mL	<0.5 EU/mL
Packaging	Package: Describe size Fill volume : Describe volume Package sterilization: Describe method	Same
Manufacturing capability	Ability to manufacture following cGMP	Same

The following overview primarily focuses on CMC aspects of ophthalmic formulations as a roadmap for developmental scientists.

3 CMC of Ophthalmic Drug Substance (DS)

3.1 Ocular Drug Candidate Developability Criteria

A critical aspect in formulation development is to assess the druggability of the molecule of interest. Physicochemical properties such as solubility, lipophilicity, ionic charge, molecular size, and polar surface area contribute to drug penetration through ocular tissues [5–9]. Topically applied drugs that penetrate through the cornea by passive diffusion usually proceed via either transcellular or paracellular pathway. Partition coefficient (log P) of the drug molecule has significant impact on drug penetration through cornea. Compounds with log P between 1 and 3 showed maximum penetration. Molecular weight and size of the drug molecule also plays a role in penetration through different ocular tissues due to different cutoff molecular weight of ocular tissues. For example, molecular weight cutoff for cornea is at approximately 500 Da, whereas for conjunctiva and sclera are approximately 40 and 150 kDa, respectively. Therefore, higher molecular weight molecules would more likely be absorbed in conjunctiva and sclera compared to cornea [9–16].

The ionization constant is an important parameter in ocular absorption of acidic and basic drugs. Although both the ionizable and the unionized forms of the drug may diffuse across ocular membranes, it is predominantly the unionized form that determines the extent of ocular drug absorption (bioavailability). Therefore, from a drruggability perspective, it is important to select functional groups that maximize the unionized fraction at physiological pH without compromising other attributes such as solubility, stability and potency. The salt form of the drug molecule can also play a significant role in ocular bioavailability as well as comfort after instillation.

A salt form of the drug may be considered to improve or modify the solubility or aqueous dissolution rate. Identification and selection of the best physical form from developability viewpoint are critical to avoid issues at a later time. Physical form and salt screening at this stage is an important step to identify the most stable form that can go to the product development [17–20]. Therefore, judicious selection of salt form is essential.

In some cases prodrug approach may be considered in drug candidate selection if there is a need to modulate certain physicochemical properties that cannot be resolved by physical methods. Prodrugs can have substantially better bioavailability and solubility characteristics than the parent compound. For example, prodrugs of various prostaglandins showed substantial higher bioavailability compared to parent compound and are used in marketed products for treatment of open-angle glaucoma. Esters of pilocarpine were developed with enhanced aqueous stability [20–25].

The characterization of the physicochemical properties of the drug substance or active pharmaceutical ingredient (API) is critical in developing a successful ophthalmic product. Drug substance storage temperature, humidity, and packaging materials require evaluation as part of formulation development. Packaging materials and storage conditions should be evaluated with the assumption that the package will be opened multiple times for sampling and subdivision at the manufacturing site. Improper storage conditions can lead to moisture uptake or product degradation, impacting potency of the formulation.

3.2 Preformulation Studies for Drug Substance

Preformulation studies are routinely carried out to characterize and profile the chemistry and pharmaceutics of the drug substance [26]. Physicochemical information on the compound of interest (API) is also needed for dossier in regulatory submission. A list of such studies is provided in Table 2.

3.3 Drug Substance Chemistry, Manufacturing, Control

Code of federal register and FDA guidance related to drug substance were issued with intention "to provide sponsors with procedures acceptable to the agency for complying with regulations pertaining to the submission of adequate information on the production and control of new drug substances" [27, 28]. Most recent guidance to industry by regulatory agencies on drug substance CMC were published in 2010 [29–35]. According to ICH e-CTD format, CMC of drug substance constitute section 3.2.S.1–3.2.S.7 (*see* Table 12), including all aspects of drug substance such as manufacturing, characterization, control, stability, impurity, and reference standard.

The DS characterization process involves structural characterization with NMR, FTIR, UV, MS, and single crystal structure determination. Physical characterization involves particle size, morphology (optical microscopy and SEM), XRPD, TGA, DSC, moisture content, moisture sorption/desorption isotherms, etc. A detailed crystal form study should be carried out as well to identify the most stable form for development. Other tests, as appropriate and as needed, would be conducted on DS to characterize properly and identify uniqueness and risk associated. According to ICH Q3A guidance, impurities in an API can be classified into three categories as mentioned below [29].

3.3.1 Organic Impurities

Organic impurities constitute process-related impurities and any associated degradation products. Reporting, identification, and qualification thresholds of impurities, as per ICH Q3A guidance [29], are provided in Table 3.

Table 2
List of preformulation studies

Study	Comment
Ionization constant (pKa)	Information helpful to improve aqueous solubility, assess BCS classification, and identify best candidate.
Partition/distribution coefficient (Log D/P)	Lipophilicity. Information helpful to assess BCS classification and identify best candidate for development.
Solubility	Intrinsic solubility. pH solubility (preferred pH 4–8).
Effect of solubilizers	Surfactant. Cosolvent. Complexing agents. Surfactant/cosolvent combination. Cosolvent/complexing agent combination. Cosolvent/surfactant/complexing agent combination.
Effect of common ions on solubility	With appropriate salts.
Solution stability	pH stability (preferred pH 4–8). Arrhenius study (pH 5 and 7). Oxidation study with oxidants.
Photostability	Under ICH light condition (preferred pH 4–8).
Crystal properties and polymorphism, solid-state characterization, evaluate relative stability of known solid forms	Conduct study to determine the most stable crystal form. Important for suspension formulation.
Excipient compatibility	With excipients commonly used in ophthalmic formulations.
Effect of sterilization	Determine the best method of sterilization (dry heat, gamma, autoclave slurry, ETO).
Packaging compatibility	Assess packaging compatibility (as appropriate and needed).

The impurities should be specified in the drug substance specification section. Furthermore, a rationale for inclusion/exclusion of impurities should also be included in the submission. A decision tree for identification and qualification of impurities is also provided in the guidance.

3.3.2 Inorganic Impurities

These are generally assessed and if necessary qualified following compendia or other suitable procedures. Discussion in the submission should be provided on inclusion/exclusion requirement of

Table 3
Reporting, identification, and qualification thresholds of impurities in drug substance

Maximum daily dose	Reporting threshold	Identification threshold	Qualification threshold
≤2 g/day	0.05 %	0.10 % or 1.0 mg per day intake (whichever is lower)	0.15 % or 1.0 mg per day intake (whichever is lower)
>2 g/day	0.03 %	0.05 %	0.05 %

inorganic impurities as well as acceptance criteria in a new drug substance. Based on pharmacopoeial standard and available safety data, acceptance criteria should also be established [34].

3.3.3 Solvents

Analysis and control of residual solvents used in manufacturing process should be discussed and need to follow guidance provided in ICH Q3C Impurities: Residual Solvents [35].

4 CMC of Drug Product (DP)

As previously mentioned in Section 2 QTPP should be considered carefully as a part of drug product design criteria. Since these products are intended for regulatory submission and obtaining marketing approval, therefore, they must meet compendia (major pharmacopeia) requirements and satisfy safety and regulatory requirements. It is advisable to adhere to ICH Q8 (R2) guidance since it encompasses most of the critical aspects of pharmaceutical development [30]. In addition, other appropriate guidelines related to stability, impurities, etc. should be adhered to as well [36, 37]. In general, the products are expected to have at least two year of shelf life at room-temperature storage. For multidose ophthalmic products, a general guideline provided in Table 4 will highlight CMC aspects that need to be considered in ophthalmic formulation design. Overall, the design process involves that development of drug product must be safe and efficacious, and that drug products should be stable with desired pharmaceutical attributes. Table 4 provides a list of the test parameters and rationale for topical ophthalmic drug products.

4.1 Comparative Assessment of Dosage Form Options

As various topical ocular formulation options may be considered it would be helpful to provide a brief description of each dosage form to get a better understanding on CMC of drug products. A decision tree for formulation selection is presented in Fig. 3.

Table 4
Test parameters, recommended targets, and test rationale for ophthalmic products

Test	Recommended target	Rationale for test	Comment
Appearance	As per compendia	Required test Control of DP	–
pH	As per target product profile	Required test Control of DP	–
Viscosity (cps)	As per target product profile	Required test Control of DP (for viscous product only)	–
Osmolality (mOsm/kg)[a]	As per target product profile	Required test Control of DP	–
Osmolality ratio[a]	0.9–1.2	Required test for Japan Per JP	Required in Japan
Particulates (for solution)	As per compendia 10 μm NMT 50/mL 25 μm NMT 5/mL 50 μm NMT 2/mL	Required test Control of DP	Unique specification for ophthalmic solution, more stringent compared to LVP
Particle size (for suspension)	D10 D50 D90	Required test Control of DP	–
Insoluble particulate material	NMT one particle of ≥ 300 μm size per mL of dosage form	Required test for Japan Per JP	Required in Japan
Sterility	Must be sterile	Required test Control of DP	Must meet requirements
Bacterial endotoxin	<0.5 EU/mL	Required test Control of DP	Only required in the USA for topical ophthalmic products Criteria similar to injectable products
Preservative effective test[b]	Must meet compendia requirements	Developmental test required for multidose products Control of DP	Not required in unit dose sterile products
Packaging	No interaction with packaging material Leachates should be justifiable Packaging integrity must be demonstrated Packaging material should meet compendia requirements	Control of DP Control of container closure system	–

(continued)

Table 4 (continued)

Test	Recommended target	Rationale for test	Comment
Drop size[a]	As per QTPP Usually 25–45 μL/drop for topical ophthalmics	Control of container closure system Control of dosage form administration	–
Weight loss	Preferably less than 5 % at 40 °C/26 weeks	Control of DP Control of container closure system For information purpose Developmental test	–

[a]Not required for ointment
[b]Not required for injectable products (IVT, intracameral, etc.)

4.1.1 Solution

Solutions are the most common dosage form for BCS class I and III compounds or their suitable salts. Most of the currently marketed ophthalmic products belong to this dosage form. The solution dosage form has several advantages including dose uniformity, ease of manufacturability and often provides better bioavailability. The limitations with solution dosage forms is rapid clearance and a short precorneal residence time after instillation. Additionally, solutions of hydrolytically labile compound may have a limited shelf life to have a marketable product.

Improvement of precorneal residence time after administration by reducing drainage can be improved by increasing viscosity of the formulation [38–40]. For this purpose, synthetic, semisynthetic, and naturally occurring polymers such as carbomer, polyvinyl alcohol, povidone, hypromellose, other cellulose derivatives, and guar gum were successfully used in various products [41]. According to current USP and work by Robinson [39] the corneal residence time of active from topically applied formulation increases proportionally with the increase of formulation viscosity up to 20 cps. Potential disadvantages of high-viscosity solution formulation include blurred vision and ocular discomfort; therefore attention should be paid before developing a high-viscosity formulation.

For a solution formulation the drug concentration that can be achieved is dependent on the pH solubility profile of the DS. If needed the strength that can be achieved by increasing solubility using suitable cosolvents and solubilizing systems. Low-dose volumes, typically less than 50 μL, are necessary for a product to be appropriate for topical ocular administration. Selection of formulation pH is driven by the drug substance's pH stability, pH solubility, and ocular tolerability data, with the typical pH range for

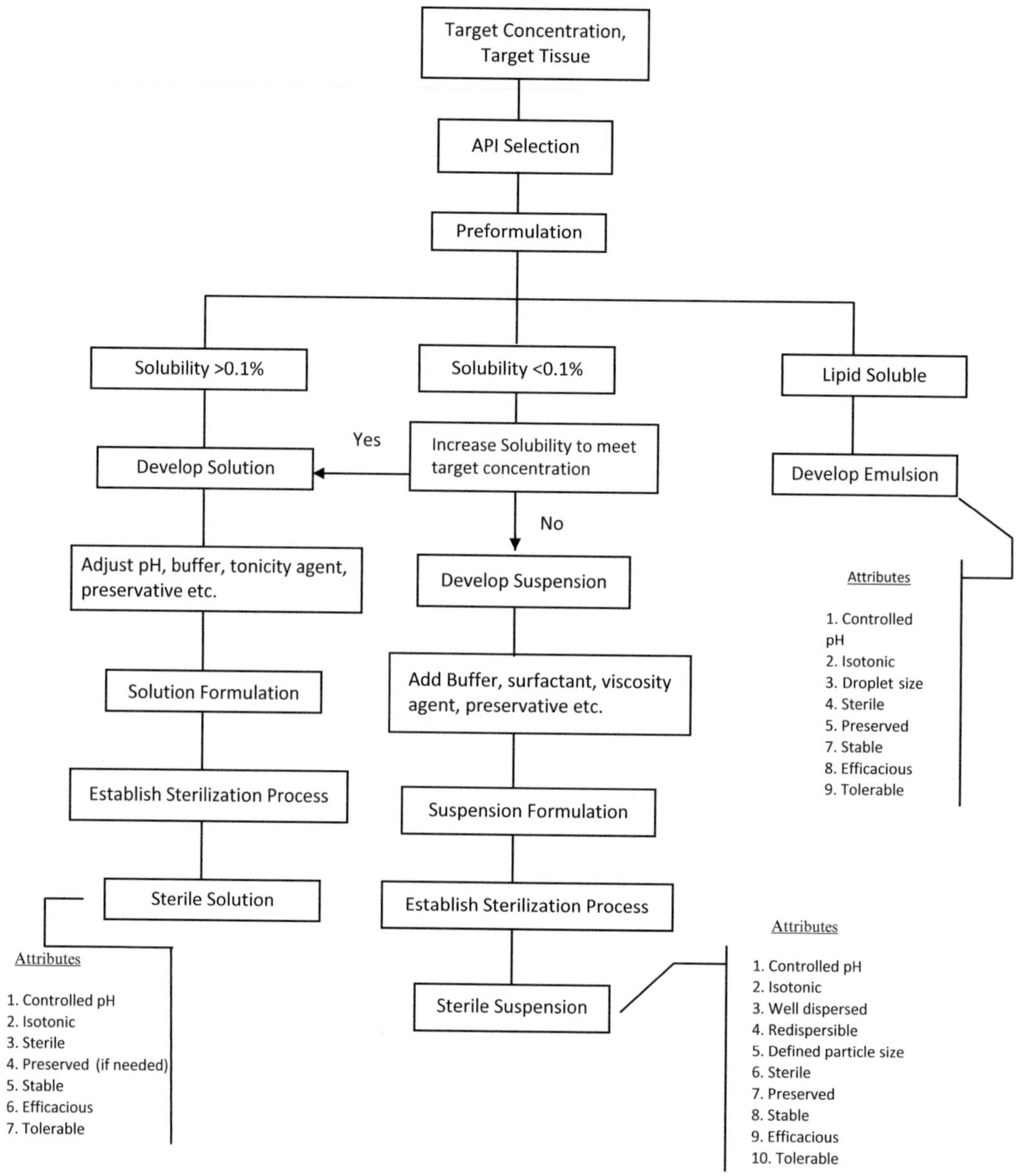

Fig. 3 Topical ocular formulation selection decision tree

topical ocular formulations of 3–8. If DS and excipient(s) stability are sensitive to pH range, then a tight pH specification is important. If DS and excipient(s) are stable and effective across a wide range, then a broader pH range is acceptable. A formulation pH range should be chosen such that there is adequate DS solubility[1] to be able to create a formulation with high enough strength to allow

[1]Rule of thumb for acceptable solubility is to formulate at not more than 75–80 % of saturation level at 5 °C.

dosing at reasonable dose volumes and adequate DS (and excipient) stability over the proposed shelf life and storage temperature.

If no pH provides adequate solubility to allow for small-dose volumes, excipients that enhance solubility of the DS may allow formulation of a solution that otherwise has insufficient solubility. Solubility studies should be conducted with the solubilizing system to determine if solubility enhancement is possible. If solubility enhancement of the API is not possible and resulting dose volumes will be too high, a solution formulation will not be possible. Likewise, if no pH provides adequate stability then a topical ocular solution may not be possible.

4.1.2 Gel

Gel formulations can be of two types: one that gels upon instillation in the eye, and the other type that is a high-viscosity gel and somewhat similar to ointment. Incorporation of stimuli-sensitive polymers in solution dosage form can provide a formulation that is a solution at ambient conditions. However, under appropriate stimuli; it undergoes phase change giving a viscous gel. Stimuli can be of various types such as temperature (poloxamer), ions (gelrite, alginic acid and its derivatives), complexation (borate/pH), pH (cellulose acetate phthalate), and lysozyme (xanthan gum). These formulations have better dispensing characteristics compared to highly viscous formulation. Moreover, they provide longer residence time compared to solution. Two currently marketed products were developed that are based on this approach. Timoptic XE® uses Gelrite (gellan gum), whereas timolol gel-forming solution (TGFS) uses xanthan gum. As an alternative to ointment, high-viscosity semisolid gel preparation of an antiglaucoma drug was developed by Alcon. This product (Pilopine HS® Gel) showed higher bioavailability compared to solution [19, 20].

4.1.3 Suspension

With extensive use of high-throughput screening new chemical entities with fewer drugs like properties are being identified. These compounds, which fall in BCS class II and IV category, have very poor aqueous solubility, and therefore cannot be formulated as a solution dosage form. Other dosage form such as suspension was often explored to achieve a pharmaceutically acceptable alternative. A suspension formulation is a coarse dispersion of insoluble solid particles of a drug substance in an aqueous vehicle containing a suitable amount of surfactant, preservative, buffering, and tonicity agents. The particle size of the suspension may vary from nanometer to micrometer range depending on the situation. Although development of suspension formulation is more complex and challenging than solution, ophthalmic suspension formulations can provide higher bioavailability by prolonging residence time of formulations in precorneal area and therefore may be desirable. In those cases suspensions satisfy two critical attributes: (1) the

Table 5
Compendial requirements of particle size specification

Regulatory jurisdiction	Acceptance criteria
EP	Particles with diameter 20–50 μm should be 20 or less per 10 μg active ingredient Particles with diameter 50–90 μm should be 2 or less per 10 μg active ingredient Particles with diameter 90 μm or more should NOT be observed per 10 μg active ingredient
JP	No particles >75 μm
USP	"Solid particles must be smaller than 5–10 μm to avoid ocular discomfort or irritation"

particles retain in cul-de-sac, and act as reservoir, and (2) dissolution rate of particles are slow enough to provide ocular tissue exposure in a significant manner [19, 20, 42].

The particle size of the suspended drug particles in an ophthalmic suspension should be such to avoid foreign body sensation and ocular tolerability issue. It is reported that formulation with particle size 95 % <10 μm is well tolerated. Suspension formulations also possess a unique advantage particularly if the DS is unstable. Since the degradation of DS in a suspension follows zero-order kinetics, and DS solubility is poor, the chemical stability of suspension formulation is always better than corresponding solution.

Suspension formulation development is more challenging compared to solution formulation. Control of particle size is a critical aspect and it may be achieved by starting with micronized DS. If micronized DS is not available, suitable milling procedure (such as wet ball mill, jet mill) can be used for particle size reduction of DS. This process has been extensively used to manufacture ophthalmic products. Irrespective of the method of manufacture, suspension formulations must meet compendia particle size requirements (measured by microscope) as provided in Table 5.

Ideally, it is desirable to develop a suspension that does not aggregate during storage and remains uniformly suspended in the vehicle. However, it is difficult to accomplish in practice since suspension systems are thermodynamically unstable even though they may be kinetically stable; therefore over time the particles will settle. The large surface area of dispersed phase attributes to high surface free energy of the system contributing to instability of the system. Even though it is known that suspensions are intrinsically unstable, it is important to be able to resuspend the particles by gentle-to-moderate shaking.

4.1.4 Emulsion

This is a good platform of developing ophthalmic formulation with liphophilic compounds which are otherwise difficult to formulate. The emulsion formulation usually consists of aqueous continuous phase in which a lipid phase (suitable oils) is dispersed. The lipid/oil phase is usually <10 % by weight ratio and DS is solubilized in oil phase. The emulsion system also contains suitable surfactants (with appropriate HLB values) which act as stabilizer [43].

The reward of developing emulsion systems is often associated with its ability to provide a superior driving force of poorly water-soluble compounds for absorption in ocular tissues. Furthermore, emulsion systems often protect a hydrolytically unstable compound. The predominant challenges of developing ocular emulsions are (1) manufacturability of sterile product with desired droplet size, (2) stability of final product, and (3) obtaining preservation.

4.1.5 Ointment

Ointments for ophthalmic use are sterile semisolid preparations and have several advantages [44]. They can offer better product stability with hydrolytically unstable and pH-sensitive API. In addition, ointments may offer better bioavailability due to longer residence time of the formulation, and dilution effect due to tear is marginal and low nasolacrimal clearance [45].

Ophthalmic ointment preparation typically involves a combination of a suitable amount of mineral oil and white petrolatum. Depending on DS solubility in vehicle, the ointment may be developed as a one-phase or a two-phase (suspension) system. In general, petrolatum used as ointment base melts between 38 and 60 °C. The melting characteristics of petrolatum are often modulated by incorporating mineral oil in the system. Usually micronized DS is used in preparation of ointments. Since the ointments do not contain water, the presence of preservative is generally not needed in ointment formulation. Further, the components of ointment base (petrolatum and mineral oil) do not have any impact on pH and tonicity upon administration in eye; therefore, buffering and tonicity agents are not necessary.

Manufacturability of sterile ointments is challenging and requires special techniques. Manufacturing can be performed using aseptic manufacturing method by using sterile components and procedures. The products can be terminally sterilized as well. The physical stability of ointment and packaging compatibility are important aspects to consider since bleeding (phase separation) and packaging compatibility issue are known for ointments. Ointments can cause blurry vision and are often preferred for nighttime and once-a-day administration.

4.2 Excipient Selection Criteria

From CMC aspect, it is a requirement to provide justification for use of each component (along with the amount used in formulation) in pharmaceutical development section (3.2.P.2) following

Table 6
Excipient selection guideline[a]

Component	Solution	Suspension	Emulsion	Gel/gelable solution	Ointment
DS	√	√	√	√	√
Buffer	√	√	√	√	–
Tonicity agent	√	√	√	√	–
Surfactant	O	√	√	O	–
Other solubilizing agent	O	–	O	O	–
Suspending agent	–	√	–	–	–
Viscosity agent	O	O	O	O	–
Gelling agent	O	O	O	O	–
Preservative	√	√	√	√	–
Preservative aid	O	O	O	O	–
Antioxidant	O	O	O	O	–
Oil	–	–	√	–	√
Water	√	√	√	√	–
Petrolatum	–	–	–	–	√
pH adjuster (acid/base)	√	√	√	√	–
Target pH	Preferred 5–7.5				–
Target osmolality	Preferred 250–350 mOsm/kg				–
Target viscosity	As required per product profile				

√: required; O: optional

[a]Adapted from Lang JC (1995) Ocular drug delivery conventional ocular formulations. Adv Drug Deliv Rev 16: 39–43

ICH Q8 guideline [30]. Table 6 provides a guidance on selection of excipients and target physical characteristics of ophthalmic formulations.

5 CMC: Development Pharmaceutics

CMC of drug product consist of several key components that are available in e-CTD format (3.2.P.1–3.2.P.8) and are summarized below. Each section has more detailed subsections to cover all pertinent aspects of product:

- 3.2.P.1: Description and Composition of the Drug Product
- 3.2.P.2: Pharmaceutical Development
- 3.2.P.3: Manufacture

- 3.2.P.4: Control of Excipients
- 3.2.P.5: Control of Drug Product
- 3.2.P.6: Reference Standards or Materials
- 3.2.P.7: Container Closure System
- 3.2.P.8: Stability

5.1 Control of Drug Products (Tests)

Final product release specifications are developed on drug product characteristics and container closure system used. Ophthalmic product quality tests were classified into two general categories namely, universal and specific tests as per USP [1]. If necessary, often performance tests may be included into test and specification to sustain quality. Universal tests consist of active assay, impurity analysis, preservative assay, pH, osmolality, appearance, particulate matter, sterility, bacterial endotoxin, etc. Specific tests include particle size, viscosity, drop size, etc. Acceptance criteria of release specifications are based on target product profile, regulatory guidance, route of administration, and dosing posology. Shelf life specifications are always developed based on real time data in final packaging. If adequate real time data is not available, stress stability results may be used as per guidance of regulatory agencies.

5.1.1 Universal Tests

Product Description (Appearance)

A qualitative description of dosage form as to how it should appear is a part of acceptance criteria of DP. While it is straightforward for suspension, ointment, and emulsion dosage forms, solution appearance test consists of four individual tests, namely, color, clarity, particulate, and precipitate tests. Visual observation should indicate solutions to be essentially particle free.

pH

Tolerability of ocular formulation to ocular tissues without causing any considerable irritation is observed in pH ranges 4–8. However, most of the marketed formulations are formulated at a pH from 5 to 8. This is a critical quality test for all ophthalmic formulations except ointment. Formulation pH drift should be studied well to set specification that would allow desired shelf life. Drift of pH in a well-buffered formulation is usually insignificant. A pH drift may be associated with leachable from packaging or from degradation of one component in the formulation. Buffer capacity of the formulation should be kept as such that it does not induce irritation. Test for pH is usually conducted according to USP <791>.

Osmolality

Ocular tissues can tolerate ophthalmic preparation with a wide range of osmolality ranging from 160 to 480 mOsm/kg corresponding to 0.5–1.5 % sodium chloride concentration. However, it is prudent to develop formulation as close as possible to isotonic (equivalent to 0.9 % sodium chloride concentration). This will assure comfort and tolerability of the product. Osmolality test is routinely performed using freezing point osmometer.

Table 7
USP criteria of particulates in topical ocular solutions

Particulates (for solution)	NMT 50 particles/mL ≥10 μm NMT 5 particles/mL ≥25 μm NMT 2 particles/mL ≥50 μm

Particulate Test

For ophthalmic solutions, emulsions and ointment particulate test are required. Particulate test can be done by light obscuration or microscopic method. According to USP <789>, an ophthalmic solution product must meet the following specification (*see* Table 7).

It is noteworthy that the particulate specification for ophthalmic solutions can be considered more stringent than LVP depending on the fill size of LVP. For ophthalmic ointments, 21 CFR Part 211.167 (b) [46] specifically mentioned that there must be proper control of foreign matter.

Active Assay

The recommended release specification is 95–105 % of label claim or even tighter, if possible. The shelf life specification for all regulatory jurisdictions should not be wider than 90–110 % of label claim at proposed storage condition in final package. Accelerated stability study with formulations should be carried out to justify storage condition and estimate shelf life for IND/CTA filing. Real-time data at proposed storage condition and three or more primary stability batches would be required to ascertain shelf life for submission in NDA/MAA [30, 31, 36].

Impurities

Most of the time drug product contains various impurities that are associated with DS. It also contains impurities arising from degradation of drug products during manufacturing and storage. A clear understanding on the nature of these impurities is essential and ICH guidelines, provided in Table 8, should be followed [47].

Preservative Assay

Multidose ophthalmic preparations must contain antimicrobial agents unless one of the following conditions exists: (1) the product consists of a radionuclide with a half-life of <24 h, (2) the active ingredient(s) is antimicrobial, and (3) vehicle allows adequate preservation. Therefore, preservative content is critical for multi-dose presentation to assure patient safety.

Preservative requirement as set forth in Ph. Eur. (chapter 5.1.3) is most difficult to meet. Although it is desirable to meet Ph. Eur. A requirement, formulations meeting Ph. Eur. B criteria are also acceptable by European agencies as long as appropriate scientific justifications are provided.

Antimicrobial preservative effectiveness is usually determined using an organism challenge test according to the methods described in the United States Pharmacopeia 36 (USP) for category 1 products. Samples are inoculated with known levels of one or

Table 8
Reporting, identification, and qualification thresholds of impurities in formulation

Maximum daily dose	Threshold
Reporting thresholds	
≤1 g	0.1 %
>1 g	0.05 %
Identification thresholds	
<1 mg	1.0 % or 5 μg TDI, whichever is lower
1–10 mg	0.5 % or 20 μg TDI, whichever is lower
>10 mg to 2 g	0.2 % or 2 mg TDI, whichever is lower
>2 g	0.10 %
Qualification thresholds	
<10 mg	1.0 % or 50 μg TDI, whichever is lower
10–100 mg	0.5 % or 200 μg TDI, whichever is lower
>100 mg to 2 g	0.2 % or 3 mg TDI, whichever is lower
>2 g	0.15 %

TDI total daily intake

more of the following: gram-positive vegetative bacteria (*Staphylococcus aureus* ATCC 6538), gram-negative vegetative bacteria (*Pseudomonas aeruginosa* ATCC 9027 and *Escherichia coli* ATCC 8739), yeast (*Candida albicans* ATCC 10231), and mold (*Aspergillus niger* ATCC 16404). The samples are then pulled at specified intervals to determine if the antimicrobial preservative system is capable of killing or inhibiting the propagation of organisms purposely introduced into the formulation. The rate or the level of antimicrobial activity determines compliance with the preservative efficacy standards for the cited categories of preparations. Preservative Standards for multidose topical ophthalmic products (Log Reduction of Organism Population at recommended test time) are presented as in Table 9.

The USP 36 Antimicrobial Effectiveness Test requires that compositions containing category 1 products have sufficient antibacterial activity to reduce an initial inoculum of approximately 10^5 to 10^6 bacteria by one log (i.e., a 90 % reduction in the microorganism population) over a period of 7 days and by three logs (i.e., a 99.9 % reduction in the microorganism population) over a period of 14 days, and requires that there cannot be any increase in the microorganism population following the conclusion of the 28-day period. Relative to fungi, the USP standards require that the compositions maintain stasis (i.e., no growth) relative to the population of the initial inoculum over the entire 28-day test period. Ophthalmic formulations are considered as a category 1 product.

The margin of error in calculating microorganism populations is generally accepted to be ±0.5 logs. The term "stasis" means that

Table 9
Preservative effectiveness test (PET) requirement for multidose topical ophthalmic products

Time pulls	6 h	24 h	7 days	14 days	28 days
For bacteria (*S. aureus*, *P. aeruginosa*, and *E. coli*)					
Ph. Eur. A (EPA)	2	3	NA	NA	NR
Ph. Eur. B (EPB)	NA	1	3	NI	NI
USP	NA	NA	1	3	NI
For fungi (*C. albicans* and *A. niger*)					
Ph. Eur. A (EPA)	NA	NA	2	NA	NI
Ph. Eur. B (EPB)	NA	NA	NA	1	NI
USP	NA	NA	NI	NI	NI

NI = no increase at this or any following time pulls, NA = time point not required for applicable standard (e.g., USP, Ph. Eur. B), NR = no organisms recovered

the initial population cannot increase by more than 0.5 log orders, relative to the initial population. A comparison of various compendia preservative effective tests has been reviewed recently [48].

Assay of antimicrobial preservative along with preservative effectiveness test assures the product safety. Since the preservatives are used in small amount, attention must be paid to potential loss of preservative due to various interactions. The recommended release specification for preservative usually is 90–110 % of label claim, or even tighter, depending on specific formulation and preservation data. The shelf life specification for all regulatory jurisdictions may be wider at proposed storage condition in final package. Lower shelf life limit can be justified by PET testing and correlating data with preservative assay value.

Unit dose products are often formulated without a preservative. Therefore, preservative test and preservation efficacy tests are not required for unit dose products.

Uniformity in Dosage Units

For unit dose products, this is a required test to assure both mass of the dosage as well as content of active in the supplied volume. This test is usually conducted as content uniformity test (USP <905>).

Uniformity in Containers

This test is usually performed during product development phase. However, it may be considered as necessary for semisolid dosage forms (ointment for example) since this dosage form has a tendency to phase separation during manufacturing and storage. It is a must to evaluate uniformity of the finished product prior to release of the batch as well as during storage period. Procedure as detailed in USP <3> may be followed.

Sterility

FDA has announced in 1953 that all ophthalmic dosage form must meet sterility requirement. However, USP has introduced the requirement only in 1972 (USP VXIII, third supplement). The manufacturing of ophthalmic formulations should be performed using terminal sterilization process, where possible. If not (for scientific reason such as instability of DS), sterile manufacturing should adhere to ICH guideline. Container closure system for ophthalmic preparation should be sterile as well, and the filled units must be sealed and tamper resistant to ensure sterility at first-time use. Required sterility test should be conducted as specified in various pharmacopeia (such as USP <71>).

Bacterial Endotoxin

According to USP, ophthalmic preparations should be manufactured in a way to have very little bacterial endotoxin. Accordingly, FDA expects ophthalmic preparations for topical use to have bacterial endotoxin <0.5 EU/mL. This requirement is very stringent and same as that of injectable preparations. The test methods are described in USP <85> and <151>. However, it should be mentioned that European and Japanese agencies do not require endotoxin test for topical ocular use.

Fill Volume

This is usually performed as in a process test. This test assures that final units contain amount consistent to package insert.

5.1.2 Specific Tests

Viscosity

Products formulated with viscosity modifiers are intended to have longer residence time upon instillation in eye and also to increase suspendibility and settling characteristics of a suspension product. Therefore, control of viscosity is important to maintain the quality of the product. Product viscosity is usually monitored using Brookfield viscometer. But other types of instruments (rheometer for example) may also be used.

Resuspendibility/Redispersibility

Physical stability of suspension is a very important part and careful thought should be directed to understand and establish physical stability of suspensions. Since the suspensions are thermodynamically unstable, eventually the particles will settle at the bottom of the container. Ophthalmic suspension must redisperse well and quickly (preferably less than 30 s) before dispensing to eye. Manual redispersibility test assures that the product is well redispersed to assure dosage uniformity.

Particle Size and Particle Size Distribution

Control of particle size and particle size distribution should be carefully evaluated during developmental stage and appropriate specification should be set for the product. In general, particle size is measured by laser light scattering method and information of particle size population at ≤10, ≤50, and ≤90 % is provided. This allows having information of not only median particle size but also overall particle size distribution in the formulation.

Drop Size

This test is recommended in order to have an idea of dispensing volume of instilled formulation. Usually the drop size of ophthalmic formulation ranges from 25 to 45 μL. Drop size is measured gravimetrically. There is no recommendation from pharmacopeia regarding the need for drop size determination.

5.1.3 Container Closure System

Container closure system has a very important place in ophthalmic formulation. FDA has classified that ophthalmic formulations have a high likelihood of packaging component–dosage form interaction; thereby the level of concern is high. Furthermore, ophthalmic drug products are intended for application to the eye; therefore, compatibility and safety should be evaluated carefully to the container closure system's potential to generate irritating substances and/or introduce particulate matter into the product.

This has necessitated identification and selection of packaging components that meet the criteria. Currently almost all marketed ophthalmic products are supplied in plastic containers which were pioneered by Alcon in the late 1940s. These packagings are prepared from low-density polyethylene with or without light blocking (opacifying) agent. Polypropylene and high-density polyethylene are also used. Packaging for ophthalmic preparations must be sufficient to protect from light (if needed), loss of moisture, microbial contamination, and damage due to handling and transportation.

Therefore, container closure system for both multidose and unit dose products must possess the following important characteristics:

1. Material should be inert and should not interact with any component of the formulation so that the quality of the drug product is compromised. Particularly they should not absorb active or preservative.
2. Meet the material requirement as set forth in various pharmacopeia. In general, tests specified in the pharmacopeia are typically considered adequate standards for establishing specified properties/characteristics of container closure system.
3. Maintain packaging integrity during storage at various stress conditions.
4. MVTR (Moisture Vapor Transmission Rate) of semipermeable material (such as LDPE, PP, PTE) used for packaging should be such that moisture loss during proposed storage is minimal.

In addition to that multidose products when properly closed and sealed must demonstrate absence of contamination (microbial and physical/chemical) from the outside. Depending on regulatory and marketing guidance, multidose products are often fitted with tamper-resistant seals enabling users to know if the container has ever been opened.

For ointments, flexible plastics or collapsible metal tubes are used. Guidance on appropriate use of container closure system is provided by regulatory agencies [49].

The American Academy of Ophthalmology (AAO) recommended to the agency that a uniform color coding system be established for the closures and labels of all topical ocular medications (*see* Table 10).

Table 10
AAO-recommended color coding of caps and labels for topical ophthalmic medications

API class	Cap color	Pantone number
Anti-infective	Tan	467
Anti-inflammatories/steroids	Pink	197,212
Mydriatics and cycloplegics	Red	485C
Nonsteroidal anti-inflammatories	Gray	4C
Miotics	Green	374,362,348
Beta-blockers	Yellow or blue[a] Yellow C	290, 281
Adrenergic agonists	Purple	2583
Carbonic anhydrase inhibitors	Orange	1585
Prostaglandin analogues	Turquoise	326C

[a]The AAO noted that coding system can be modified in the future as new classes of drugs are developed by reassigning blue color to a new class of drugs while maintaining yellow for beta-blockers

If an applicant does not wish to follow the guidance, sufficient justification needs to be provided to the agency.

5.2 Manufacturing

FDA and USP have recommended that all multidose ophthalmic preparations must be prepared sterile and since then all ophthalmic formulations are manufactured according to that direction. A detailed description of sterile product manufacturing methods is beyond the scope of this chapter and has been the subject of many books and articles. However, a brief description will be given for general understanding of the reader. The Committee for Medicinal Products for Human Use (CHMP) has provided guidelines with a decision tree that was issued in 2000 on selection of appropriate method of sterilization [50]. There are other guidance available on types of processes, facilities, manufacturing procedure, etc. (USP, <797>, <1211>, ISO11137-3, CFR211.25, CFR211.80, 211.84, 211.86, etc.).

In general, sterilization process employed should destroy bacterial, fungal (yeast/mold), and viral organism that may be present in the drug product but definitely would not compromise product quality or integrity. Therefore, proper studies should be carried out to ascertain the most suitable sterilization method to manufacture ophthalmic drug products. Marketed sterile ophthalmic preparations are manufactured in two ways.

- Terminal sterilization: This is the most preferred route of sterilization and should be used whenever possible. The product is manufactured and packaged in an environment as per guidance.

Terminal sterilization can be accomplished by moist heat or by exposure to gamma radiation of suitable intensity. Although this is most preferred, due to stability issues of DP and container closure systems, often this method possesses technical challenges and could not be realized.

- Aseptic processing: This would require very tight control on environment used in manufacturing product. Usually the formulations are prepared in an environmentally sealed vessel and sterilized (such as sterile filtration, autoclaving) prior to filling. For suspension products, however, autoclaving can induce many changes in formulation characteristics including crystal form change of DS, agglomeration, particle morphology, particle size, and particle size distribution. Therefore, often the DS is sterilized (and may be micronized) first and then is mixed aseptically with the other part of vehicle which was presterilized. This process allows avoiding exposure of DS particle to high temperature.

Various books and reviews on sterile product manufacturing are available in literature [51, 52].

5.3 Typical Stability Study and Protocol

Topical ophthalmic formulations (solution, gels, and suspensions) contain >95 % water as formulation vehicle and are packaged in semipermeable plastic containers. Table 11 provides a stability guideline for conducting stability study.

It should be noted that stability study should be designed by keeping characteristics of drug substance, drug product, and QTPP in mind. The stability study should be carried out in final packaging. Table 11 provides a guideline only and should be modified depending on the situation by including additional storage condition and timepoints.

Table 11
A general guideline to develop stability protocol for ophthalmic formulations

Storage condition	Pull time (week)	Comment
−20 °C	1	Excursion criteria
5 °C/35%RH	26, 52	NA
25 °C/40 % RH	13, 26, 39, 52, 78, 104	Standard condition
30 °C/65 % RH	13, 26, 39, 52, 78, 104	Intermediate condition
40 °C/<25 % RH	6, 13, 26	Accelerated condition
55 °C	1	Excursion criteria
Cycle (5 °C/25 °C)	–	NA
Cycle (−20 °C/30 °C)	–	NA
Light (ICH condition)	6	NA

5.4 Expiration Date

Setting of proper expiration date in final presentation at desired storage condition is very critical and is an important part of CMC. The stability data of multiple lots should be carefully reviewed to understand the behavior of the product at storage condition. Statistical data analysis of stability results would help to ascertain shelf life of the product. Although it is desirable to have 2-year shelf life of the product at room temperature storage, on many occasions sufficient data is not available; at that time requested shelf life would be based on available stability data and regulatory guidance.

6 Regulatory Aspects

The contents of CMC section for eCTD submission consist of all pertinent information including DS, DP, manufacturing, test procedure, specifications, and control, and a detailed list is provided in Table 12.

Table 12
Contents of eCTD sections—module 3 (quality)

3.1	**MODULE 3 TABLE OF CONTENTS**
3.2	**BODY OF DATA**
3.2.S	**DRUG SUBSTANCE**
3.2.S.1	**General Information**
3.2.S.1.1	*Nomenclature*
3.2.S.1.2	*Structure*
3.2.S.1.3	*General Properties*
3.2.S.2	**Manufacture**
3.2.S.2.1	*Manufacturer(s)*
3.2.S.2.2	*Description of Manufacturing Process and Process Controls*
3.2.S.2.3	*Control of Materials*
3.2.S.2.4	*Controls of Critical Steps and Intermediates*
3.2.S.2.5	*Process Validation and/or Evaluation*
3.2.S.2.6	*Manufacturing Process Development*
3.2.S.3	**Characterization**
3.2.S.3.1	*Elucidation of Structure and Other Characteristics*
3.2.S.3.2	*Impurities*
3.2.S.4	**Control of Drug Substance**
3.2.S.4.1	*Specification*
3.2.S.4.2	*Analytical Procedures*
3.2.S.4.3	*Validation of Analytical Procedures*
3.2.S.4.4	*Batch Analyses*
3.2.S.4.5	*Justification of Specification*
3.2.S.5	**Reference Standards or Materials**
3.2.S.6	**Container Closure System**

(continued)

Table 12 (continued)

3.2.S.7	**Stability**
3.2.S.7.1	*Stability Summary and Conclusions*
3.2.S.7.2	*Post-Approval Stab Protocol and Stability Commitment*
3.2.S.7.3	*Stability Data*
3.2.P	**DRUG PRODUCT**
3.2.P.1	*Description and Composition of the Drug Product*
3.2.P.2	*Pharmaceutical Development*
3.2.P.2.0	*Pharmaceutical Development—Inclusive*
3.2.P.2.1	*Components of the Drug Product*
3.2.P.2.1.1	Drug Substance
3.2.P.2.1.2	Excipients
3.2.P.2.2	*Drug Product*
3.2.P.2.2.1	Form Development
3.2.P.2.2.1.1	Overages
3.2.P.2.2.1.2	Physiochemical and Biological Properties
3.2.P.2.3	*Manufacturing Process Development*
3.2.P.2.4	*Container Closure System*
3.2.P.2.5	*Microbiological Attributes*
3.2.P.3	**Manufacture**
3.2.P.3.1	*Manufacturer(s)*
3.2.P.3.2	*Batch Formula*
3.2.P.3.3	*Description of Manufacturing Process and Process Controls*
3.2.P.3.4	*Controls of Critical Steps and Intermediates*
3.2.P.3.5	*Process Validation and/or Evaluation*
3.2.P.4	**Control of Excipients—Compendial**
3.2.P.4.1	*Specifications*
3.2.P.4.2	*Analytical Procedures*
3.2.P.4.3	*Validation of Analytical Procedures*
3.2.P.4.4	*Justification of Specifications*
3.2.P.4	**Control of Excipients**
3.2.P.4.5	*Excipients of Human or Animal Origin*
3.2.P.4.6	*Novel Excipients*
3.2.P.5	**Control of Drug Product**
3.2.P.5.1	*Specification(s)*
3.2.P.5.2	*Analytical Procedures*
3.2.P.5.3	*Validation of Analytical Procedures*
3.2.P.5.4	*Batch Analyses*
3.2.P.5.5	*Characterization of Impurities*
3.2.P.5.6.	Justification of Specifications
3.2.P.6	**Reference Standards or Materials**
3.2.P.7	**Container Closure System**
3.2.P.8	**Stability**
3.2.P.8.1	*Stability Summary and Conclusion*
3.2.P.8.2	*Post-Approval Stability Protocol and Stability Commitment*
3.2.P.8.3	*Stability Data*

(continued)

Table 12 (continued)

3.2.A	APPENDICES
3.2.A.1	Facilities and Equipment
3.2.A.2	Adventitious Agents Safety Evaluation
3.2.A.3	Novel excipients
3.2.R	REGIONAL INFORMATION
3.3	LITERATURE REFERENCES

7 Conclusions

Ophthalmic formulation development presents unique challenges to formulation scientists. The design space for ophthalmic formulations is constrained by safety, tolerability, regulatory, and market requirements. The complex physiology and anatomy of the eye limit the amount of drug that can be effectively delivered to intraocular targets via the topical ocular route. As such, physicochemical drug and formulation factors have a profound impact on the safety and efficacy of ophthalmic formulations. Although ophthalmic formulations are sterile products there are notable differences in specifications and controls for ophthalmology drug products versus parenteral drug products with respect to particulates, preservatives, and packaging. Another defining challenge in ophthalmic product development is the drug payload and posology. The instilled volume limitation (25–45 μL) for topical ocular delivery as well as the injection volume limitation (50–100 μL) for intraocular injection severely limit the deliverable dose. Likewise, there is a practical limitation on the number of eye drops that may be administered and the frequency of dosing. Hence, the formulation impact on the drug's pharmacokinetics and pharmacodynamics needs to be carefully investigated and optimized to ensure optimal delivery, safety, and efficacy. This overview summarizes the design strategy of a topical ophthalmic formulation particularly from the viewpoint of CMC. A rationale-based formulation design approach should lead to development of safe, stable, and efficacious ophthalmic formulations meeting regulatory requirements.

References

1. To be presented at US Pharmacopeial Forum 39 (5) Oct 2013 for inclusion into USP, section <771>, Ophthalmic Preparations–Quality Tests
2. Edelhauser HF, Rowe-Rendleman C-L, Robinson MR, Dawson DG, Chader GJ, Grossniklaus HE, Rittenhouse KD, Wilson CG, Weber DA, Kuppermann BD, Csaky KG, Olsen TW, Kompella UB, Holers VM, Hageman GS, Gilger BC, Campochiaro PA, Whitcup SM, Wong WT (2010) Ophthalmic

drug delivery systems for the treatment of retinal diseases: basic research to clinical applications. IOVS 51(11):5403–5020. doi:10.1167/IOVS.10-5392
3. Lang JC (1995) Ocular drug delivery conventional ocular formulations. Adv Drug Deliv Rev 16:39–43
4. Yu LX (2008) Pharmaceutical quality by design: product and process development, understanding and control. Pharm Res 25 (4):781–791
5. Urtti A (2006) Challenges and obstacles of ocular pharmacokinetics and drug delivery. Adv Drug Deliv Rev 58:1131–1135
6. Davies NM (2000) Biopharmaceutical considerations in topical ocular drug delivery. Clin Exp Pharmacol Physiol 27:558–562
7. Kidron H, Vellonen K-S, del Amo EM, Tissari A, Urtti A (2010) Prediction of the corneal permeability of drug-like compounds. Pharm Res 27(7):1398–407
8. Liaw J, Rojanasakul W, Rojanasakul JR (1992) The effect of drug charge type and charge density on corneal transport in rabbits. Int J Pharm 88:111–124
9. Shirasaki Y (2008) Molecular design for enhancement of ocular penetration. J Pharm Sci 97(7):2462–2496. doi:10.1002/jps.21200
10. Schoenwald RD, Ward WR (1978) Relationship between steroid permeability across rabbit cornea and octanol-water partition coefficients. J Pharm Sci 67:786–788
11. Kishida K, Otori T (1980) A quantitative study on the relationship between transcorneal permeability of drugs and their hydrophobicity. Jpn J Ophthalmol 24:251–259
12. Schoenwald RD, Huang HS (1983) Corneal penetration behavior of β blocking agents I: physicochemical factors. J Pharm Sci 72:1266–1272
13. Huang AJ, Tseng SC, Kenyon KR (1989) Paracellular permeability of cornea and conjunctival epithelia. IOVS 30(4):684–689
14. Schoenwald RD (1993) Ocular pharmacokinetics/pharmacodynamics. In: Mitra AK (ed) Ophthalmic drug delivery system. Marcel Decker, New York
15. Wang W, Sasaki H, Chien DS, Lee VHL (1991) Liphophilicity influence on conjuctival drug penetration in pigmented rabbit: a comparison with corneal penetration. Curr Eye Res 10:571–579
16. Burstein NL, Anderson JA (1985) Review: corneal penetration and ocular bioavailability of drugs. J Ocu Pharmacol 1:309–326
17. Prausnitz MR, Noonan JS (1998) Permeability of cornea, sclera and conjunctiva: a literature analysis for drug delivery to the eye. J Pharm Sci 87(12):1479–1488
18. Lee VHL, Robinson J (1986) Topical ocular drug delivery: recent developments and future challenges. J Occup Pharmacol 2(1):67–108
19. Fiscella RG (2008) Ophthalmic drug formulations. In: Bartlett JD, Jaanus NL (eds) Clinical ocular pharmacology, 5th edn. Elsevier, New York, pp 17–37
20. Gibson M (2009) Ophthalmic dosage forms. In: Gibson M (ed) Pharmaceutical preformulation and formulation. Informa Healthcare, New York, pp 431–455
21. Lee VHL, Li VHK (1989) Prodrugs for improved ocular drug delivery. Adv Drug Deliv Rev 3:1–38
22. Jarvinen T, Jarvinen K, (1996) Prodrugs for improved ocular drug delivery. Adv Drug Deliv Rev 19(2): 203–224, doi: http://dx.doi.org/10.1016/0169-409X(95)00107-I
23. Tammara VK, Crider MA (1996) Prodrugs: a chemical approach to drug delivery. In: Reddy IK (ed) Ocular therapeutics and drug delivery. Technomic, Lancaster, PA, pp 285–334
24. Kwatra D, Vaishya R, Gaudana R, Jwala J, Mitra AK (2011) Ocular delivery using prodrugs. In: Rautio J (ed) Prodrugs and targeted delivery, vol 47. Wiley-VCH, Weinheim, pp 181–205
25. Barot M, Bagui M, Gokulgandhi MR, Mitra AK (2012) Prodrug strategies in ocular drug delivery. Med Chem 8(4):753–768
26. Niazi SK (ed) (2007) Handbook of preformulation. Informa Healthcare, New York
27. Center for Drug Evaluation and Research Guideline (1987) Submitting supporting documentation in drug applications for the manufacture of drug substances
28. Code of Federal Regulations, 21CFR314.50 (Revised 2012)
29. ICH Harmonized Tripartitite Guidelines (2006) Guidance for industry, Q3A impurities in new drug substances
30. ICH Harmonized Tripartitite Guidelines (2009) Guidance to industry, Q8 (R2) pharmaceutical development
31. ICH Harmonized Tripartitite Guidelines (1998) Q6A specifications: test procedures and acceptance criteria for new drug substances and new drug products: chemical substances
32. Center for Drug Evaluation and Research Guidance (2000) NDAs: impurities in drug substances
33. ICH Harmonized Tripartitite Guidelines (2006) Q3A (R2), Impurities in drug substances

34. ICH Harmonized Tripartitite Guidelines (2011) Q3D, Metal impurities
35. ICH Harmonized Tripartitite Guidelines (2011) Q3C (R5), Impurities: residual solvents
36. ICH Harmonized Tripartitite Guidelines (2003) Q1A (R2), Stability testing of new drug substance and products
37. ICH Harmonized Tripartitite Guidelines (1996) Q1C, Stability testing of new dosage forms
38. Chari SS, Robinson JR (1974) Ocular evaluation of methyl cellulose vehicle in albino rabbits. J Pharm Sci 63:1218–1223
39. Li VHK, Robinson JR (1989) Solution viscosity effects on the ocular disposition of cromolyn sodium in the albino rabbit. Int J Pharm 88:111–124
40. Rozier A, Mazuel C, Grove J, Plazonnet B (1989) Gelrite®: A novel, ion-activated, in-situ gelling polymer for ophthalmic vehicles. Effect on bioavailability of timolol. Int J Pharm 57(2):163–168
41. Kuno N, Fujii S (2011) Recent advances in ocular drug delivery systems. Polymers 3:193–221. doi:10.3390/polym3010193
42. Bandyopadhyay P, Coffey M, Shawer M (2010) Development of ophthalmic formulations. In: Nema S, Ludwig JD (eds.) Pharmaceutical dosage forms, parenteral medications, vol. 1. 3rd ed. Formulation and packaging. pp. 254–286
43. Tamilvanam S, Benita S (2004) The potential of lipid emulsion for ocular delivery of lipophilic drugs. Eur J Pharm Biopharm 58(2): 357–368
44. Robin JS, Ellis PP (1978) Ophthalmic ointments. Surv Ophthalmol 22(5):335–340
45. Robin JS, Wilson CG, Birmingham AT (1993) Assessment of the precorneal residence of an ophthalmic ointment in healthy subjects. Br J Clin Pharmacol 35(2):188–192
46. Code of Federal Regulations (2012) 21 CFR 211.167, Special Testing requirements
47. ICH Harmonized Tripartitite Guidelines (2006) Q3B (R2), Impurities in drug products
48. Moser CL, Meyer BK (2011) Comparison of compendial antimicrobial effectiveness tests: a review. AAPS PharmSciTech 12(1): 222–226
49. FDA (1999) Guidance to industry, container closure systems for packaging
50. CPMP (2000) Decision tree for selection of sterilization methods (CPMP/QWP/054/98)
51. Akers MJ (ed) (2010) Sterile drug products: formulation, packaging, manufacturing and quality. Informa Healthcare, New York
52. Nizai SK (ed) (2005) Handbook of pharmaceutical manufacturing formulations, sterile products, vol 6. CRC, New York

Methods in Pharmacology and Toxicology (2014): 81–89
DOI 10.1007/7653_2013_12

Published online: 19 September 2013

ADME and Ocular Therapeutics: Retina

Cornelis J. Van der Schyf, Samuel D. Crish, Christine Crish, Denise Inman, and Werner J. Geldenhuys

Abstract

Ocular diseases such as glaucoma and macular degeneration can greatly impact the quality of patients' lives, with the possibility of loss of vision. The development of orally available drugs that can reach the posterior segment of the eye is hampered by the anatomy of the eye. In this chapter, we describe methods for obtaining and analyzing retina and associated optic tract structures for drug levels. These techniques can be used in drug development paradigms as well as for regulatory approval processes.

Key words ADME, Drug analysis, Glaucoma, Macular degeneration, Ocular therapeutics, Optic nerve, Retina, Superior colliculus, Tissue harvesting, Transporters

1 Introduction

Ocular drug delivery faces many challenges in obtaining adequate therapeutic levels of agents at their respective sites of action [1, 2]. Historically, the major drug delivery route to the eye has been topical application of drugs [1, 3]. Unfortunately several limitations occur for formulation using this route, such as the volume instilled in the eye, as well as limitations on excipients that are compatible with the sensitive nature of the eye, not to mention reaching the posterior segment of the eye/retina [4]. With drug discovery of ocular diseases gaining momentum [5, 6], there is significant need to accurately assess the distribution of drugs into the eye. Previous chapters have covered the general scope of absorption, metabolism, distribution, and excretion into the eye. This chapter will focus on the techniques necessary to obtain and measure drug levels in the retina.

The eye has several features that challenge drug delivery, in that the vasculature of the eye is similar in nature to the blood–brain barrier (BBB) [7]. The blood–retinal barrier (BRB) constitutes a microvascular unit in the eye, which is selectively permeable, therefore restricting access of organic compounds to the retina [7–11]. The vasculature of the retina has several tight junctions that largely prevent paracellular uptake of compounds. Additionally, there are several efflux transporters located in the retina, similar to those in the BBB, that are largely responsible for removal of compounds from the retina. It is this combination of selective permeability and highly active efflux transporters [7, 8], that has led to a lag in the development of orally active compounds which can be used to treat and prevent major ocular diseases including glaucoma and macular degeneration. ADME analysis for ocular drug delivery will require examining various transporters and metabolites in the retina, the optic nerve, and optic tract targets in the brain. The following method covers the removal of these tissues from experimental rodents after perfusion with phosphate-buffered saline. Non-fixed tissues (absent blood products) are necessary for downstream analysis by LC-MS/MS or HPLC.

2 Materials and Methods

2.1 Materials

1. Peristaltic pump with tubing and needle appropriate for PBS delivery (25–18G).
2. Straight scissors for trimming fascia, fat, muscle.
3. Hemostat for grasping xiphoid process.
4. Bone cutting shears for head removal.
5. Curved toothed forceps for eye and optic nerve removal.
6. Straight smooth or 45° smooth forceps for lens and retina removal.
7. Curved scissors for eye removal [alternative].
8. Small surgical spring scissors [Vannas, Moria, or Castroviejo] for corneal removal.
9. Rongeurs for brain dissection.

2.2 Methods: Dissection

Figure 1 shows representation of main steps to obtain tissue.

1. Make 0.1 M phosphate-buffered saline (PBS; pH 7.4).
2. Purge the peristaltic pump then fill its tubing with PBS. Affix a needle (25G is sufficient for mouse, 18G for rat) to the end of the pump tubing. This needle will be placed into the exposed heart to deliver the PBS throughout the body, eliminating all blood.
3. Subject the rodent to an overdose of injectable or inhalant anesthetic.
4. Once the diaphragm has stopped contracting, but prior to cessation of the heartbeat, use straight scissors to make a horizontal incision through the skin and then the fascia directly posterior to the rib cage.

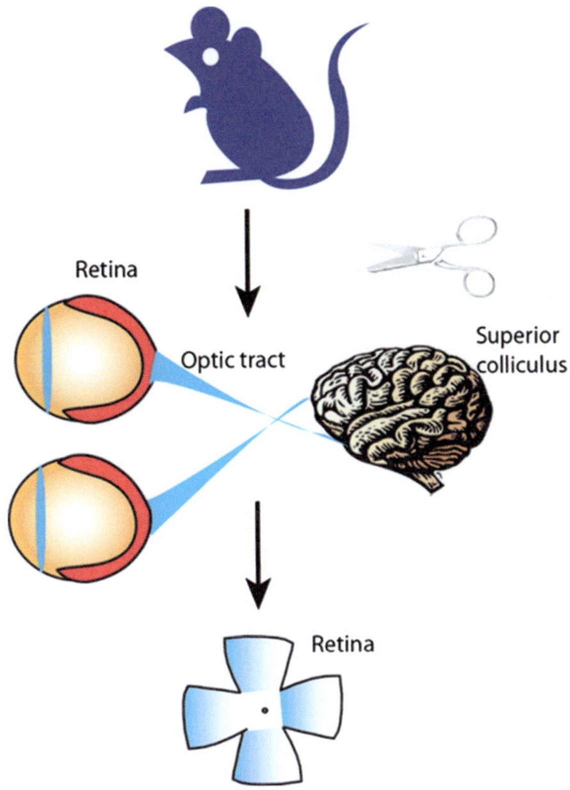

Fig. 1 To analyze drug concentrations in the eye, the key is to accurately dissect the correct tissue types. For the retina, the eye is removed after which the retina is dissected out. Similarly, the optic tracts and the superior colliculus can be dissected to analyze the distribution of drug in these areas

5. Use hemostats in one hand grasp the xiphoid process and elevate the anterior rib cage in order to cut across the diaphragm with the scissors using the other hand. This protects the heart from possible damage by the scissors.
6. Make cuts perpendicular to the ribs that extend up toward the neck, creating a thorax flap that can be laid open to expose the heart. Lay the hemostats in such a way as to keep the thorax flap open.
7. Use scissors to cut into the right anterior chamber of the heart.
8. Use forceps to hold the heart while placing the pump needle into the apex of the left ventricle.
9. Turn on the pump. Monitor the pump tubing so that no air bubbles are delivered to the heart.
10. Mouse blood volume is 77–80 μL/g; rat blood volume is 55–70 mL/kg. Run the pump so the volume of PBS through the rodent is at least two times the blood volume, but bear in mind that liver clearance is always a better indicator of quality of

exsanguination. The liver is a well-perfused organ that is clearly visible during the PBS perfusion. Liver clearance, the paling color change that results from blood leaving the liver, will indicate the quality of the exsanguination. Once liver clearance is achieved, stop the pump.

Mouse	
Weight (g)	**Blood volume (mL)**
20	1.6
25	2.0
30	2.4

11. Use the bone cutting shears to remove the rodent head at the neck.
12. To collect retina and optic nerve tissue, curved toothed forceps are used to enucleate the eye. With either the left or right eye pointed up, press down the flesh above and below the eye socket to proptose the eye.
13. Place the curved toothed forceps behind the globe and close them. Pull straight up, bringing the eye and optic nerve out of the socket.

Rat	
Weight (g)	**Blood volume (mL)**
250	17.5
300	21.0
400	28.0

14. While still holding the eye clamped in the enucleating forceps, use spring scissors to enter the cornea anterior to the ora serrata. Cut along the circumference of the cornea; discard the cornea.
15. The iris is often removed as a result of corneal removal. Use forceps to pull out the lens.
16. Finally, with the globe pressed against a flat surface (gloved fingertip or sterile surface) place forceps at the back of the globe, press down and forward. This action will ease the retina out of the eyecup so that it can be collected. Place the retina in PBS for further dissection or until ready for the pre-analysis processing.
17. Once the retina is removed, use scissors to cut the optic nerve off the posterior eyecup. Place it in PBS for further dissection or until ready for the pre-analysis processing.

18. To remove the brain, split the scalp from neck to nose using straight scissors.
19. Peel back the scalp to expose the skull. Grasp the rodent skull between thumb and forefinger then use straight scissors to remove the muscle from around the brainstem.
20. Use Rongeurs to remove the topmost vertebrae and then chip away at the casing around the cerebellum.
21. Continuing with the Rongeurs (especially with rat) or with strong straight scissors (with mouse), split the braincase along the midline, pulling bone to either side to expose the brain. Continue to remove bone until the top of the brain is free.
22. If removing the entire brain, use closed scissors or spatula to free brain from any remaining dura connections, and then lift the brain from the braincase, cutting through the large trigeminal nerve bands at the base of the brain caudal to the cerebellum.
23. If simply removing the superior colliculus, use closed scissors to push the posterior edge of the cortex forward, exposing the structure. Use scissors or scalpel to cut the superior colliculus away from the inferior colliculus (anterior) and pretectum/cerebellum (posterior) then cut below, roughly 500 μm deep. Remove the superior colliculus to tube with PBS until ready for pre-analysis processing.

3 Drug Analysis

The analysis of drug levels in tissue can be done using several standard analytical methods. The choice of analytical method depends on the availability of equipment as well as the chemical nature of the compounds tested. With complex matrixes of tissue, it is necessary that a method of extraction and quantification be determined before the full study is started. Generally, the main choices of analysis include HPLC or LC-MS/MS techniques. The latter is generally more sensitive and not influenced by the ability of a compound to absorb in the UV range or have fluorescent characteristics. Secondly, the LC-MS/MS method is generally thought to be more sensitive.

A typical flow of events during analysis is described below (see Fig. 2 for visual workflow). A first step is determining which conditions are required for analysis on either HPLC or LC-MS/MS systems. Normal considerations are used for column chromatography, e.g. selection of normal phase or C-18 reverse phase columns. The solvent system should be designed to optimize separation in the column, and often is a combination of methanol, acetonitrile, and water. The advantage of using an MS/MS system over conventional HPLC systems is the availability of the electrospray method.

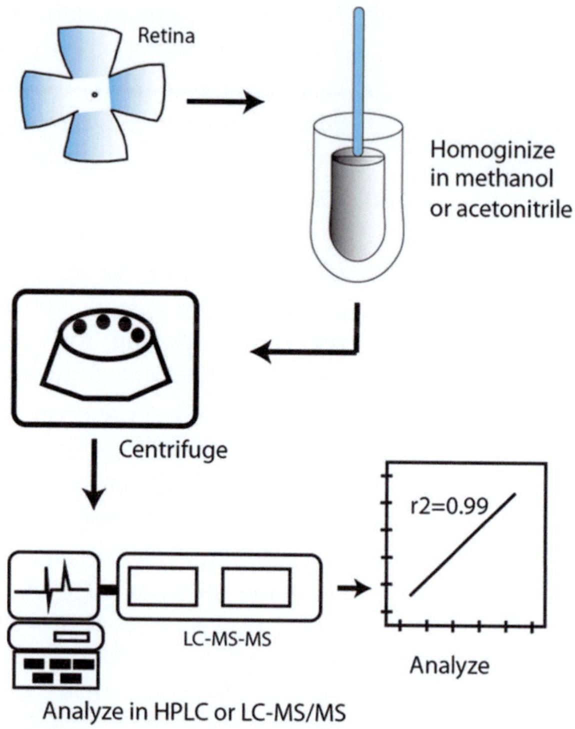

Fig. 2 After tissue is dissected, it is homogenized in organic solvent to extract the drug. After the method is correctly worked out by which the concentration of the drug is going to be measured, the tissue extract can be analyzed to determine the concentration of drug in the tissue preparation

In electrospray, the sample can be directly introduced into the MS/MS system in cases where there is excessive compound retention by the column or significant interference by the matrix. Additional parameters that have to be optimized include calibration linearity as well as determining the lower limits of quantification. In these cases, comparative evaluation over several days will give insight into the overall variability of the analysis system.

The matrix from which the drug is extracted plays an important role in the ability to accurately measure drug concentrations. For instance, serum and brain have different lipid compositions, which would alter their extraction as well as possible interference with drug extraction and detection. Therefore, it is generally necessary to thoroughly evaluate recovery from these different matrices, that are studied. Several companies sell mouse serum in adequate volumes for ease of method development and evaluation of matrix effect. The use of different batches of mouse sera facilitates adequate quality control and reproducibility in method development stages. This latter approach is very important if the method is going to be used for regulatory approval purposes.

The internal standard chosen for the experiments plays a role in determining the accuracy of the extraction process. As a matter of standard practice a compound that is structurally similar to the analyte is chosen, such that their retention times on the HPLC column are similar. Similar solubility characteristics ensure concurrent extraction with the drug under analysis. The role of the internal standards is to verify the degree of extraction, as well as for normalization.

3.1 Extraction of Drug from Tissue

3.1.1 Materials

Dounce homogenizer or Potter-Elvehjem homogenizer.

Methanol and/or acetonitrile.

Phosphate-buffered saline (PBS) pH 7.4.

Micro-centrifuge tubes.

Table top centrifuge.

3.1.2 Methods

1. Place tissue into a Dounce homogenizer or in a Potter-Elvehjem homogenizer.
2. Add 1 volume of the tissue PBS, and add the appropriate amount of internal standard and homogenize the tissue completely and no more tissue chunks are visible.
3. Add 2 volumes of acetonitrile or methanol and mix well. Transfer mixture to a centrifuge tube.
4. Centrifuge 10,000 × g for 10 min at room temp or at 4 °C if drug is thermolabile.
5. Transfer the organic phase to a clean tube.
6. Inject an appropriate amount into HPLC or LC-MS/MS or use the electrospray method.

4 Transporters

Several transporters exist in the vasculature of the BRB. These transporters play a central role in the influx and efflux of several substrates including drugs, toxins, metabolites, and nutrients into the retinal spaces [7, 12, 13]. Table 1 shows a summary of the transporters commonly found in the BRB and their main metabolites. For drug discovery purposes, several methods are available to measure substrate affinity for a specific transporter. The simplest form is the use of radiolabeled substrates known to be high affinity substrates for specific transporters. In such cases, competition with the novel drug will show any potential interaction. These types of studies can be done in vitro using a cell line such as TR-iBRB2 cells [14] or using the carotid artery single injection method [14]. Additionally, these types of experiments can be done using an LC-MS/MS instrument if available.

Table 1
List of major transporters in the BRB [15]

Transporter	Common name	Major substrate	Direction of transport
ABCB1	PGP/MDR1	Lipophilic drugs Organic cations	Efflux
ABCC3	MRP4	Organic anions	Efflux
ABCG2	BCRP/MTX	Organic anions	Efflux
SLC2A1	GLUT1	D-Glucose	Influx
SLC5A6	SMVT	Biotin	Influx
SLC6A6	TAUT	Taurine/GABA	Influx
SLC6A8	CRT	Creatine	Influx
SLC6A9	GLyT	Glycine	Influx
SLC7A1	CAT1	L-Arginine	Influx
SLC7A5	LAT1	L-Leucine	Influx
SLC7A11	xCT	L-Cystein/L-glutamine	Influx
SLC16A1	MCT1	L-Lactate	Influx
SLC19A1	RFC1	Methyltetrahydrofolate	Influx
SLC22A5	OCTN2	L-Carnitine	Influx
SLC22A8	OAT3	Organic anions	Efflux
SLC29A2	ENT2	Nucleosides	Influx
SLC38A2	ATA2/SNAT2	L-Proline/L-alanine	Efflux
SLO1A4	OATP1A4/oatp2	Organic anions	Efflux

Acknowledgment

This work was funded in part by the Bloomberg Foundation, Youngstown, OH.

References

1. Molokhia SA, Thomas SC, Garff KJ, Mandell KJ, Wirostko BM (2013) Anterior eye segment drug delivery systems: current treatments and future challenges. J Ocul Pharm Therap 29(2):92–105
2. Alqawlaq S, Huzil JT, Ivanova MV, Foldvari M (2012) Challenges in neuroprotective nanomedicine development: progress towards noninvasive gene therapy of glaucoma. Nanomedicine (Lond) 7(7):1067–1083
3. Rawas-Qalaji M, Williams CA (2012) Advances in ocular drug delivery. Curr Eye Res 37 (5):345–356
4. Thrimawithana TR, Young S, Bunt CR, Green C, Alany RG (2011) Drug delivery to the posterior segment of the eye. Drug Discov Today 16(5–6):270–277
5. Zhang K, Zhang L, Weinreb RN (2012) Ophthalmic drug discovery: novel targets and

mechanisms for retinal diseases and glaucoma. Nat Rev Drug Discov 11(7):541–559

6. Clark AF, Yorio T (2003) Ophthalmic drug discovery. Nat Rev Drug Discov 2(6):448–459
7. Hosoya K, Tachikawa M (2012) The inner blood-retinal barrier: molecular structure and transport biology. Adv Exp Med Biol 763:85–104
8. Hosoya K, Yamamoto A, Akanuma S, Tachikawa M (2010) Lipophilicity and transporter influence on blood-retinal barrier permeability: a comparison with blood-brain barrier permeability. Pharm Res 27(12):2715–2724
9. Runkle EA, Antonetti DA (2011) The blood-retinal barrier: structure and functional significance. Methods Mol Biol 686:133–148
10. Simo R, Villarroel M, Corraliza L, Hernandez C, Garcia-Ramirez M (2010) The retinal pigment epithelium: something more than a constituent of the blood-retinal barrier—implications for the pathogenesis of diabetic retinopathy. J Biomed Biotechnol 201:190724
11. Stewart PA, Tuor UI (1994) Blood-eye barriers in the rat: correlation of ultrastructure with function. J Comp Neurol 340 (4):566–576
12. Kubo Y, Kusagawa Y, Tachikawa M, Akanuma S, Hosoya K (2013) Involvement of a novel organic cation transporter in verapamil transport across the inner blood-retinal barrier. Pharm Res 30(3):847–856
13. Hosoya K, Tachikawa M (2009) Inner blood-retinal barrier transporters: role of retinal drug delivery. Pharm Res 26(9):2055–2065
14. Kubo Y, Shimizu Y, Kusagawa Y, Akanuma SI, Hosoya KI (2013) Propranolol transport across the inner blood-retinal barrier: potential involvement of a novel organic cation transporter. J Pharm Sci 102(9): 3332–3342
15. Kubo Y, Hosoya K (2012) Inner blood-retinal barrier transporters: relevance to diabetic retinopathy. In: Ols MS (ed) Diabetic retinopathy. InTech, Croatia, pp 91–108

Methods in Pharmacology and Toxicology (2014): 91–118
DOI 10.1007/7653_2013_10

Published online: 30 August 2013

Compositions, Formulation, Pharmacology, Pharmacokinetics, and Toxicity of Topical, Periocular, and Intravitreal Ophthalmic Drugs

Kishore Cholkar, Aswani Dutt Vadlapudi, Hoang M. Trinh, and Ashim K. Mitra

Abstract

The unique anatomy and physiology of the eye make it a highly protected organ. Drug delivery to the eye has become a major challenge to ocular pharmacologists and drug delivery scientists. Designing an effective therapy for ophthalmic disorders, especially for the chronic posterior segment diseases, has been considered a formidable task. Ocular static, dynamic, and precorneal barriers prevent administered drug from reaching the target site at therapeutic concentrations. Topical drops occupy a majority of the marketed ophthalmic products because of easy self-administration, cost-effectiveness, and most importantly patient compliance, whereas other routes of drug administration such as periocular and intravitreal routes require attention of a medical specialist to administer the dose. Drug delivery via periocular and intravitreal routes demonstrated better therapeutic outcomes in front and back of the eye diseases. Though intravitreal route appears to be promising to attain high drug concentrations in back of the eye tissues, however, this route is often limited by postdosing adverse effects such as retinal detachment and endophthalmitis. Periocular injections are associated with fairly high patient compliance relative to intravitreal injections. This chapter provides an overview of various routes of drug administration to anterior and posterior ocular tissues such as topical, periocular (subconjunctival, subtenon, peribulbar, retrobulbar, and juxtascleral), and intravitreal injections. These routes are currently widely recommended in clinics as effective treatment modalities for ocular pathologies. Further this chapter emphasizes drug product composition, dosage regimen, pharmacodynamic and pharmacokinetic profiles, and adverse effects associated with the use of selected drug products administered by these routes.

Key words Eye, Topical drops, Periocular injections, Intravitreal injections, Formulations

1 Introduction

Human eye is a very sensitive organ, which responds to the surrounding stimulus. Eye is a multicompartmental system with various tissues and fluids. For ease of understanding, human eye is divided into two segments as (1) anterior and (2) posterior (Fig. 1). Anterior segment (cornea, conjunctiva, aqueous humor, iris ciliary body, and lens) occupies 1/3rd and the remainder is occupied by posterior segment (vitreous humor, retina, retinal pigment epithelium, choroid, and sclera). The blood-retinal and blood-aqueous barriers impede effective drug delivery to ocular

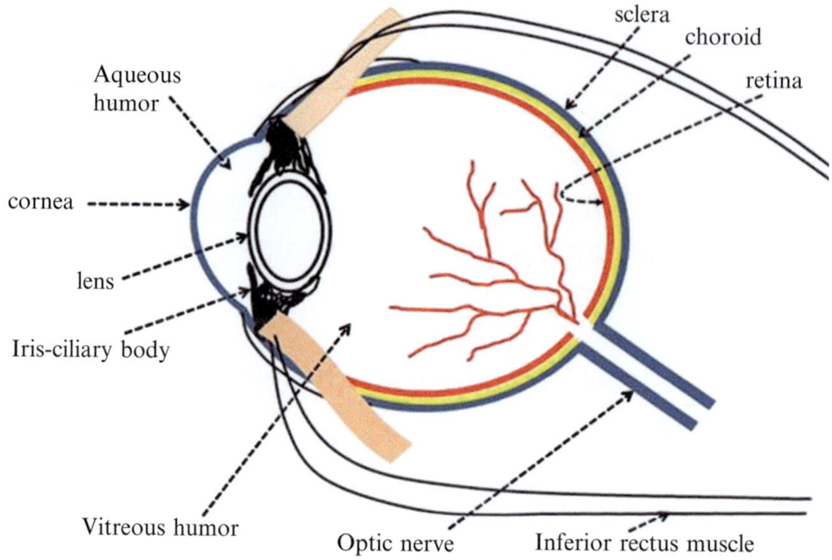

Fig. 1 Structure of human eye

tissues [1]. Conventional routes of drug administration via oral or intravenous are not efficient in delivering drugs to diseased ocular tissues due to ocular static and dynamic barriers. Ocular static barriers include corneal and conjunctival epithelial tight junctions, blood-aqueous barrier, sclera, retinal pigment epithelia, and blood capillary endothelial cells. On the other hand, ocular dynamic barriers that impede deeper ocular drug permeation include conjunctival and choroidal blood and lymph circulation and precorneal barriers such as tears [2]. Therefore to deliver drugs in therapeutic amounts local routes of drug administration need to be explored. Despite precorneal, static, and dynamic barriers, local drug administration remains the mainstay routes to deliver drugs and treat ocular pathologies. For anterior segment disease treatment topical drop formulations are recommended. For posterior segment ocular disease treatment, intravitreal injections are commonly used. In this chapter, we have discussed various routes of drug administration followed by selected drug products administered by these routes. Moreover this chapter emphasizes drug product composition, dosage regimen, pharmacodynamic and pharmacokinetic profiles, and adverse effects associated with the use of such drug products.

2 Routes of Drug Administration

Drug administration to the eye can be broadly classified into three categories, namely, topical (drops, emulsions, suspensions, ointment, and gels), systemic (oral or intravenous), and intraocular injection/implants following periocular (subconjunctival, subtenon,

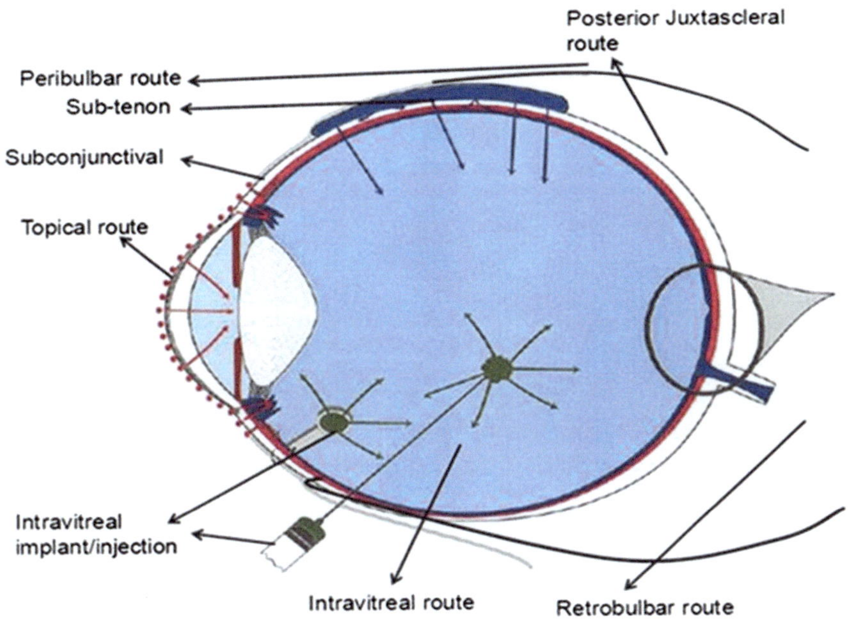

Fig. 2 Routes of drug administration to the eye

retrobulbar, and posterior juxtascleral) and intravitreal route (Fig. 2). The most commonly employed and recommended routes for treating ocular diseases include topical drops for anterior chamber and intraocular injections/devices (implants) for posterior chamber. These routes of drug administration are discussed in the following sections. Readers are directed to Chapter 7 for intravitreal implants/devices.

2.1 Topical Route

Topical eye drops may be solution, emulsion, or suspension consisting of water, active pharmaceutical ingredient, excipients, and preservatives. Advantages of topical drop administration to eye include patient convenience, self-administrable, efficacious, and cost-effective treatment strategy. It is noninvasive, avoids first-pass metabolism, and allows selective delivery of drugs to anterior ocular tissues. Therefore, topical eye drops remain the mainstay for the treatment of anterior ocular pathologies. Ophthalmic solutions are prepared in glass/LDP plastic container for single- or multi-dose administrations (Fig. 3). These devices are specially designed and fitted with different types of dropper tips such that a defined volume of drug solution is dispensed with each application. Commercially available topical medications dispense a range from 25.1 to 70 μL with an average drop size of 39 μL [3, 4]. In a healthy human, the tear volume is 7–9 μL with a turnover rate of 0.5–2.2 μL/min. Topical formulations are intended for instillation as a drop into the lower conjunctival sac (cul-de-sac) [5]. Topical drops may be administered by lowering the eyelid or by pinching

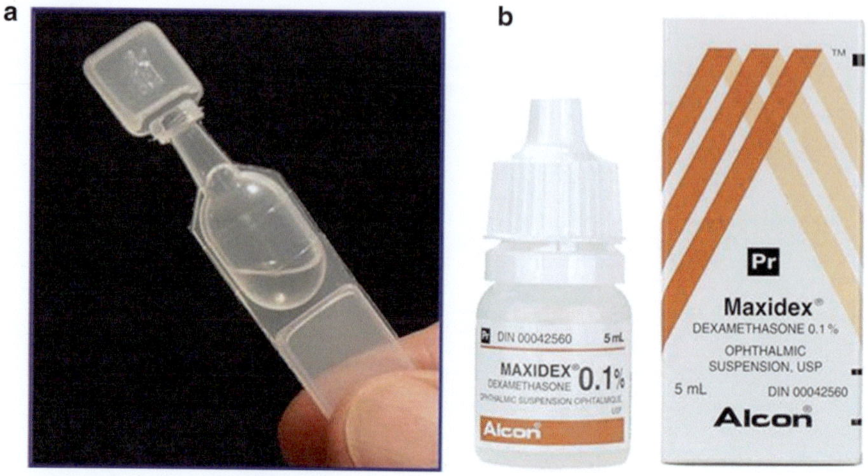

Fig. 3 Topical ocular drug delivery devices, (**a**) single-dose and (**b**) multi-dose delivery device (Maxidex®, Alcon Laboratories Inc., Fort Worth, TX, USA)

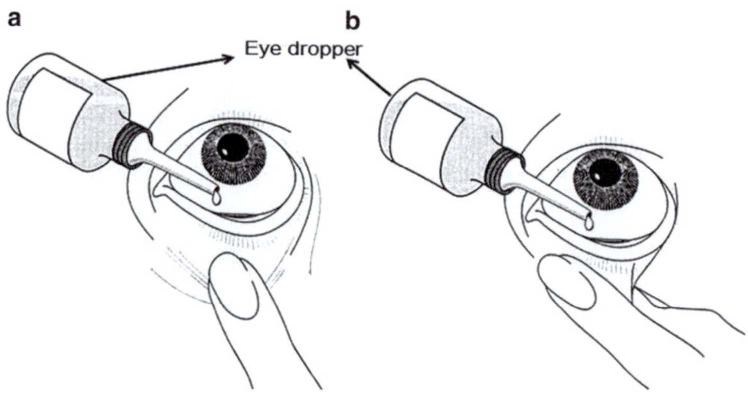

Fig. 4 Modes of topical drop administration by (**a**) pulling down the lower eyelid, (**b**) pinching out the lower eyelid

the lower eyelid as shown below (Fig. 4). Application of topical drop causes increase in tear volume and rapid reflex blinking. Of the dose instilled ~50 % is retained in the cul-de-sac and the remainder is drained into systemic circulation via nasolacrimal duct or spilled onto the cheeks. Of the administered dose, only 1–7 % of drug reaches aqueous humor. The inefficiency of drug delivery may be attributed to anterior chamber ocular static barriers (corneal and conjunctival epithelial tight junctions) and dynamic barriers (tear production and conjunctival lymph and blood flow). Also, the difficulty that elderly patients have with dosing topical drops to the eye may lead to insufficient amounts of drug delivered to ocular tissues [6]. Further, to minimize loss of dosage during drop administration, ocular drop delivery holders have been developed.

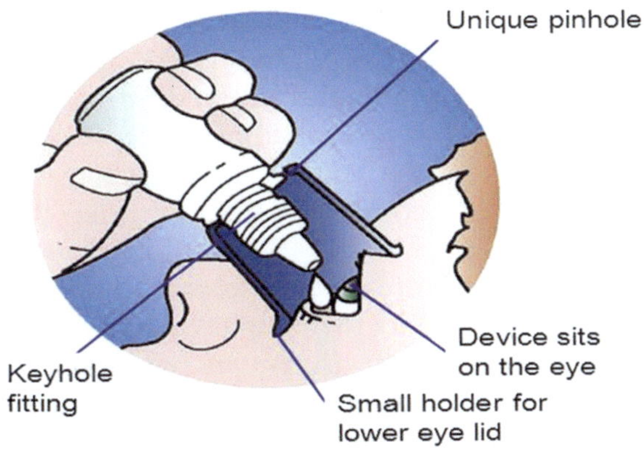

Fig. 5 Autodrop® device delivering topical drops into cul-de-sac of the eye (Owen Mumford Ltd, Woodstock, Oxfordshire, UK) (modified and reproduced from [71]

Example of such holder includes "Autodrop®" (Owen Mumford Ltd, Woodstock, Oxfordshire, UK) (Fig. 5). These holders help in directing gaze away from descending drops, hold lower eyelid, prevent eye blinking, and efficiently deliver topical drop into the cul-de-sac. Such devices may improve patient compliance and minimize drug loss due to blinking while drop application.

2.2 Intravitreal Route

During past two decades considerable momentum has been gained by intravitreal injection. This technique is an invasive method of drug delivery involving direct administration of drug solutions into the vitreous humor via pars plana using a 30 gauge needle. High drug concentrations are achieved in vitreous/retina following intravitreal injection relative to periocular injections. The procedure for intravitreal injection involves several steps. Initially the pupil is dilated and the individual is reclined. Topical anesthetics such as proparacaine 0.5 % and an antibiotic (Zymar™) (Allergan, Inc., Irvine, CA) are applied to the eye. The outer ocular skin, eye lashes, caruncle, and upper and lower eyelids are swabbed with 10 % povidone-iodine followed by insertion of a lid speculum. A preservative-free 4 % lidocaine is applied for 30 s with a cotton tip applicator, followed by two drops of artificial tears (Systane®) (Alcon Laboratories Inc., Fort Worth, TX) to cornea. A drop of 5 % betadine solution is applied in conjunctival cul-de-sac. The injection site is located at 6–7 o'clock of the right eye or at 5–6 o'clock of the left eye. The injection site is selected at 3.0–3.5 mm posterior to the limbus, inferotemporally, and the needle is directed towards the center of the vitreous humor to a depth of 4–6 mm. A volume of ~200 μL may be administered with a 30 or a 32 gauge needle, over a period of 0.5–2.0 s. Post injection the needle is slowly retracted and removed. Patients are subjected to retinal perfusion by indirect ophthalmoscopy followed by application of an antibiotic such as Zymar™ (Allergan, Inc., Irvine, CA) or Vigamox® (Alcon Laboratories, Fort Worth, TX) [7]. Following this technique small-molecule drugs and linear and globular shaped macromolecules with high molecular weights may be injected. Intravitreal elimination was found to depend on the molecular weight of drug candidates. Macromolecules such as proteins (40 and 70 kDa) may tend to cause longer retention in vitreous body leading to slower elimination relative to small molecules [8]. In spite of offering high drug concentrations in the back of the tissues (vitreous humor, retina, and choroid), this technique is associated with various short-term complications. Ocular complications such as endophthalmitis, retinal detachment, and intravitreal hemorrhages have been reported.

2.3 Periocular Route

Periocular is a broad term which refers to the region surrounding the eye. Periocular route includes subconjunctival, peribulbar, posterior juxtascleral, retrobulbar, and subtenon routes (Fig. 2). Drug administration via this route is considered as one of the most promising mode for posterior ocular drug delivery, i.e., to retina. Solutions are administered in close proximity to sclera which results in high drug concentrations in deeper neural retina and vitreous body. Sclera is a fibrous tissue made of collagen fibers derived from dura mater of central nervous system. This tissue offers very low resistance to drug permeability [9]. Hence, increased drug permeability into deeper ocular tissues is achievable.

2.3.1 Subconjunctival Injection

Conjunctiva is a thin, semitransparent, mucous-secreting tissue which forms the loose inner lining of the eye. It is continuous with cornea and forms a thin membranous layer (bulbar conjunctiva) above the white part of the eye called "sclera." Administration into the space between conjunctiva and sclera, i.e., beneath the conjunctiva, is called as "subconjunctival injection." This mode of drug administration is considered minimally invasive. In general, a 25–30 gauge and 30 mm long needle is selected for drug administration. During administration the beveled edge of needle is faced towards sclera ($\geq$3 mm beyond sclera) and is slowly penetrated across bulbar conjunctiva until the fold appears [10]. A volume of 500 μL drug solution may be administered by this method.

2.3.2 Subtenon Injection

Subtenon injection implies administration of solutions into tenon's capsule. It is a fibrous membrane that envelopes the eye from limbus to the posterior optic nerve [11]. Subtenon's space is a virtual cavity that is bound by tenon's capsule and sclera [12]. Initially a small surgical dissection is made into conjunctiva and subtenon space. To administer drug solution into subtenon's space, the individual is directed to look downwards with simultaneous retraction of upper eyelid. A sharp-tipped 26-gauge and ~1.6 cm long needle is inserted into posterior subtenon space [12]. Vision threatening complications may be observed with the use of sharp needles [13]. Therefore, to avoid complications during drug administration to subtenon's space, cannulated needles have been introduced. Following small incision across conjunctiva into subtenon space, the individual is directed to look downwards. Subsequently, a blunt-tipped, 2.5 cm long cannulated needle is passed into tenon's capsule at temporal edge of superior rectus muscle. The injection is directed posteromedially to deliver ~4 mL of drug solution around the ocular muscles behind the equator [14]. Subconjunctival hemorrhage may be observed during this procedure due to tearing of conjunctival blood vessels in tenon's space. Commonly observed complications with this procedure include ocular pain and swelling of conjunctiva (chemosis). As the advantages overweigh side effects for this procedure, this technique is widely employed for ocular anesthesia during ocular surgeries.

2.3.3 Peribulbar Injection

Peribulbar is also referred to as extraconal injection. This mode of drug administration is safer but less effective relative to other techniques such as retrobulbar. In this technique the injection is made at the location external to the four rectus muscles and intramuscular septa (Fig. 2) [15]. Peribulbar injection can be divided into two categories depending on the location of drug delivery, i.e., injection site—anterior and posterior peribulbar injection. A 25 gauge, 1.25 in. needle is recommended and is directed beyond the equator of the eye. It is performed by one of the two procedures such as (a) injection at the inferotemporal position and (b) injection at the superonasal position. Inferior peribulbar injections are given at the junction of outer third and inner two-thirds of lower orbital rim by directing the needle away from the eye and towards orbital floor [14]. On the other hand, superior injections are given nasally or temporally towards orbital roof. Following these techniques a volume of 8–10 mL of anesthetic may be administered.

2.3.4 Retrobulbar Injection

Retrobulbar injections are also referred as intraconal injections. In this technique drug solutions are placed inside the conical compartment within the confines of four rectus muscles and their intermuscular septa [15]. Retrobulbar route of drug administration is more effective than peribulbar in anesthetizing the eye. To perform the injection, a 25–27 gauge blunt needle is employed. The needle is inserted at the inferotemporal orbital margin aimed at lower edge of superior orbital fissure with the globe in primary gaze position [16]. The needle is directed from the sagittal plane and superiorly at 45° and 10°, respectively. Therefore, care must be taken when the needle is penetrated until this depth has been reached from the point of injection, i.e., from corneal surface. This technique may cause optic nerve trauma. In order to avoid such complications needles may be placed in the temporal half of the orbit with penetration no deeper than 1.5 cm behind the eye [17].

2.3.5 Posterior Juxtascleral Injection

This technique utilizes a blunt-edged, specially designed 56° curved cannula placed on the syringe to deliver drug solutions/formulations in direct contact with outer scleral surface without puncturing the eyeball [18]. With this technique drug solution is placed above macula as a depot. This technique allows efficient and prolonged drug delivery to retinal cells in macula. For the injection procedure, the individual is laid in the supine position, 5 % povidone-iodine is applied to the periocular skin and cul-de-sac, and a lid speculum is inserted. Post topical anesthesia application, a 1–1.5 mm incision is made in superotemporal quadrant to expose sclera. The incision is made through midway between the superior and lateral rectus muscles through conjunctiva and tenon's capsule ~8 mm posterior to limbus. When sclera is visualized, the cannula is inserted with direct contact to the scleral surface. Once the cannula is completely inserted, a volume of 500 μL drug solution/formulation is injected. Post injection the cannula is slowly retracted and removed. The procedure is completed by lid speculum removal and application of topical antibiotic with light patching of eye.

Several drug products are available to treat ocular pathological conditions. In the following sections we discuss some of the commercially available products administered by topical drop and intravitreal and periocular injections. Further, we discuss dosage regimen, route of administration, pharmacokinetics, pharmacodynamics, and associated adverse effects.

3 Topical Products

In this section we describe topical ocular products such as drops (Ciloxan®) (Alcon Laboratories, Inc., Fort Worth, TX), suspensions (Maxidex®) (Alcon Laboratories, Inc., Fort Worth, TX), emulsions (RESTASIS®) (Allergan, Inc. Irvine, CA), gels (Zirgan®) (Bausch & Lomb Incorporated, Tampa, FL), and ointments (Lotemax®) (Bausch & Lomb Incorporated, Tampa, FL). Each formulation is associated with its own advantages and disadvantages. As this discussion is beyond the scope of this chapter, we have described only the important aspects related to drug composition, pharmacology, pharmacodynamics, pharmacokinetics, and adverse effects of CILOXAN®, MAXIDEX®, RESTASIS®, ZIRGAN®, and LOTEMAX®.

3.1 Ciloxan®

Indications and Usage: Ciloxan® is a synthetic, sterile, multi-dose, antimicrobial topical ophthalmic drop of ciprofloxacin (0.3 %). Ciloxan® is indicated in the treatment of infections caused by susceptible strains of microorganisms (broad spectrum of gram-positive and gram-negative ocular pathogens) [19].

Dosage and Administration: The recommended dosage regimen includes two drops into the affected eye every 15 min for the first 6 h followed by two drops every 30 min for the remainder of the first day. Second-day dosage schedule includes instillation of two drops every hour. From third to fourteenth day, two drops in the affected eye every 4 h is recommended. The dosage regimen may vary depending upon the type of microbial infection affecting the eye. For example in case of bacterial conjunctivitis, the recommended dosage regimen is one- to two-drop administration into cul-de-sac every 2 h while awake for 2 days and one or two drops every 4 h while awake for next 5 days.

Drug Composition: Each milliliter of Ciloxan® consists of active drug ingredient, ciprofloxacin HCl 3.5 mg equivalent to 3 mg of base (ciprofloxacin, 0.3 %). Other excipients include sodium acetate, acetic acid, mannitol (4.6 %), edetate disodium (0.05 %), sodium hydroxide/hydrochloric acid (pH adjusted to 4.5), and purified water. Benzalkonium chloride (0.05 %) is used as a preservative.

Pharmacodynamic Profile: Ciprofloxacin has in vitro activity against a wide range of gram-negative and gram-positive organisms. The antibacterial activity results from interference of ciprofloxacin with enzyme DNA gyrase which is required for bacterial DNA synthesis. Results demonstrated active performance of Ciloxan® against most strains of the gram-positive and gram-negative bacteria both in vitro and in clinical infections. Ciprofloxacin is active against gram-positive bacteria such as *Staphylococcus* (*S*) *aureus*, *S. epidermidis*, *S. pneumoniae*, viridans group, and gram-negative bacteria such as *Enterococcus faecalis*, *S. haemolyticus*, *S. hominis*, *S. saprophyticus*, and *S. pyrogenes*. Clinical studies with Ciloxan® drops in patients with corneal ulcers and positive bacterial cultures demonstrated re-epithelialization in ulcers (92 %). Treatment with Ciloxan® demonstrated eradication of causative pathogens by the end of treatment regimen.

Pharmacokinetic Profile: Ciloxan® topical drop instillation in each eye is recommended every 2 h while awake for 2 days followed by every 4 h for an additional 5 days. Drug concentrations in the systemic circulation were measured. Cmax for ciprofloxacin was 4.7 ng/mL (approx. 450 times less than simple 250 mg oral administration). The mean concentration was below 2.5 ng/mL. Similarly, pharmacokinetic study conducted in equine eyes demonstrated similar pharmacokinetic profile to those of rabbits and humans. Post topical application, mean tear concentrations of the drug remained above the minimum inhibitor concentration (MIC90) for most pathogenic bacteria in 6 h [20].

Adverse Reactions: Most frequently observed adverse reactions include local ocular burning or discomfort and development of white crystalline precipitate in 17 % of patients. Adverse events include lid margin crusting, foreign body sensation, itching, conjunctival hyperemia, and bad taste. Also, other adverse reactions include keratoplasty, allergic reactions, tearing, photophobia, corneal infiltrates, nausea, and decreased vision.

3.2 Maxidex®

Indications and Usage: Maxidex® is a sterile, topical ophthalmic adrenocortical steroid suspension indicated for steroid-responsive inflammatory conditions of palpebral and bulbar conjunctiva, cornea, and anterior ocular tissues.

Dosage and Administration: The recommended dose of Maxidex® suspension is one or two drops into the conjunctival sacs for every 30–60 min as initial therapy. Depending upon the response the dosage is reduced every 2–4 h. In case patients do not respond to therapy and predicted outcomes are not achieved, additional systemic or conjunctival therapy may be recommended.

Drug Composition: Each milliliter of Maxidex® contains active drug substance (dexamethasone, 0.1 %), hydroxypropyl methylcellulose (0.5 %) as vehicle, polysorbate 80, dibasic sodium phosphate, citric acid, edentate disodium, sodium chloride, purified water, sodium hydroxide (to adjust pH), and benzalkonium chloride (0.01 %) as a preservative.

Pharmacodynamic Profile: Dexamethasone is a synthetic corticosteroid (9-fluoro-16-methyl-substituted hydrocortisone) with approximately 6–7 times more potency than prednisolone and at least 30 times more potent than cortisone. The addition of methyl radical and a fluorine atom to prednisolone can be attributed to enhanced potency. After inducing lensectomy and vitrectomy, anti-inflammatory effects of topical ocular Maxidex administration to rabbits were studied [21]. Study results indicate that topical application of 0.1 % Maxidex lowered aqueous prostaglandin E2 levels and reduced corneal edema. Also, topical drops demonstrated reduced clinical scores, blood-aqueous barrier breakdown to fluorescein, and reduced particle flare in rabbits [21].

Adverse Reactions: Adverse effects with topical application of Maxidex® have been reported. Adverse reactions such as optic nerve damage, visual acuity and field defects, cataract formation, secondary ocular infections, and perforation may occur.

3.3 RESTASIS®

Indications and Usage: RESTASIS® is a sterile, preservative-free, single-use topical ophthalmic emulsion that is currently indicated as an immunomodulator to increase tear production in subjects suffering from keratoconjunctivitis sicca [22].

Dosage and Administration: RESTASIS® contains 0.05 % of cyclosporine in the form of topical ophthalmic suspension.

The recommended dosing regimen for infected eye is one drop twice a day in each eye approximately 12 h apart. Single-center, masked, prospective, randomized, longitudinal trial was conducted for 12 months with 0.05 % cyclosporine (RESTASIS®) and artificial tears twice daily. Dry eye signs and symptoms have been evaluated at baseline and months 4, 8, and 12. Baseline sign and symptoms were proportional with the disease severity level 2 and 3 comparable in both groups ($P > 0.05$). Results demonstrated an improvement in Schirmer test scores, tear breakup time, and ocular surface disease scores ($P < 0.01$) relative to artificial tears at 8 and 12 months, respectively. Study results indicated that RESTASIS® may slow or prevent disease progression in patients with dry eye at severity level 2 or 3 [23].

Drug Composition: Each milliliter of RESTASIS® emulsion contains 0.5 mg of active drug (0.05 % cyclosporine), glycerin, castor oil, polysorbate 80, carbomer copolymer type A, purified water, and sodium hydroxide (to adjust pH between 6.5 and 8.0).

Pharmacodynamic Profile: Cyclosporine is a cyclic undecapeptide, an active metabolite from *Tolypocladium inflatum*. In individuals suffering from poor tear production due to ocular inflammations associated with keratoconjunctivitis sicca, cyclosporine acts as an immunomodulator. The exact mechanism by which the active induces tear production is unclear.

Pharmacokinetic Profile: Following topical application of RESTASIS® 0.05 % twice daily, blood concentrations were below the quantitation limit of 0.1 g/mL in humans. Results demonstrated that there was no detectable drug accumulation in blood for the entire study period. Similarly, ocular tissue distribution ofcyclosporine post topical administration to albino rabbits and beagle dogs was studied [24]. Results demonstrated rapid absorption of cyclosporine into conjunctiva (Cmax: dogs, 1,490 ng/g; rabbits, 1,340 ng/g) and cornea (Cmax: dogs, 311 ng/g; rabbits, 955 ng/g). Lower drug concentrations were detected in the deeper ocular tissues. Topical ophthalmic cyclosporine penetrated deeper into extraocular tissues to generate therapeutic immunomodulatory effect with very low or minimal absorption into the blood circulation [24].

Adverse Reactions: Although the drug product is effective in treating dry eye, several adverse effects have been reported. Adverse reactions include ocular burning (17 %), conjunctival hyperemia, discharge, epiphora, eye pain, foreign body sensation, pruritus, stinging, and visual disturbances in 1–5 % of subjects. Also, few subjects reported hypersensitivity and superficial eye injury.

3.4 ZIRGAN®

Indications and Usage: ZIRGAN® is a topical ophthalmic gel that is currently indicated for the treatment of acute herpetic keratitis (dendritic ulcers). This product was approved by the FDA in September 2009 [25].

Dosage and Administration: ZIRGAN® contains 0.15 % of ganciclovir in the form of a sterile preserved topical ophthalmic gel. The recommended dosing regimen for infected eyes is one drop five times a day (i.e., approximately every 3 h while awake) until the corneal ulcer heals and then one drop three times a day for 7 days. Topical ganciclovir gel in herpetic keratitis is preferred because of its prolonged corneal contact time, similar tonicity to tears, pH adjusted to a physiologic range, sterilizability (autoclavable), long and stable shelf life, selectivity to virus-infected cells, lubricant effects for corneal anesthesia, aqueous humor penetration following topical instillation, effectiveness as acyclovir at 20 times lower concentration, and minimal/no systemic adverse effects. This formulation was generally well tolerated and associated with a significantly lower incidence of visual disturbances than 3 % acyclovir ointment [26].

Drug Composition: Each gram of gel contains 1.5 mg of active drug substance (ganciclovir 0.15 %). Other inactive ingredients include carbopol, water for injection, sodium hydroxide (for pH adjustment to 7.4), and mannitol. Benzalkonium chloride (0.075 mg) is used as a preservative.

Pharmacodynamic Profile: Ganciclovir, a guanosine nucleoside analogue, is selectively phosphorylated to its monophosphate derivative by viral thymidine kinases of the herpes virus family [27–29]. Subsequently, this monophosphate derivative is phosphorylated by viral and cellular thymidine kinases of virus-infected cells to ganciclovir triphosphate, the active metabolite. This derivative then competes with deoxyguanosine triphosphate for binding to DNA polymerases, inhibits de novo synthesis of viral DNA, and also causes chain termination by incorporation into viral strand primer DNA [30, 31]. Ganciclovir exhibits potent in vitro antiviral activity against HSV-1 and -2. The reported half maximal inhibitory concentration of antiviral activity falls in the range of 0.2–2.0 mmol/L for HSV-1 and 0.3–10.0 mmol/L for HSV-2 [30].

Pharmacokinetic Profile: According to the recommended dosing regimen which is one drop five times a day, the estimated maximum daily dose of ganciclovir is 0.375 mg. This is approximately 0.04 % of the oral (900 mg valganciclovir) and 0.1 % of the intravenous dose (5 mg/kg ganciclovir). Thus systemic exposure is likely to be minimal by topical ocular administration of 0.15 % ganciclovir ophthalmic gel. Following topical instillation of 0.15 % radiolabeled ganciclovir ophthalmic gel in rabbits, the radioactive compound was found to accumulate in external ocular tissues followed by anterior and posterior internal tissues. Drug concentrations in the intact cornea remained above IC50 for both HSV-1 and HSV-2 over 4 h after application [28].

Adverse Reactions: Although effective, the most common adverse reactions reported were blurred vision (60 %), eye irritation (20 %), punctate keratitis (5 %), and conjunctival hyperemia (5 %).

3.5 Lotemax®

Indications and Usage: Lotemax® ointment contains a corticosteroid, loteprednol etabonate, indicated for the treatment of postoperative inflammation and pain following ocular surgery [32].

Dosage and Administration: Lotemax® contains 0.5 % loteprednol etabonate in the form of an ointment. Beginning 24 h after surgery, application of this ointment is recommended in very small amounts (approximately ½ in. ribbon) into the conjunctival sac four times daily. Application needs to continue through the first 2 weeks of the postoperative period.

Drug Composition: Each gram of ointment contains 5 mg of loteprednol etabonate (0.5 %) and inactives such as mineral oil and white petrolatum.

Pharmacodynamic Profile: Loteprednol etabonate is a "soft" steroid belonging to a unique family of glucocorticoids [33]. This compound has good ocular and skin permeation properties similar to "hard" steroids [34, 35]. It is synthesized via structural modifications of prednisolone-related compounds to facilitate transformation to an inactive metabolite. This compound initially binds to the type II glucocorticoid receptor. In general, corticosteroids inhibit the inflammatory response to a variety of drugs which possibly delay or slow healing. This class of compounds inhibits edema, fibrin deposition, dilation of capillaries, leukocyte migration, capillary and fibroblast proliferation, collagen deposition, and scar formation associated with inflammation. The molecular mechanisms involved in modulation of inflammation by corticosteroids are not clearly delineated. However, these compounds are believed to act by inducing phospholipase A2 inhibitory proteins, collectively called lipocortins. It is postulated that these proteins regulate biosynthesis of potent mediators of inflammation such as prostaglandins and leukotrienes via inhibition of release of their common precursor arachidonic acid which is released from membrane phospholipids by phospholipase A2. Also, corticosteroids are known to inhibit prostaglandin production through several independent mechanisms [36, 37].

Pharmacokinetic Profile: A randomized, double-masked, placebo-controlled, single-center trial was conducted in human volunteers to determine the systemic exposure to loteprednol etabonate suspension following its chronic, ocular instillation. Volunteers were instructed to instill one drop in each eye eight times daily on days 0 and 1 and four times on days 2–42. However, plasma levels of loteprednol etabonate and its major metabolite PJ-91 were below the limit of quantitation (1 ng/mL) at all sampling times [38]. Similar study to evaluate the systemic exposure to loteprednol etabonate following topical administration of Lotemax® ointment has not been undertaken. Furthermore, administration of the ointment product dosed four times daily may not exceed loteprednol etabonate systemic exposures as compared to Lotemax® suspension. A recent study reported that loteprednol etabonate ointment was efficacious and well tolerated in the treatment of ocular inflammation and pain following cataract surgery [36].

Adverse Reactions: A common adverse effect associated with ophthalmic steroids is elevation in intraocular pressure, which may be accompanied with optic nerve damage, visual acuity and field defects, posterior subcapsular cataract formation, secondary ocular infection from pathogens including HSV, and globe perforation where corneal or scleral thinning occurs. In particular, clinical reports indicate that anterior chamber inflammation is usually observed with Lotemax® ointment. Other adverse events include conjunctival hyperemia, corneal edema, and ocular pain (less incident) [36].

4 Intravitreal Injectable Products

Drug delivery to the posterior ocular tissues (retina–choroid) is impeded due to ocular static and dynamic barriers. Topical drug administration was unable to deliver therapeutic concentrations to back of the eye tissues. In order to overcome these barriers and deliver therapeutic drug concentrations, intravitreal injections have become the primary mode of administration. This mode of drug administration is invasive, requires medical specialist to inject the drug product, and is not particularly favored by patients. Readers are directed to intravitreal route under routes of drug administration section in this chapter for deeper understanding of drug product injection and associated side effects. In the following section we describe drug product composition, pharmacology, pharmacodynamics, pharmacokinetics, and adverse effects associated with the commercially marketed products such as Macugen® (Eyetech Inc., Palm Beach Gardens, Florida), Avastin® (Genentech, Inc., South San Francisco, CA), Lucentis® (Genentech, Inc., South San Francisco, CA), and Triesence® (Alcon Laboratories Inc., Fort Worth, TX).

4.1 Macugen®

Indications and Usage: Macugen® is a sterile, clear, preservative-free ophthalmic solution indicated for the treatment of subfoveal choroidal neovascularization (CNV) secondary to age-related macular degeneration (AMD) [39].

Dosage and Administration: Macugen® is recommended for administration once every 6 weeks by intravitreal injection. To inject the drug product, prefilled staked needle syringe or luer lock syringe with excess volume of drug product is dispensed. Injecting the drug product with staked needle syringe involves attaching the threaded plastic plunger rod to the rubber stopper (inside the syringe barrel). The syringe end cap is removed to allow intravitreal administration. On the other hand, for luer lock syringe, the last ribe or plunger stopper needs to be pushed past the dose line on the syringe. Prior to injection, the last rib of the plunger needs to be aligned to the dose line to ensure proper dose dispensing. The dose is injected intravitreally. In both the syringes excess drug product is prefilled. The excess volume is removed to adjust the injectable dose before intravitreal administration.

Drug Composition: Each syringe contains active drug (pegaptanib, 0.3 mg; as free acid form of the oligonucleotide), sodium chloride, monobasic sodium phosphate, monohydrate, dibasic sodium phosphate heptahydrate, hydrochloric acid, and sodium hydroxide in water for injection.

Pharmacodynamic Profile: Macugen® (pegaptanib sodium, 0.3 %) is an RNA aptamer directed against vascular endothelial growth factor-165 (VEGF-165) [40]. VEGF is a secreted protein that selectively binds and activates receptors located on the surface of vascular endothelial cells. Activation of vascular endothelial cells contributes to the progression of neovascular form of AMD [41]. Pegaptanib sodium is a pegylated aptamer (a modified oligonucleotide) which adopts three-dimensional conformation to bind and antagonize the action of extracellular VEGF with high affinity (Kd = 200 pM). Hence, it inhibits binding of free VEGF to endothelial cells [42]. A comparative study for pegaptanib sodium and pan-VEGF demonstrated high and selective binding of pegaptanib sodium to abnormal vasculature and suppressing pathological neovascularization. On the other hand, pan-VEGF inhibition had similar activity but also binds to normal vasculature [43]. Currently, the drug is being evaluated for the treatment of retinopathy of prematurity (ROP). Recently, intravitreal pegaptanib has been shown to be effective for stage 3+ ROP in a prospective, randomized, controlled multicenter clinical trial [44]. The use of anti-VEGF therapy for ROP has been shown to be efficacious without any toxicity. However, the dose which allows maximum efficacy with least recurrences and devoid of toxicity must be determined.

Pharmacokinetic Profile: Pharmacokinetics of Macugen® is not well characterized in humans. However, preclinical studies in rabbits have been conducted. Intravitreal injection of pegaptanib sodium in animals demonstrated slow absorption (rate-limiting step) into systemic circulation. This rate-limiting step may be similar in humans. After dosing 3 mg of pegaptanib (ten times the recommended dose) the average apparent plasma half-life was 10 days [45]. The mean plasma Cmax of 80 ng/mL occurs within 1–4 days in man. The mean area under the curve (AUC) is 25 μg h/mL. Absolute bioavailability studies after intravenous administration demonstrated 70–100 % in rabbits, dogs, and monkeys [45]. Intravenous administration of pegaptanib sodium causes the drug to distribute mainly in plasma and not to peripheral tissues. In vivo studies in rabbits with intravenous and intravitreal administration of radiolabeled pegaptanib sodium were conducted. Intravenous injections demonstrated highest radioactivity in kidneys, whereas no radioactivity was detected in kidneys for animals receiving intravitreal injection. In rabbits pegaptanib is excreted as a parent compound, while the metabolites are primarily eliminated in urine [45]. Clinical trials with pegaptanib 0.3 mg exhibited statistically significant benefits, at the end of one-year study.

Adverse Reactions: Ocular adverse events in the study groups reported include anterior uveitis, blepharitis, conjunctivitis allergic, corneal abrasion, corneal deposits, corneal erosion, diplopia, endophthalmitis, eye inflammation, swelling, bleeding, eyelid disorder, irritation, retinal artery spasm, retinal and vitreous hemorrhage, retinal scar, and retinal telangiectasia. In phase II clinical trials subjects receiving 0.3 mg pegaptanib sodium had better visual acuity outcomes with significant reduction in central retinal thickness. These subjects are deemed to be less likely to need additional therapy with follow-up photocoagulation [46].

4.2 Avastin®

Indications and Usage: Avastin (bevacizumab) is a recombinant humanized monoclonal IgG1 antibody that binds and inhibits the biological activity of VEGF similar to Macugen®.

Dosage and Administration: Avastin® is an immunoglobulin (IgG) composed of two identical light chains (214 amino acids and 453 residue heavy chains) containing N-linked oligosaccharide. It has a molecular weight of approx. 149 kDa. The intravitreal dose is empirically derived in comparison to molar concentrations of each drug with 1.25 mg of bevacizumab being considered equivalent to 0.5 mg ranibizumab. The optimal dose frequency is not clear. Clinical studies reported different dosing schedules with monthly injection or as needed [47–49]. On an average, it is estimated that six to nine injections in the first year and five injections in the second year for each eye are required. Some patients may even require injections in both eyes [50].

Drug Composition: The monoclonal antibody is supplied at a concentration of 100 mg/4 mL or 400 mg/16 mL. These concentrated drug products are further diluted in 0.9 % saline solution to achieve a concentration of 1.25 mg for intravitreal injection. The entire procedure is recommended to be conducted under aseptic conditions. Currently, prefilled syringes are available that need to be used within 4–6 weeks.

Pharmacodynamic Profile: Bevacizumab specifically binds to VEGF and prevents the interaction of VEGF to Flt1 and KDR receptors on the surface of endothelial cells. Interaction of VEGF with the receptors leads to cell proliferation and formation of new immature blood vessels in in vitro models of angiogenesis. Therefore, the biological activity of VEGF is inhibited with bevacizumab which can also inhibit ocular tumor growth. Administration of bevacizumab to xenotransplant nude mice models demonstrated an extensive antitumor activity in human cancers. Also, metastasis of disease was inhibited and microvascular permeability was reduced. Choroidal neovascular AMD patients treated with intravitreal bevacizumab were reported to gain mean number of letters with diminution in central retinal thickness. Further studies are being conducted to determine the efficacy and safety of intravitreal bevacizumab to treat neovascular AMD [51].

Adverse Reactions: Intravitreal bevacizumab had no adverse effects on the growth and development of young rabbit eye [52]. Short-term studies suggested that intravitreal bevacizumab is well tolerated. No significant ocular or systemic adverse effects were observed [53]. Another study evaluated the short-term effect of intravitreal bevacizumab for subfoveal CNV in pathologic myopia. There were no short-term safety concerns. However, further long-term studies are warranted to determine the efficacy and toxicity of the drug product [54].

4.3 Triesence®

Indications and Usage: Triesence® (triamcinolone acetonide suspension, 40 mg/mL) is indicated for the treatment of sympathetic ophthalmia, temporal arteritis, uveitis, and ocular inflammatory conditions where patients do not respond to topical corticosteroids. Also, it has been used for visualization during vitrectomy [55].

Dosage and Administration: Triamcinolone acetonide is initially recommended at a dose of 100 μL (40 mg/mL suspension) administered as intravitreal injection. The other recommended intravitreal dose for visualization is 1–4 mg, i.e., 25–100 μL of 40 mg/mL suspension.

Drug Composition: Triesence® (triamcinolone acetonide injectable suspension, 40 mg/mL) forms a milky suspension. This product is supplied as 1 mL sterile suspension at a concentration of 40 mg/mL in a flint type 1 single-use glass vial.

Pharmacodynamic Profile: Triamcinolone acetonide is a water-insoluble glycocorticosteroid indicated for the treatment of various ocular inflammatory disorders. Following intravitreal injection, triamcinolone particles disperse in the vitreous body and thereby provide contrast between the transparent vitreous and membranes. Two phase II studies were conducted in the USA and Japan to evaluate the safety and efficacy of Triesence®. Results demonstrated a statistically significant improvement in the degree of visualization of posterior segment structures. Both the study outcomes were in agreement that Triesence® enhanced visualization of posterior segment structures during pars plana vitrectomy, both vitreous and membranes [56, 57]. Triesence® pharmacodynamic studies were not conducted in a clinical setting. However, several reports demonstrate the utility of triamcinolone acetonide for this indication [58, 59].

Pharmacokinetic Profile: Triesence® pharmacokinetic and ocular tissue distribution has been studied following intravitreal injection of 2.1 mg unilateral dose to male New Zealand albino rabbits. Highest activity was achieved in retina and choroid. Other ocular tissues had seven times lower radiolabeled drug accumulation than retina. The vitreous radioactivity remained high until day 60 followed by substantial decline till day 88. Drug elimination from the ocular tissues appeared to be rapid initially followed by a slower elimination phase. Systemic levels of triamcinolone acetonide were not quantifiable (<5 ng eq/g) post 4-h dosing. Aqueous humor pharmacokinetics of triamcinolone has been evaluated in five patients following a single intravitreal administration (4 mg) of triamcinolone acetonide. Aqueous humor samples were collected via an anterior chamber paracentesis on days 1, 3, 10, 17, and 31 post injections. Peak aqueous humor concentrations of triamcinolone ranged from 2,151 to 7,202 ng/mL, half-life 76–635 h, and AUC_{0-t} 231 to 1,911 ng h/mL following single intravitreal administration. The mean elimination half-life was 18.7 ± 5.7 days in four nonvitrectomized eyes (four patients). In a patient who had undergone vitrectomy (one eye), the elimination half-life of triamcinolone from the vitreous was much faster (3.2 days) relative to patients without vitrectomy.

Adverse Reactions: The most commonly observed adverse effects in 20–60 % subjects with triamcinolone acetonide intravitreal administration are elevation of intraocular pressure and cataract progression. Other less common side effects include endophthalmitis, hypopyon, injection site reactions, glaucoma, vitreous floaters, and retinal detachment.

5 Periocular Administered Drugs

Periocular routes such as subtenon and subconjunctival routes can also be employed to deliver drugs to the back of the eye. The periocular routes place the active drug adjacent to the sclera for transscleral delivery, thus minimizing the risks associated with the intravitreal route of administration. Periocular injections are associated with fairly high patient compliance relative to intravitreal injections. Below is an overview of drug composition, pharmacodynamic and pharmacokinetic profiles, and adverse events associated with RETAANE® (Alcon Laboratories Inc., Fort Worth, TX).

5.1 RETAANE®

Indications and Usage: RETAANE® is an investigational treatment containing an angiostatic steroid indicated for the prevention and treatment of ocular disorders, in particular AMD.

Dosage and Administration: RETAANE® contains 15 mg of anecortave acetate injected as a depot formulation via a specialized cannula in a posterior juxtascleral position (subtenon's space). The blunt-tipped, curved cannula follows the scleral surface without puncturing the globe. As soon as the cannula is in place, the composition is injected into the juxtascleral space overlying the macula. Drug release to choroid is expected to be slow over a 6-month period. This method is anticipated to avoid the most common side effects with frequent injections such as the risk of intraocular infections, inflammations, and retinal detachment.

Drug Composition: RETAANE® contains 15 mg of anecortave acetate in the form of suspension. RETAANE® suspension requires less frequent dosing (once every 6 months) compared to other investigational drugs.

Pharmacodynamic Profile: Anecortave acetate is an angiostatic cortisene that can inhibit the abnormal growth of blood vessels, known as angiogenesis. Anecortave acetate differs from cortisol structure by the removal of 11-beta hydroxyl, addition of a double bond at the C9-11 position, and addition of an acetate group at the C21 position [60, 61]. These substitutions tend to improve the physicochemical properties ultimately leading to enhanced bioavailability. Although the compound exhibits angiostatic activity, it does not display typical glucocorticoid receptor-mediated activity. Besides retaining antiangiogenic potency, such substitutions are engineered to reduce major side effects of steroid drugs such as cataract formation and elevated intraocular pressure.

Anecortave acetate acts by inhibiting the expression of urokinase plasminogen activator (uPA) and matrix metalloproteinases, extracellular proteases required for the breakdown of basement membrane and extracellular matrix essential for subsequent migration of vascular endothelial cells to stroma during growth of blood vessels [60, 62]. Furthermore, this compound can stimulate the production of plasminogen activator inhibitor-1 (PAI-1) which is a specific inhibitor of uPA activity [63]. Following intravitreal injection in a rat model of ROP, retinal levels of PAI-1 and mRNA level elevated six- to ninefold in 24–72 h [64]. Also, this compound reduced the expression of proangiogenic insulin-like growth factor (IGF-1) and IGF-1 receptor by 36.9 and 50.5 %, respectively [65]. Interestingly, anecortave acetate inhibited VEGF mRNA, a major upregulated gene during angiogenesis [66]. Efficacy of anecortave acetate was evaluated in patients with subfoveal CNV secondary to exudative AMD [67]. Figure 6 represents a fluorescein angiogram of a patient in 15 mg group at baseline and at month 24. A significant

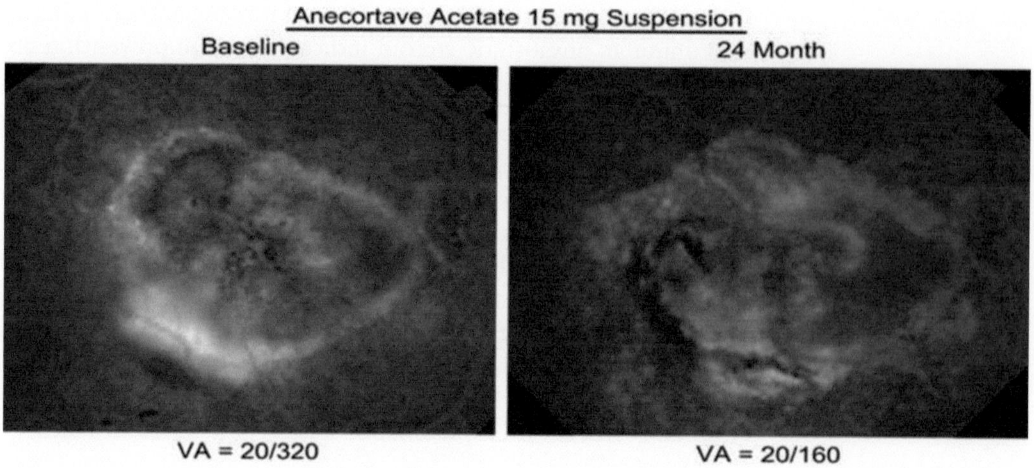

Fig. 6 Fluorescein angiogram of a patient treated with anecortave acetate 15 mg at baseline and month 24. A reduction in intensity and extent of leakage within a CNV region is depicted. Reproduced with permission from [67]

reduction in the intensity and extent of fluorescein leakage from the CNV region was observed. This improvement in the blood-retinal barrier corresponds to the visual acuity improvement.

Pharmacokinetic Profile: A pharmacokinetic study was carried out in 20 wet AMD patients following two posterior juxtascleral depot injections of RETAANE® suspension over a 12-month period [68]. The peak plasma levels were well correlated with observed reflux. Results showed that the patients for whom reflux was observed had plasma levels fourfold lower than patients without reflux, highlighting the need for a counterpressure device (CPD). Subsequent pharmacokinetic studies were undertaken to examine the ability of a CPD to eliminate reflux. The reflux was efficiently controlled in 100 % of patients, with a reflux score of 0 for all eyes. A notable observation is that there was no loss of dose upon administration using the CPD. A fourfold rise in mean plasma drug levels was observed relative to levels observed in the initial pharmacokinetic study without a CPD [68].

Adverse Reactions: Anecortave acetate 15 mg is safe and well tolerated when administered as a posterior juxtascleral depot at 6-month intervals for primary therapy or as adjunctive therapy with photodynamic therapy. This compound has been reported to possess comparable or even superior angiostatic activity of glucocorticoids without the adverse side effects associated with glucocorticoid therapy [69, 70].

Finally, a list of other commercially available ophthalmic formulations with their trade names, active ingredient, dosage form strength, inactive ingredients, type of dosage form, and indicated ocular diseases is summarized in Table 1.

Table 1
List of other commercially available ophthalmic formulations with their trade names, active ingredient, dosage from strength, inactive ingredients, type of dosage form, and indicated ocular diseases

Trade name	Active ingredient	% dosage of active ingredient	Inactive ingredients	Dosage form	Recommended for disease treatment	Reference
Azasite®	Azithromycin	1.0	Polycarbophil	Eye drops/ solution	Bacterial conjunctivitis	http://www.merck.com/product/usa/pi_circulars/a/azasite/azasite_ppi.pdf
Betoptic S® and Betoptic	Betaxolol	0.25 and/or 0.5	Poly(styrene-divinyl benzene) sulfonic acid, carbomer-934P	Eye drops/ solution	Glaucoma	http://www.medsafe.govt.nz/profs/datasheet/b/Betoptic&Betoptic%20Ssoln.pdf
TobraDex®	Tobramycin/ dexamethasone	0.3/0.1	Tyloxapol and hydroxyethyl cellulose	Ophthalmic suspension	Ocular infections and inflammations	http://ecatalog.alcon.com/pi/TobraDexSusp_us_en.pdf
TobraDex® ST	Tobramycin/ dexamethasone	0.3/0.05	Xanthan gum	Gel-forming eye drops	Blepharitis	http://ecatalog.alcon.com/pi/TobraDexST_us_en.pdf
Timoptic-XE®	Timolol maleate	0.25 and/or 0.5	Gellan gum	Eye drops/ solution	Glaucoma	http://www.merck.com/product/usa/pi_circulars/t/timoptic/timoptic_xe_pi.pdf
Durezol™	Difluprednate	0.05	Polysorbate-80 and castor oil	Emulsion eye drops	Anterior uveitis and for inflammation and pain associated with ocular surgery	http://ecatalog.alcon.com/pi/Durezol2012_us_en.pdf
Cationorm®	–	–	Light mineral oil, glycerol, tyloxapol, poloxamer-188	Eye drops	Mild dry eye	http://www.santen.eu/eu/products/therapyareas/dryeye/Pages/Cationorm.aspx
Nevanac®	Nepafenac	0.1	carbomer 975P and Tyloxapol	Suspension	Pain and inflammation after cataract surgery	http://www.accessdata.fda.gov/drugsatfda_docs/label/2011/021862s008lbl.pdf

(continued)

Table 1 (continued)

Trade name	Active ingredient	% dosage of active ingredient	Inactive ingredients	Dosage form	Recommended for disease treatment	Reference
Triesence®	Triamcinolone acetonide	4.0	CMC sodium and polysorbate-80	Suspension	Sympathetic ophthalmia, temporal arteritis, uveitis, and ocular inflammations	http://ecatalog.alcon.com/pi/Triesence_us_en.pdf
RESTASIS®	Cyclosporine-A	0.05	Glycerin, castor oil, polysorbate-80, carbomer copolymer type A	Emulsion eye drops	Severe chronic dry eye syndrome	http://www.allergan.com/assets/pdf/restasis_pi.pdf
Refresh dry eye therapy®	Carboxymethyl cellulose (CMC)	0.5	–	Emulsion eye drops	Dry eye syndrome	http://www.refreshbrand.com/html/practitioner/formulation.asp
Lipimix™	Huile de soja	1.25	Phospholipids, medium-chain triglycerides (MCT)	Emulsion eye drops	Dry eye syndrome	http://www.has-sante.fr/portail/upload/docs/application/pdf/2008-07/cepp_1705_lipimix.pdf
Acuvail	Ketorolac tromethamine	0.45	CMC	Eye drops/solution	Pain and inflammation after cataract surgery	http://www.allergan.com/Assets/pdf/acuvail_pi.pdf
Voltarin	Diclofenac sodium	0.10	Polyoxyl 35 castor oil, tromethamine, sorbic acid	Eye drops/solution	Pain and inflammation after cataract surgery	http://www.pharma.us.novartis.com/cs/www.pharma.us.novartis.com/product/pi/pdf/voltaren_ophthalmic.pdf
Chlorptic	Chloramphenicol	0.5	Polyethylene 300, polyoxyl 40 stearate	Eye drops/solution	Bacterial ocular infections	http://www.ruaipharmaceuticals.com/index.php/pharmacy-a-m-pesa-franchise/852-chloroptic

Zirgan	Ganciclovir	0.15	Carbopol	Gel-forming eye drops	Acute herpetic keratitis (dendritic ulcers)	http://www.bauschlocal.com/zirgan/Zirgan-JosephColinMD.pdf
Zymar	Gatifloxacin	0.30	Edetate disodium	Eye drops/solution	Bacterial conjunctivitis	http://www.allergan.com/assets/pdf/zymar_pi.pdf
Betaxon™	Levobetaxolol	0.5	Mannitol, poly(styrene-divinyl benzene) sulfonic acid, carbomer 974P, boric acid, *N*-lauroylsarcosine	Suspension	Lowering intraocular pressure in patients with chronic open-angle glaucoma or ocular hypertension	http://www.accessdata.fda.gov/drugsatfda_docs/label/2010/021114s003lbl.pdf
Bipreve™	Bepotastine besilate	1.5	Monobasic sodium phosphate dihydrate	Eye drops/solution	Itching associated with allergic conjunctivitis	http://www.accessdata.fda.gov/drugsatfda_docs/label/2009/022288lbl.pdf
Besivance™	Besifloxacin	0.6	Polycarbophil, mannitol, poloxamer 407	Suspension	Bacterial conjunctivitis	http://www.accessdata.fda.gov/drugsatfda_docs/label/2009/022308lbl.pdf
Ciloxin	Ciprofloxacin hydrochloride	0.3	Mannitol, edetate disodium	Eye drops/solution and ointment	Ocular infections such as conjunctivitis	http://www.alcon.ca/pdf/Product_pharma/Product_pharma_ciloxan_eng.pdf
Pred forte	Prednisolone acetate	1.0	Boric acid; edetate disodium, hypromellose, polysorbate 80	Suspension	Steroid-responsive inflammation of the palpebral and bulbar conjunctiva, cornea, and anterior segment of the globe	http://www.allergan.com/assets/pdf/pred_forte_pi.pdf
Macugen	Pegaptanib sodium	0.03	Phosphate buffer	Intravitreal injection	Neovascular (wet) age-related macular degeneration	http://www.macugen.com/macugen_PI.pdf

(continued)

Table 1 (continued)

Trade name	Active ingredient	% dosage of active ingredient	Inactive ingredients	Dosage form	Recommended for disease treatment	Reference
Visudyne	Verteporfin	0.2	Lactose, egg phosphatidylglycerol, dimyristoyl phosphatidylcholine, ascorbyl palmitate, and butylated hydroxytoulene	Intravenous injection	Photodynamic therapy for choroidal neovascularization	http://www.vidyya.com/2pdfs/visudyne.pdf
Rysmon® TG	Timolol maleate	0.25 and/or 0.5	Methylcellulose	Eye drops/solution	Glaucoma	

6 Conclusions

Effective treatment of ocular diseases is a challenging task because of the complex nature of diseases and presence of ocular barriers which hinder delivery of therapeutic agents in required levels. Age-related chronic ophthalmic disorders are expected to rise dramatically in the next two decades. Hence, there is an unmet need to develop new ophthalmic formulations that meet the multi-medication needs of the elderly patients. An ideal ophthalmic formulation would be easy to manufacture, permit noninvasive self-administration, and attain and sustain effective drug concentrations at the target site for desired time periods. It must also produce negligible systemic exposure and afford good patient well-being, acceptance, and compliance. Over the last two decades there has been a significant growth in the development of formulations which would efficiently incorporate agents and sustain release following topical ocular administration. But none of these formulations have advanced into clinic. Eye drops still account for 90 % of all ophthalmic formulations and are considered ideal for treating anterior segment disorders. However, these formulations may not be able to deliver drugs to the back of the eye. An ideal therapy should maintain effective levels for a longer duration following a single application. Drug delivery by intravitreal routes cannot be particularly considered safe, effective, and patient friendly. Drug delivery by periocular route can potentially overcome many of these limitations and can provide sustained drug levels in ocular pathologies affecting both segments. Nevertheless, the selection of an administration route is also dependent on the severity of the disease and the target ocular tissue. A clear understanding of the complexities associated with normal and diseased conditions, physiological barriers, and pharmacokinetics would significantly improve drug development in this field. Currently there is no product approved for treating back-of-the-eye diseases via noninvasive topical drug administration. Much emphasis should be given to noninvasive sustained drug delivery for both front- and back-of-the-eye disorders. Development of noninvasive delivery techniques will revolutionize retinal drug delivery. Advances in noninvasive drug delivery techniques will remain in the forefront of new ophthalmic formulations.

Acknowledgements

This work was supported by NIH grants R01EY09171 and R01EY010659.

References

1. Cunha-Vaz JG (1997) The blood-ocular barriers: past, present, and future. Documenta ophthalmologica. Adv Ophthalmol 93(1–2):149–157
2. Cholkar KPA, Vadlapudi AD, Mitra AK (2012) Novel nanomicellar formulation approaches for anterior and posterior segment ocular drug delivery. Recent Pat Nanomed 2(2):82–95
3. Kumar S, Karki R, Meena M, Prakash T, Rajeswari T, Goli D (2011) Reduction in drop size of ophthalmic topical drop preparations and the impact of treatment. J Adv Pharm Technol Res 2(3):192–194
4. Lederer CM Jr, Harold RE (1986) Drop size of commercial glaucoma medications. Am J Ophthalmol 101(6):691–694
5. Van Santvliet L, Ludwig A (2004) Determinants of eye drop size. Surv Ophthalmol 49(2):197–213
6. Schoenwald RD (1997) Ocular pharmacokinetics. In: Zimmerman TJ (ed) Textbook of ocular pharmacology. Lippincott-Raven Publishers, Philadelphia, PA, pp 119–138
7. Frenkel RE, Haji SA, La M, Frenkel MP, Reyes A (2010) A protocol for the retina surgeon's safe initial intravitreal injections. Clin Ophthalmol 4:1279–1285
8. Marmor MF, Negi A, Maurice DM (1985) Kinetics of macromolecules injected into the subretinal space. Exp Eye Res 40(5):687–696
9. Raghava S, Hammond M, Kompella UB (2004) Periocular routes for retinal drug delivery. Expert Opin Drug Deliv 1(1):99–114
10. Roper-Hall MJ (ed) (1989) Anesthesia and akinesia for eye operations. Stallard's eye surgery, 7th edn. UK Wright & Sons Ltd, Bristol, pp 44–63
11. Fatt WB (ed) (1992) Physiology of the eye: an introduction to the vegetative functions, 2nd edn. Butterworth-Heinemann Inc, Stoneham, pp 2–3
12. Canavan KS, Dark A, Garrioch MA (2003) Sub-Tenon's administration of local anaesthetic: a review of the technique. Br J Anaesth 90(6):787–793
13. Kumar CM, Eid H, Dodds C (2011) Sub-Tenon's anaesthesia: complications and their prevention. Eye 25(6):694–703
14. Jaffe NSJM, Jaffe GF, Craven L (eds) (1997) Cataract surgery and its complications, 6th edn. Mosby-Year Book, Inc., St. Louis, pp 20–25
15. Hamilton RC (2004) Retrobulbar and periocular anesthesia for cataract surgery. In: Steinert RF (ed.) Cataract surgery: techniques, complications and management. Elsevier Health Sciences, Philadelphia, PA. pp. 79–95
16. Stead S, Miller KM (2003) Anesthesia for ophthalmic surgery. In: Spaeth GL (ed) Ophthalmic surgery: principles and practice. W.B. Saunders Company, Philadelphia, PA, pp 15–25
17. Eisner G (1990) Eye surgery: an introduction to operative technique. Springer Limited, London
18. D'Amico DJ, Goldberg MF, Hudson H, Jerdan JA, Krueger DS, Luna SP et al (2003) Anecortave acetate as monotherapy for treatment of subfoveal neovascularization in age-related macular degeneration: twelve-month clinical outcomes. Ophthalmology 110(12):2372–2383, discussion 84–85
19. http://www.accessdata.fda.gov/drugsatfda_docs/label/2006/019992s020lbl.pdf.
20. Hendrix DV, Stuffle JL, Cox SK (2007) Pharmacokinetics of topically applied ciprofloxacin in equine tears. Vet Ophthalmol 10(6):344–347
21. Scheib SA, Garner WH (2004) Anti-inflammatory effects of topical ocular MAXIDEX administration to rabbits following vitrectomy or lensectomy. Exp Eye Res 79(6):893–902
22. http://www.allergan.com/assets/pdf/restasis_pi.pdf.
23. Rao SN (2010) Topical cyclosporine 0.05% for the prevention of dry eye disease progression. J Ocul Pharmacol Ther 26(2):157–164
24. Acheampong AA, Shackleton M, Tang-Liu DD, Ding S, Stern ME, Decker R (1999) Distribution of cyclosporin A in ocular tissues after topical administration to albino rabbits and beagle dogs. Curr Eye Res 18(2):91–103
25. http://www.bauschlocal.com/zirgan/zirgan PackageInsert.pdf
26. Hoh HB, Hurley C, Claoue C, Viswalingham M, Easty DL, Goldschmidt P et al (1996) Randomised trial of ganciclovir and acyclovir in the treatment of herpes simplex dendritic keratitis: a multicentre study. Br J Ophthalmol 80(2):140–143
27. Vadlapudi AD, Vadlapatla RK, Mitra AK (2012) Current and emerging antivirals for the treatment of cytomegalovirus (CMV) retinitis: an update on recent patents. Recent Pat Antiinfect Drug Discov 7(1):8–18
28. Croxtall JD (2011) Ganciclovir ophthalmic gel 0.15%: in acute herpetic keratitis (dendritic ulcers). Drugs 71(5):603–610

29. Crumpacker CS (1996) Ganciclovir. New Engl J Med 335(10):721–729
30. Kaufman HE, Haw WH (2012) Ganciclovir ophthalmic gel 0.15%: safety and efficacy of a new treatment for herpes simplex keratitis. Curr Eye Res 37(7):654–660
31. Matthews T, Boehme R (1988) Antiviral activity and mechanism of action of ganciclovir. Rev Infect Dis 10(Suppl 3):S490–S494
32. http://www.bausch.com/en/ECP/Our-Products/Rx-Pharmaceuticals/Rx-Pharmaceuticals-ECP/Lotemax-Ointment-ECP
33. Druzgala P, Hochhaus G, Bodor N (1991) Soft drugs–10. Blanching activity and receptor binding affinity of a new type of glucocorticoid: loteprednol etabonate. J Steroid Biochem Mol Biol 38(2):149–154
34. Bodor N, Loftsson T, Wu WM (1992) Metabolism, distribution, and transdermal permeation of a soft corticosteroid, loteprednol etabonate. Pharm Res 9(10):1275–1278
35. Druzgala P, Wu WM, Bodor N (1991) Ocular absorption and distribution of loteprednol etabonate, a soft steroid, in rabbit eyes. Curr Eye Res 10(10):933–937
36. Comstock TL, Paterno MR, Singh A, Erb T, Davis E (2011) Safety and efficacy of loteprednol etabonate ophthalmic ointment 0.5% for the treatment of inflammation and pain following cataract surgery. Clinical Ophthalmol 5:177–186
37. Samudre SS, Lattanzio FA Jr, Williams PB, Sheppard JD Jr (2004) Comparison of topical steroids for acute anterior uveitis. J Ocul Pharmacol Ther 20(6):533–547
38. Howes J, Novack GD (1998) Failure to detect systemic levels, and effects of loteprednol etabonate and its metabolite, PJ-91, following chronic ocular administration. J Ocul Pharmacol Ther 14(2):153–158
39. http://www.macugen.com/macugenUSPI.pdf
40. Ng EW, Shima DT, Calias P, Cunningham ET Jr, Guyer DR, Adamis AP (2006) Pegaptanib, a targeted anti-VEGF aptamer for ocular vascular disease. Nat Rev Drug Discov 5(2):123–132
41. Krzystolik MG, Afshari MA, Adamis AP, Gaudreault J, Gragoudas ES, Michaud NA et al (2002) Prevention of experimental choroidal neovascularization with intravitreal anti-vascular endothelial growth factor antibody fragment. Arch Ophthalmol 120(3):338–346
42. Klein R (1999) Epidemiology. In: Berger JW, Fine SL, Maguire MG (eds) Age-related macular degeneration. Mosby, St. Louis, MO, pp 31–56
43. Gragoudas ES, Adamis AP, Cunningham ET, Feinsod M, Guyer DR (2004) Pegaptanib for neovascular age-related macular degeneration. N Eng J Med 351(27):2805–2816
44. Mintz-Hittner HA (2012) Intravitreal pegaptanib as adjunctive treatment for stage 3+ ROP shown to be effective in a prospective, randomized, controlled multicenter clinical trial. Eur J Ophthalmol 22(5):685–686
45. http://www.pfizer.ca/en/our_products/products/monograph/142
46. Cunningham ET Jr, Adamis AP, Altaweel M, Aiello LP, Bressler NM, D'Amico DJ et al (2005) A phase II randomized double-masked trial of pegaptanib, an anti-vascular endothelial growth factor aptamer, for diabetic macular edema. Ophthalmology 112(10):1747–1757
47. Schouten JS, La Heij EC, Webers CA, Lundqvist IJ, Hendrikse F (2009) A systematic review on the effect of bevacizumab in exudative age-related macular degeneration. Graefes Arch Clin Exp Ophthalmol 247(1):1–11
48. Cleary CA, Jungkim S, Ravikumar K, Kelliher C, Acheson RW, Hickey-Dwyer M (2008) Intravitreal bevacizumab in the treatment of neovascular age-related macular degeneration, 6- and 9-month results. Eye 22(1):82–86
49. Pedersen R, Soliman W, Lund-Andersen H, Larsen M (2007) Treatment of choroidal neovascularization using intravitreal bevacizumab. Acta Ophthalmol Scand 85(5):526–533
50. Colquitt JL, Jones J, Tan SC, Takeda A, Clegg AJ, Price A (2008) Ranibizumab and pegaptanib for the treatment of age-related macular degeneration: a systematic review and economic evaluation. Health Technol Assess 12(16):iii–iv, ix-201
51. El-Mollayess GM, Noureddine BN, Bashshur ZF (2011) Bevacizumab and neovascular age related macular degeneration: pathogenesis and treatment. Semin Ophthalmol 26(3):69–76
52. Axer-Siegel R, Herscovici Z, Hasanreisoglu M, Kremer I, Benjamini Y, Snir M (2009) Effect of intravitreal bevacizumab (avastin) on the growing rabbit eye. Curr Eye Res 34(8):660–665
53. Avery RL, Pearlman J, Pieramici DJ, Rabena MD, Castellarin AA, Nasir MA et al (2006) Intravitreal bevacizumab (Avastin) in the treatment of proliferative diabetic retinopathy. Ophthalmology 113(10):1695e1–1695e15
54. Hernandez-Rojas ML, Quiroz-Mercado H, Dalma-Weiszhausz J, Fromow-Guerra J, Amaya-Espinosa A, Solis-Vivanco A et al (2007) Short-term effects of intravitreal bevacizumab for subfoveal choroidal neovascularization in pathologic myopia. Retina 27(6):707–712

55. http://dailymed.nlm.nih.gov/dailymed/lookup.cfm?setid=3f045347-3e5e-4bbd-90f8-6c3100985ca5
56. Dyer D, Callanan D, Bochow T, Abraham P, Lambert HM, Lee SY et al (2009) Clinical evaluation of the safety and efficacy of preservative-free triamcinolone (triesence [triamcinolone acetonide injectable suspension] 40 mg/ml) for visualization during pars plana vitrectomy. Retina 29(1):38–45
57. http://www.alcon.ca/pdf/Product_pharma/Product_pharma_triesence_eng.pdf
58. Bardak Y, Cekic O, Tig SU (2006) Comparison of ICG-assisted ILM peeling and triamcinolone-assisted posterior vitreous removal in diffuse diabetic macular oedema. Eye 20(12):1357–1359
59. Peyman GA, Cheema R, Conway MD, Fang T (2000) Triamcinolone acetonide as an aid to visualization of the vitreous and the posterior hyaloid during pars plana vitrectomy. Retina 20(5):554–555
60. Clark AF (2007) Mechanism of action of the angiostatic cortisene anecortave acetate. Surv Ophthalmol 52(Suppl 1):S26–S34
61. Blei F, Wilson EL, Mignatti P, Rifkin DB (1993) Mechanism of action of angiostatic steroids: suppression of plasminogen activator activity via stimulation of plasminogen activator inhibitor synthesis. J Cell Physiol 155(3):568–578
62. DeFaller JM, Clark AF (2000) A new pharmacological treatment for angiogenesis. In: Taylor HR (ed) Pterygium. Kugler Pub, The Hague, Netherlands, pp 159–181
63. Penn JS, Rajaratnam VS, Collier RJ, Clark AF (2001) The effect of an angiostatic steroid on neovascularization in a rat model of retinopathy of prematurity. Invest Ophthalmol Vis Sci 42(1):283–290
64. BenEzra D, Griffin BW, Maftzir G, Sharif NA, Clark AF (1997) Topical formulations of novel angiostatic steroids inhibit rabbit corneal neovascularization. Invest Ophthalmol Vis Sci 38(10):1954–1962
65. Liu C, Gu X, Wang W-H, Bingaman D (2005) Local delivery of anecortave acetate inhibits the expression of retinal IGF-1/IGF-1 receptor in the rat OIR model. Invest Ophthalmol Vis Sci 46(5):4135
66. Yang R, McCollum GW, Bingaman DP, Penn JS (2005) The effect of anecortave acetate on VEGF message and protein levels in hypoxic muller cells and in rat OIR. Invest Ophthalmol Vis Sci 46(5):4177
67. Russell SR, Hudson HL, Jerdan JA (2007) Anecortave acetate for the treatment of exudative age-related macular degeneration–a review of clinical outcomes. Surv Ophthalmol 52(Suppl 1):S79–S90
68. Augustin A (2006) Anecortave acetate in the treatment of age-related macular degeneration. Clin Interv Aging 1(3):237–246
69. Stalmans I, Callanan DG, Dirks MS, Moster MR, Robin AL, Van Calster J et al (2012) Treatment of steroid-induced elevated intraocular pressure with anecortave acetate: a randomized clinical trial. J Ocul Pharmacol Ther 28(6):559–565
70. Regillo CD, D'Amico DJ, Mieler WF, Schneebaum C, Beasley CH, Sullins GT (2007) Clinical safety profile of posterior juxtascleral depot administration of anecortave acetate 15 mg suspension as primary therapy or adjunctive therapy with photodynamic therapy for treatment of wet age-related macular degeneration. Surv Ophthalmol 52(Suppl 1):S70–S78
71. http://www.pocd.com.au/files/pdfs/OM_Autodrop_AutoSqueeze_POCDbrochure.pdf

Methods in Pharmacology and Toxicology (2014): 119–142
DOI 10.1007/7653_2013_3

Published online: 29 August 2013

Sustained-Release Ocular Drug Delivery Systems: Bench to Bedside Development

Susan S. Lee, Michael R. Robinson, and Scott M. Whitcup

Abstract

The process of bringing a drug through early development and on through a successful clinical trials campaign is long and complex. This chapter provides an overview of the drug development process and some of the challenges and pitfalls that can be encountered on the path to marketing approval for a sustained-release intraocular drug delivery system. In general, the drug development process proceeds from exploratory analyses of new compounds, through preclinical and clinical testing of promising drug candidates, to application for marketing approval in one or more markets. Although the application for marketing approval is the final step, success depends on taking the requirements for obtaining marketing approval into consideration early in the process and initiating communication with the relevant regulatory agency(s) while the candidate drug is still in preclinical testing. A successful preclinical development program should be designed to provide all the information needed to determine if the drug is appropriate for further testing in human subjects. Approval to begin human testing (phase I trials) is only granted if there is sufficient evidence of drug safety, if the pharmacologic profile of the drug is appropriate for the condition it is proposed to treat, and the clinical trial design submitted is sufficient to ensure the safety of the human subjects. Clinical testing, if approved, proceeds through phase I (to evaluate safety and dosing considerations), to phase II (early investigations of efficacy and further exploration of dose–response), and finally to phase III (definitive investigations of safety and efficacy in the intended patient population). If the results of the clinical trials demonstrate sufficient safety and efficacy, the drug developer can apply for marketing approval in the United States (US) through the Food and Drug Administration (FDA) or in the European Union (EU) through one of three separate pathways to approval—the centralized, decentralized, or mutual recognition procedures. In all cases, the success of an application will depend not only on the merits of the drug itself but also on how well the drug development program was designed to meet the concerns and requirements of the appropriate regulatory agency(s). The single most effective way to ensure that a drug application meets these requirements and concerns is through early and frequent consultation with the appropriate regulatory agency contacts.

Key words Clinical trials, Ocular drug delivery, Regulatory, FDA, EMA, Sustained-release, Marketing approval, Drug approval

1 Introduction

As our understanding of normal physiology and pathophysiological processes improves, new targets for therapeutic intervention become apparent and begin to be investigated by drug developers.

How novel compounds are chosen as candidates for drug development is complex and influenced by ongoing basic research in a variety of disciplines. The vast majority of compounds investigated are found to lack the appropriate pharmacologic or pharmacokinetic properties suitable for therapeutic use and never move beyond preclinical testing in animals. Those compounds that do appear promising need to be paired with the appropriate drug delivery system—chosen based on a thorough understanding of the real-world needs of patients as well as the properties of the candidate drug—before the drug can move into the final stages of preclinical testing and, if appropriate, begin clinical trials in humans. Advances in drug delivery can not only allow new compounds to be delivered more efficiently but also create opportunities to develop novel therapeutics from compounds that have been in clinical use for decades.

In the case of localized, chronic diseases, the challenge is to deliver sustained, effective drug therapy to the target tissues while limiting drug exposure in non-target tissues. Sustained-release implantable drug delivery systems loaded with the appropriate drug offer an elegant solution to this problem, but are accompanied by their own unique drug development challenges. This approach to drug delivery dramatically changes the pharmacokinetics and pharmacodynamics of the therapy; often improving the safety profile of the drug treatment, but introducing other safety and logistical concerns relating to the implant itself.

The process of bringing any drug from initial development through approval for clinical use is long and complex. The United States Food and Drug Administration (US FDA) estimates that it takes, on average, approximately 8 ½ years to study and test a new drug before it is approved for use by the general public. This process starts with a rigorous preclinical development program that must provide strong evidence of safety, as well as clinical potential before human testing is allowed to begin. In the case of sustained-release implants, it is critical that the preclinical development program and resultant data package be complete and provide information about all of the unique aspects of the drug delivery technology as well as the active agent itself.

The purpose of this chapter is to provide drug developers with an overview of the drug development process and some of the challenges and pitfalls that can be encountered on the path to the successful clinical debut of a sustained-release drug delivery system for the treatment of chronic retinal diseases. This chapter will begin with an overview of the drug development process with an emphasis on what is required to support a successful application for marketing approval. This will include a detailed discussion of some of the issues of specific interest to those developing medicines for ophthalmic applications. The final section will provide a brief sketch of the bench to bedside journey for Ozurdex® (dexamethasone intravitreal implant 0.7 mg; Allergan, Inc.) which is approved for use in both the US and the European Union (EU).

2 A Successful Drug Development Process

In general, the drug development process proceeds from exploratory analyses of new compounds, through preclinical and clinical testing of promising drugs, to application for marketing approval in one or more markets (Fig. 1). Although the application for marketing approval is the final step, drug developers should begin familiarizing themselves with the requirements for obtaining marketing approval and begin communicating with the relevant regulatory agency(s) as soon as a compound is identified as "promising" [1].

Both the US Food and Drug Administration (US FDA) and the European Medicines Agency (EMA) provide detailed guidance on the nature of the preclinical and clinical studies that should be conducted during the drug development process in order to support a successful application for marketing approval. The specific requirements differ depending on the type of therapeutic and may change over time as regulations change, so it is important to consult with the relevant agency(s) early and often as drug development proceeds. This should start with a visit to the relevant agency website while the candidate drug is still in preclinical development [2, 3]. In Europe, there are three pathways to marketing approval (described in detail below) [4] and drug developers should begin considering which will be the most appropriate pathway for their drug long before the drug is ready for early clinical testing, so that consultation with the most appropriate contacts can begin as soon as appropriate.

In addition, the regulatory agencies in the US, EU, and Japan have been working through the International Conference on Harmonisation (ICH) to develop consensus guidelines (on drug quality, safety, efficacy, and medical terminology) that are acceptable across agencies so that developers can bring quality therapeutics to market in a more resource-efficient manner [5]. The FDA and EMA also offer the opportunity for drug sponsors to request "parallel scientific advice"—in the form of a teleconference or video conference with representatives from both agencies—on aspects of study design that could be critical to achieving marketing approval [5]. The importance of taking advantage of all available guidance and opportunities for early communication with regulatory agencies cannot be over-emphasized.

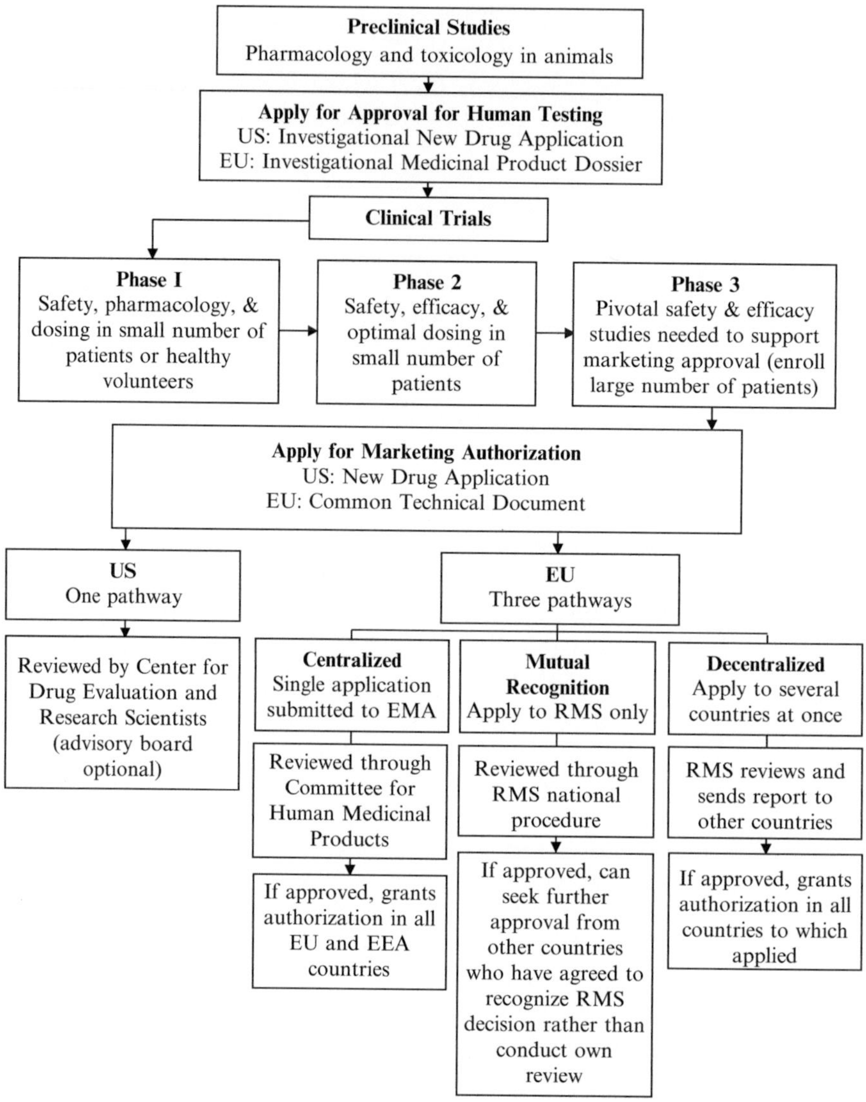

Fig. 1 Drug Development and Approval Process in the United States (US) and the European Union (EU). EMA: European Medicines Agency; RMS: Reference member state; EEA: European Economic Area

2.1 Preclinical Development

Worldwide, a candidate clinical therapeutic begins the drug development process with extensive in vitro and in vivo testing in non-human models. A successful preclinical development program should provide all the information needed to determine if the drug is appropriate for further testing in human subjects [6]. To obtain approval for human testing in either the US or the EU, preclinical testing should establish a detailed pharmacologic profile of the drug, including pharmacokinetics, pharmacodynamics, and mechanism of action [6, 7]. It should also determine the acute toxicity of the drug in at least two species of animals (usually one rodent and one non-rodent species) chosen for similarities to humans with regard to the organ system of interest and susceptibility to drug class (if known). The toxicity studies may range from 2 weeks to 3 months of drug exposure, depending on the proposed duration of use of the drug in clinical studies [6, 7].

It is important that the drug sponsor (drug developer seeking to bring a drug to market) requests a meeting with the appropriate contacts in either the FDA or the EMA before preclinical testing is complete. There should be sufficient pilot data in hand to guide decisions about further testing, but enough flexibility in the development plan that modifications can be made if the agency requests changes [1]. The drug sponsor should come to the meeting with a list of questions about whether specific aspects of their development plan and study designs are considered sufficient to support a successful application to proceed with clinical testing. For example, in the testing of intraocular implants it is common to use rabbits and monkeys rather than rodents because of the need to use animal models with large enough eyes to accommodate the implant. Agency preapproval of this approach should always be obtained, however, to ensure that the preclinical package is acceptable.

It is common knowledge that most candidate drugs never make it out of this stage of development. Any sign of unfavorable pharmacology, excessive toxicity, or other safety issues can and, in most cases, should cause a drug to be removed from further development activities; exceptions are drugs intended for conditions with a high rate of morbidity/mortality for which there is no effective treatment. If, however, preclinical testing has demonstrated that the product is safe for initial use in humans and exhibits pharmacological activity that justifies commercial development, the drug developer can apply for approval to proceed with human testing.

2.2 Obtaining Approval to Proceed with Clinical Testing in Humans

The vehicle through which a drug sponsor advances their product to clinical testing in the US is called the Investigational New Drug Application (IND) [6]. The IND does not specifically authorize clinical trials to begin, but rather allows an investigational product to be shipped across state lines to reach the appropriate clinical investigational sites. After the IND is submitted, the sponsor must wait 30 calendar days before initiating any clinical trials [6]. During this time, the Center for Drug Evaluation and Research (CDER) at the FDA will review the IND for safety to assure that research subjects will not be subjected to unreasonable risk [6]. If the CDER is not convinced that clinical trials can be conducted without unreasonable risk to human subjects, they will initiate a clinical hold (within the 30-day review period) to stop the clinical trial. The sponsor must then address the issue(s) that the CDER identifies as the reason for the clinical hold before the hold can be lifted and clinical trials can continue [6].

Before clinical trials can commence in Europe, an Investigational Medicinal Product Dossier (IMPD) must be submitted to the relevant Competent Authority in the country in which the clinical trial will be conducted [8]. Each authority will have its own procedures for the processing of these applications but, like the IND, these applications must contain all of the information needed to demonstrate that clinical trials can be safely conducted in humans [8].

If the drug sponsor has received advice from the regulatory agency during preclinical testing, they should have received the guidance needed to put together an IND/IMPD with a high likelihood of success.

2.2.1 Content of a Successful IND or IMPD

To assure approval to proceed with clinical trials, the application must contain (a) results of animal pharmacology and toxicology studies, (b) drug manufacturing information, and (c) clinical protocols and investigator information. The emphasis of all of the information provided at this point must be on safety. Descriptions of the type of detailed information required can be found in guidelines published by the ICH [9], the FDA [6], and the EMA [7]. Adherence to the principles of good clinical practices (GCPs) in the clinical protocols, including adequate human subject protection (HSP), is critical.

In brief, the preclinical data provided must be sufficient to determine if the new drug is reasonably safe for initial testing in humans [7]. Information from preclinical studies should also be augmented by any information about previous use of the drug in humans—either in other countries or for other indications. Information about the drug manufacturing process should be sufficient to assure regulatory agencies that a consistently high quality and stable drug with consistent potency can reliably be produced, as well as describing the nature of the drug itself. This includes information about the composition of the drug, the manufacturer, and the manufacturing process (including control procedures) [6, 7]. The protocols proposed for initial clinical trials should have been developed in consultation with the appropriate agency contacts and be designed to assure the safety of the human subjects/ patients enrolled. More details on clinical trials are provided below, but, in general, initial clinical trials should enroll a fairly small number of healthy volunteers or patients and propose to treat them with a range of clinically relevant doses over a relatively short period of time. The clinical investigators chosen should be well qualified to administer the experimental drug and to assess patient outcomes. As part of the clinical protocol section, the sponsor should also provide assurances that they will obtain informed consent from all research subjects and approval from the Institutional Review Board at each study site before initiating any clinical trial [6].

2.3 Clinical Development

The clinical development of a new drug proceeds through three key phases on the way to obtaining marketing approval (Fig. 1). A fourth phase of clinical testing (Phase IV) is usually conducted after the drug is approved for marketing in order to obtain information important for optimizing effective use of the drug. The descriptions of the different phases of clinical trials are very similar in both FDA and EMA documents [10, 11] and are summarized below.

2.3.1 Phase I Studies

A phase I study represents the first use of a new drug in human subjects and is designed to evaluate the pharmacologic effects, metabolism, and mechanism of action of the drug in humans, as well as the tolerability of the dose range expected to be used in later clinical studies. The goal is to generate sufficient information to permit the design of well-controlled and scientifically valid phase II studies (to investigate drug efficacy) [10, 11].

Phase I studies usually do not have any therapeutic objectives and are often conducted in healthy volunteer subjects rather than patients, but they can be conducted in patients if deemed appropriate. For example, the insertion of an intravitreal implant into an otherwise healthy eye may not be considered appropriate; therefore, phase I studies of such treatments are generally conducted in patients. When conducted in patients, phase I trials may provide some preliminary insight into the efficacy of the new drug. The total number of patients enrolled in phase I studies typically ranges from 20 to 80 [10, 11].

2.3.2 Phase II Studies

Phase II studies represent the first investigation of the therapeutic efficacy of a new drug for a particular indication. They are well-controlled trials conducted in patients with the disease or condition for which the treatment is intended. These studies are usually randomized and the investigators and/or patients are masked with regard to study treatment, though this is not always appropriate or feasible (as in the placement of an intraocular implant, for example). The sample size is usually small (<200) [10, 11], often narrowly defined, and well-monitored throughout the study for any safety signals. In addition to determining the potential efficacy of the new drug, other important goals of phase II studies are to determine the short-term adverse effects and risks associated with the drug, as well as the most appropriate dose and dosing regimen for phase III clinical trials [10, 11].

Accurate dose–response information is important for understanding how the drug should be administered to maximize clinical benefits while minimizing undesirable effects. Dose selection for phase II and phase III trials is challenging for many drug developers, as a poor choice of dosing regimen may lead to trial failure. Consequently, the use of several different doses or dose-escalation protocols is common in phase II trials. The US FDA has a long-standing interest in defining dose–response relationships and agency guidance with this can be obtained by scheduling an "end of phase IIA meeting" after the completion of phase I trials and the first set of exposure–response trials in patients [12].

Phase II studies can be subdivided into phase IIA and phase IIB trials. The purpose of a phase IIA trial is to gain a better understanding of the safety of a potential drug and to obtain a preliminary impression of drug efficacy and optimal dosing. These trials are sometimes combined with a phase I trial and are usually conducted in a small group of patients. The results help inform the design of the phase IIB trial, which is usually randomized, masked, well-controlled, and conducted in a larger group of patients [12].

Additional objectives of phase II trials may include an evaluation of potential study endpoints, therapeutic regimens (including concomitant medications), and target populations. Consequently, these studies may include multiple endpoints, exploratory analyses, or prospectively defined subgroup analyses [10, 11]. For example, phase II testing of the Ozurdex® dexamethasone intravitreal implant enrolled patients with macular edema due to a variety of causes (allowing for exploratory subgroup analyses) and included a variety of efficacy outcome measures [13].

The results of all studies conducted during phase II should provide the information needed to design a rigorous and focused phase III trial.

2.3.3 Phase III Studies

Phase III studies are designed to provide the pivotal safety and efficacy data needed to support marketing approval. Phase III studies are conducted after preliminary evidence of therapeutic effectiveness has been demonstrated in phase II clinical trials, and are designed to gather sufficient evidence about overall safety and efficacy to allow an evaluation of the overall benefit–risk relationship of the drug. The results of these studies will also provide the basis of the product labeling should the drug receive marketing approval, so the efficacy endpoints should be chosen with care. As in phase II studies, additional objectives may include an evaluation of different treatment regimens or target populations [10, 11].

Phase III studies must be randomized and well-controlled (either placebo or active-controlled, as appropriate for the indication). Investigators (and patients, if possible) should be masked as well as possible to reduce the risk of bias. If the treating physician cannot be masked (e.g., because a surgical procedure is involved), then a different physician should be responsible for follow-up assessments. The study population may include several hundred to several thousand people [10, 11].

2.3.4 Important Protocol Considerations

Study objectives. It is essential that the objectives of all clinical studies be clearly stated and the protocol be clearly designed to fulfill the study objectives. The patient population should also be chosen to be appropriate to the type of study being conducted, and phase III studies should include those patients that preliminary studies suggest will be most likely to benefit from the new drug. The size of the study population should be large enough to allow for accurate statistical analysis; adequately powered to detect a clinically meaningful difference between the treatment groups in the primary outcome measure [11].

Control group. The choice of control treatment should be chosen to ensure both an adequate test of the safety and efficacy of the drug, as well as to ensure the well-being of patients. The use of a placebo is common, but may be impossible or inappropriate. In the case of an intraocular implant, for example, there may not be a comparable placebo, so either observation, a sham procedure, or an active control must be used. An active control is chosen if there is significant risk of disease progression if the patient is left untreated, and is usually the standard-of-care for the indication under study (if a widely accepted standard-of-care exists) [11].

Primary outcome measures and endpoints. It is important that the efficacy endpoints chosen are both readily quantifiable and clinically relevant to patient health and quality of life. Well-validated surrogate endpoints can be used for health outcomes that take years to manifest (such as blindness, paralysis, or death). Surrogate endpoints are not a direct measure of how a patient feels, functions, or survives, but are considered likely to predict a long-term therapeutic benefit for the patient [10, 11]. A commonly used surrogate endpoint in ophthalmology, for example, is intraocular pressure (IOP), which has been shown to correlate with the risk of eventual loss of visual function in patients with glaucoma [14, 15].

Outcome measures relevant to ophthalmology were recently discussed at an international workshop convened by the EMA [16]. In the fall of 2011, approximately 200 experts in eye diseases from Europe, Australia, Japan, and the US gathered to discuss the regulatory and scientific challenges in developing medicines for eye disorders. Participants included representatives from the pharmaceutical industry, patient and physician groups, academia, and European regulatory agencies. The regulatory viewpoint expressed was that visual function endpoints are fundamental to the assessment of ophthalmic products, but that measurements of anatomical structure (e.g., changes in retinal or retinal vascular anatomy) can also be valuable. Measurements of visual function can include visual acuity, visual field, contrast sensitivity, and color vision, as well as complex visual tasks such as reading, orientation, activities of daily living, and even more complex concepts such as vision-related quality of life (social skills, self confidence, coping skills). The primary endpoint in clinical trials for retinal disease, however, is usually some measurement of visual acuity, with an emphasis on

Table 1
Clinical outcome measures relevant to ophthalmology (16)

Endpoint	Notes
Best corrected visual acuity (BCVA)	Repeated measurements over time to a prespecified primary time point (often 12 months) should be made. Providing data from a single time point might be considered questionable, although a specific time point should be indicated as the primary endpoint.
% of patients who gained ≥15 letters BCVA	Common primary outcome measure. Often referred to as "responders." Needs to be backed up by other secondary visual outcome measures because dichotomizing a continuous variable will result in a loss of information.
% of patients with gain/loss/no change	Valuable secondary outcome measures. A change of ≥10 letters is often considered the minimally clinically relevant improvement that can be perceived by patients and may be used to define visual gain/loss/no change. Loss of BCVA should be included in definition of treatment failure.
Mean BCVA	May be acceptable as primary outcome if suitable secondary outcome measures are included.
Mean change in BCVA	Common secondary outcome measure. May be acceptable as primary outcome if suitable secondary outcome measures included. May be preferred as the primary outcome in noninferiority studies.
Visual fields	Rarely proposed as primary endpoint, but has been accepted as such in some cases if supported by test–retest reliability, sensitivity, and feasibility in the actual patient group as well as information to support the clinical relevance of any changes seen.
Contrast sensitivity	Generally a secondary outcome measure.
Automatic perimetry	Generally a secondary outcome measure.
Anatomical assessments	Generally secondary outcome measures. Example: macular thickness.
Patient-reported outcomes	Generally secondary or exploratory outcome measures. Need to be well validated to be accepted by regulatory agencies.

identifying clinically relevant changes (the minimal improvement that can be perceived by patients or has an impact on vision-related tasks). The definition of clinically relevant improvement should be prospectively defined. A list of potential specific endpoints is provided in Table 1 [16].

Patient-reported outcome measures (PROs) should be used with care in phase III clinical trials. Patient-reported outcomes are of increasing interest to physicians because, if well-designed, these outcome measures can provide an important measure of both patient satisfaction with their treatment and the impact of the disease and its treatment on patient's daily lives. Regulatory agencies, however, have been critical of PROs in the past and demand that any PRO used be developed and evaluated with a high level of scientific rigor, especially if it is to be used to support regulatory approval [17]. An acceptable PRO should be developed with extensive input from patients and thoroughly evaluated in the appropriate patient population. The PRO instrument should be properly validated and the definition of "responder" determined a priori based on input from patients regarding what they consider to be a meaningful change in the outcome to be measured [17]. Most PROs, however, do not meet these requirements. For example, a recent systematic review that evaluated 27 PRO instruments for glaucoma, found that most demonstrated only partial adherence to predefined quality standards [18].

Other protocol considerations. The protocol should specify how missing data will be handled [11]. The most conservative approach should be used and it may be appropriate to do a second analysis with another method to confirm the results. Last observation carried forward is a common method, but may not be appropriate in a rapidly progressing disease. The protocol should also specify what rescue treatments or concomitant medication will be allowed and how the impact of these treatments on key outcome measures will be determined [11].

2.3.5 Regulatory Agency Oversight

In the US, the CDER can halt a phase I clinical trial if there are concerns about safety or if the sponsor failed to accurately disclose the treatment risks to study investigators. Phase II or III clinical trials can also be halted if the CDER determines the study to be unsafe or that the design is clearly insufficient to meet the stated objectives of the study [10].

3 Applying for Marketing Approval

3.1 The New Drug Application/Marketing Authorization Application

The first formal step in initiating a request for marketing approval is the compilation of a New Drug Application (NDA) for submission to the FDA [19] or a Marketing Authorization Application (MAA) for submission to an EU regulatory agency [4, 20]. Since 2003, the mandatory format for all MAAs in the EU and Japan has been the Common Technical Document (CTD) developed by the participants in the ICH [20]. The CTD is also the strongly recommended format of choice for all NDAs submitted to the US FDA [20]. The wide acceptance of this common format makes it easier for drug sponsors to submit applications for marketing approval to multiple regulatory agencies.

The NDA/MAA should provide a complete profile of the drug itself, its manufacturing, chemistry and pharmacology as well as the results of preclinical testing and clinical trials. A successful NDA/

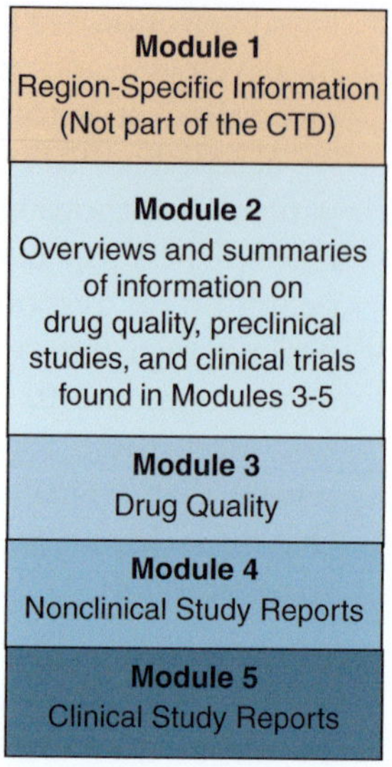

Fig. 2 Organization of the Common Technical Document (CTD). The CTD is organized into 5 modules. Module 1 is region-specific and modules 2 through 5 are common for all regions. Modified from [20]

MAA must demonstrate that the new drug is effective for its intended use and that the benefits of its use outweigh the known risks. It should also provide enough information to determine if the proposed labeling for the drug is appropriate and what additional information the labeling may need to contain. It should also provide sufficient information about the manufacturing process to allow regulatory agencies to determine if the methods and controls used are sufficient to maintain drug quality, identity, strength, and purity. Some of this information may be adapted from the IND or Clinical Trial Application submitted earlier in the process [19, 20].

The general format of the CTD is shown in Fig. 2. The CTD is divided into five modules. The first module contains region specific information (required by the specific regulatory authority receiving the document), while modules 2 through 5 are intended to be common for all regions. Module 2 contains overviews and summaries of the detailed information found in modules 3, 4, and 5 on drug quality, non-clinical studies, and clinical trials, respectively. Detailed guidelines for each section of the CTD can be downloaded from the ICH website [20].

The US FDA also provides detailed guidance documents that can be used to put together an NDA for regulatory approval in the US [19]. As mentioned above, a CTD prepared for submission for regulatory approval in the EU should also be an acceptable format for an FDA NDA. Nonetheless, all of the relevant guidance documents provided by the FDA should also be consulted to make sure that all of the specific details that the FDA requires in each section (e.g. microbiology, toxicology, manufacturing, etc.) for your specific drug class are included in your application.

3.2 The Drug Approval Process in the US

After an NDA is submitted, the FDA has 60 days to decide whether to file it so it can be reviewed; the FDA may decide not to file an application if it is incomplete. Once the NDA is filed, a team of CDER scientists (including, but not limited to, physicians, statisticians, chemists, and pharmacologists) reviews the data and proposed labeling. The review team determines if the data provided support the conclusions of the study sponsor regarding safety and efficacy or if additional information is needed [21].

The CDER may convene an advisory committee to assist in the evaluation of NDAs [22]. These committees consist of physicians and academicians, as well as representatives from the pharmaceutical industry and consumer advocacy groups. All members of a given committee, however, must be technically qualified experts in their field and have experience interpreting complex data. The recommendations of such advisory committees are not binding on the CDER, but the agency considers the recommendations carefully when deciding whether or not to grant marketing approval [22]. The FDA tries to act on the majority of applications within 10 months after the NDA is received [23].

The CDER usually communicates often and promptly with sponsors about scientific, medical, and procedural issues that arise during the review process so that the sponsor has an opportunity to address any relatively minor deficiencies or elaborate on anything that is not clear [10].

After all members of the review team have completed their evaluations, the team leader and/or division director makes the final decision regarding drug approval and one of three possible action letters is issued: (1) not approvable, (2) approvable, or (3) approved. The drug is approved if the data provided in the NDA support the conclusion that the new drug is effective for its intended use, that it has an acceptable risk/benefit profile, and can be manufactured according to the highest standards. An "approvable" letter is issued if the CDER determines that the drug can be approved if minor deficiencies are corrected. A "not approvable" letter is issued if the review team finds insufficient evidence of drug safety, efficacy, or quality to justify marketing approval. The "not approval" letter will list any deficiencies and explain exactly why the application cannot be approved [10].

Some of the reasons that a drug may be considered "not approvable" include (1) the lack of adequate tests, using well accepted methods, demonstrating that the drug can be used safely as indicated in the proposed labeling, (2) the lack of sufficient demonstration of efficacy, or (3) deficiencies in the manufacturing process sufficient to raise concerns about drug quality and reliability [24]. Because of all the opportunities for drug sponsors to receive guidance and advice from their FDA contacts throughout the drug development process, failure to obtain marketing approval this far into the process is fairly unusual [24]. Once a drug is approved, the FDA publishes the Summary Basis of Approval (SBA) and most of the other reports and letters generated during the approval process on the "drugs@fda" page of its website [2].

3.2.1 Special FDA Regulatory Designations

Drugs that treat conditions of particular concern may receive one of several special designations that affect how the drug is approved and/or regulated [25, 26].

Orphan product designation. This designation is granted to drugs intended to treat uncommon diseases (those affecting <200,000 people in the US) and was developed to help motivate pharmaceutical companies to develop drugs for markets that might otherwise be considered too small to be profitable. Orphan drug status does not change the regulatory requirements that the drug must meet for approval, but it may result in the manufacturer being allowed to waive certain fees, or being granted additional marketing exclusivity or eligibility for drug development grants [26, 27].

Fast track designation. This designation is granted to drugs intended to treat a serious or life-threatening condition (e.g., cancer, diabetes, AIDS, and Alzheimer's) and fill an important unmet medical need (e.g., improved efficacy or safety, decreasing the toxicity of another treatment, or allowing earlier disease diagnosis). It allows the drug sponsor to access various mechanisms designed to accelerate the drug approval process, such as more frequent and interactive communication between the sponsor and the FDA and the ability to request accelerated approval (see below) or submit a "rolling submission." A rolling submission allows the sponsor to submit each section of the NDA as it is completed rather than requiring the entire application to be complete before submission. This allows the preclinical and quality portions of the application to be reviewed while the clinical studies are being finalized [25, 26].

Priority review. A priority designation is granted at the time of NDA submission to those drugs intended to treat a disease for which there is no satisfactory therapy, or to drugs that offer a significant improvement over existing therapies. Drugs that receive a priority designation are reviewed within 6 months rather than the usual 10 months. It is not unusual for a fast track designation during the development process to be followed by a priority designation during the review process [25, 26].

Accelerated approval regulation. This regulation allows the approval of a drug based on a surrogate endpoint rather than a final clinical endpoint. It is reserved for those drugs intended to treat a serious disease and to fill an unmet medical need, and is important when the impact of treatment on the final clinical outcome (e.g., longevity or blindness) may take many years to manifest. IOP is a commonly used surrogate endpoint for glaucoma therapies, for example. The willingness of the FDA to accept a surrogate endpoint depends on the availability of strong scientific evidence of a clear relationship between the surrogate and the appropriate clinical endpoint [25, 26].

3.3 The Drug Approval Process in the EU

A new drug has three potential routes to multicountry marketing approval in the EU: the Centralized Procedure, the Mutual Recognition Procedure, and the Decentralized Procedure [4]. Applications submitted through the Centralized Procedure are reviewed by the EMA (*Sidebar 1*) [28]. Applications submitted through the Mutual Recognition and Decentralized Procedures are facilitated by the Co-ordination Group for Mutual Recognition and Decentralised Procedures—Human (CMDh) (*Sidebar 2*) [29, 30] In addition, marketing authorization for single countries can be sought through the National Competent Authority in each country.

Sidebar 1.
The European Medicines Agency (EMA)

Each country in the European Union (EU) has its own national drug regulatory agency, but all member states also participate in the EMA—a decentralized agency of the EU with main offices in London [42]. Most of the scientific evaluations conducted under the EMA are carried out by its scientific committees. These committees are composed of members from European Economic Area (EEA) countries and include representatives from patient, consumer, and healthcare professional organizations as well as regulatory bodies. The EMA works with a total of more than 4,500 European experts, made available to the EMA by the medicines regulatory authorities in EEA countries.

The EMA is directly involved in the evaluation of the drugs submitted for marketing authorization through the centralized procedure. The EMA only becomes involved in the approval of drugs submitted for approval through other pathways if the application has been referred to the EMA due to a disagreement between two or more member states or some other issue that requires resolution in the interest of protecting public health.

The EMA also plays a role in stimulating innovation and research in the pharmaceutical sector by giving scientific advice and other assistance to companies in the process of developing new medicines, and by publishing guidelines on quality, safety, and efficacy testing.

Sidebar 2.
The Coordination Group for Mutual Recognition and Decentralised Procedures—Human (CMDh)

The CMDh was established for the examination of any question relating to marketing authorization of a medicinal product in two or more European Union (EU) Member States via the mutual recognition or decentralized procedure [43]. It consists of one representative per EU Member State. An observer from the European Commission and European Medicines Agency (EMA) may also participate at meetings of the CMDh, and the EMA provides a secretariat to the group. The CMDh does not review new drug applications, but exists to help resolve any disagreements between any member states with regard to an application, and works to promote harmonization of marketing authorization procedures across the European Community. The CMDh started its activities in 2005 and replaced the informal Mutual Recognition Facilitation Group that had been meeting since 1995.

3.3.1 Centralized Procedure

In the centralized procedure, a single marketing-authorization application is submitted to the EMA for review and approval [4, 28]. If a new drug application is approved through this procedure, the drug is granted marketing authorization in all EU member states as well as in the European Economic Area (EEA) countries Iceland, Liechtenstein, and Norway. Not all drugs, however, qualify for the centralized procedure. This procedure is required for all drugs for HIV/AIDS, cancer, diabetes, neurodegenerative diseases, auto-immune and other immune dysfunctions, and viral diseases; medicines derived from biotechnology processes (such as genetic engineering); advanced-therapy medicines (such as gene therapy, somatic cell therapy, or tissue-engineered medicines); and officially designated orphan medicines [4, 28]. Other types of drugs may be submitted through the centralized procedure if they represent a significant therapeutic, scientific, or technical innovation. The marketing application for Ozurdex®, for example, was processed through the centralized procedure [4, 28].

The journey of a drug through the centralized procedure begins with the submission of a letter announcing the intent to submit an MAA (usually sent several months prior to the intended MAA submission date) [4]. This letter triggers the appointment of the Rapporteur and Co-Rapporteur from the Committee for Human Medicinal Products (CHMP; formerly known as the Committee for Proprietary Medicinal Products). The CHMP is composed of members from each of the member states in the EU plus Iceland and Norway, and up to five co-opted members chosen among experts nominated by Member States or the Agency and recruited, when necessary, to provide additional expertise in a particular scientific area [31]. The Rapporteur and Co-Rapporteur are always from two different EU member states and are charged with leading and coordinating an analysis of the MAA and presenting the results of their analysis (in two separate reports) to the CHMP. The Rapporteur and, when appropriate, Co-Rapporteur recruit an assessment team from among the experts included in the European experts list available from the EMA [32]. The analyses provided by the Rapporteurs and their assessment team will form the basis of the conclusions of the CHMP regarding any questions they may have for the drug sponsor and the final decision regarding marketing approval [4, 33].

Evaluation by the Agency's scientific committees takes up to 210 working days, with the "clock" starting when the MAA dossier is validated by the EMA and delivered to the Rapporteurs. The Rapporteurs are to complete their analyses and send their reports to the CHMP by day 70, which will have 30 days to provide their comments. The reports are then sent to the drug sponsor and the clock stopped at day 120. The drug sponsor has 180 days to respond to any questions or concerns raised in the reports or the CHMP comments. After the drug sponsor responds, the Rapporteurs prepare a joint assessment report (within 30 days) which is then evaluated by the CHMP. The final assessment by the CHMP must be completed within 210 days on the "clock," but the clock may be stopped again before an opinion is reached if it there are outstanding issues that need to be addressed by the drug sponsor. If the opinion is positive, it is transmitted to the European Commission and marketing authorization is issued within 67 days after receipt of the CHMP opinion [33].

3.3.2 Mutual Recognition Procedure

The mutual recognition procedure is to be used to obtain wider marketing approval for a drug that has already received marketing approval in one EU member state. It is based on the assumption that the evaluation criteria for drug safety, efficacy, and quality are now sufficiently harmonized across countries that a drug that has been approved in one member state will also meet the requirements for approval throughout the EU [33].

In this procedure, authorization is first sought in one EU country according to the national procedures in that country; this is referred to as the reference member state (RMS). Further marketing authorizations are then sought from other EU countries who have agreed to recognize the decision of the RMS rather than conducting their own review [33].

This process under this procedure (Concerned Member States; CMSs) while the RMS sends out a copy of its assessment report to the CMSs and the drug sponsor [29]. The "clock" begins when all documents have been received by each CMS and they have validated the dossier. Each CMS should communicate their position on the application to the drug sponsor and the RMS by day 50. In principal, each CMS should rely on the assessment of the RMS. If a CMS is concerned that the new drug presents a serious public health concern, it will communicate this objection in detail to the RMS and drug sponsor. The RMS will then coordinate the dialogue between the sponsor and the National Competent Authority raising the objection. If any objections cannot be resolved satisfactorily, the issue is referred to the CMDh for further negotiations. The drug sponsor should circulate their response document by day 60. This response should address all comments and propose any changes to the drug labeling deemed appropriate to gain wider authorization for the new drug. Once the response document is received, the RMS circulates a report on the applicant's response to all CMSs; a response is generally requested by approximately day 75. If needed, the RMS may schedule a meeting with the CMSs and the CMDh to resolve any outstanding issues. The entire procedure should be complete by day 90. If consensus on approval of the application cannot be reached among the CMSs by day 90, the application is referred to the CMDh for moderation. All CMSs and the CMDh endeavor to reach consensus within 60 days after referral to the CMDh. Once the process is complete, the National Competent Authority in each CMS should adopt a national decision within the next 30 days [29].

3.3.3 Decentralized Procedure

This procedure was introduced in late 2005 as an alternative to the mutual recognition procedure for drugs that do not qualify for submission for marketing authorization through the centralized procedure. This allows drug sponsors to apply for simultaneous authorization in more than one EU country provided that marketing authorization does not yet exist in any of the EU member states [29, 30, 33].

In this procedure, identical MAAs are submitted to all member states in which authorization is sought. An RMS, selected by the drug sponsor, prepares a draft assessment which is then sent to all of the other concerned member states designated by the drug sponsor. Each concerned member state can then either approve the assessment or request arbitration of any differences of opinion through the CMDh [29, 33].

The regulations regarding this process are very similar to those for the Mutual Recognition Procedure, but the timeline is longer. The RMS has until day 70 to prepare a preliminary assessment report (PrAR), and the CMSs have until day 100 to respond. Discussions between the RMS, CMSs, and the drug sponsor occur from day 100 through day 105. If consensus is not reached during this time, the clock is stopped to allow the applicant time to respond to any questions and supplement the dossier as needed. The clock restarts after the response is received by the RMS. The RMS then prepares a revised assessment, draft summary of product characteristics, and a draft of the labeling and package leaflet and sends them to each CMS. If consensus is reached among the CMSs, the procedure can close at this time and proceed to national authorization (within 30 days as described for the Mutual Recognition Procedure). If consensus is not reached, further discussion and modification of the dossier can continue with the assistance of the CMDh for an additional 130 days [29, 30].

4 Case Study: The Path to Marketing Approval for Ozurdex®

Ozurdex® is a sustained delivery, bioerodable dexamethasone intravitreal implant containing 0.7 mg dexamethasone in a solid polymer drug delivery system. It is inserted into the eye using a preloaded, single-use, custom-designed applicator that allows injection of the implant directly into the vitreous (Fig. 3) [34, 35]. Ozurdex® was approved for the treatment of macular edema (ME) following branch or central retinal vein occlusion (BRVO or CRVO) in June 2009 in the US and in July 2010 in the EU. Ozurdex® was approved for the treatment of noninfectious uveitis affecting the posterior segment of the eye in September 2010 in the US and in June 2011 in the EU [36–38]. It should be noted that the same studies were used to support the application for marketing approval in both the US and the EU.

Marketing approval for the BRVO/CRVO indication was based on the results of two identical, multicenter, double-masked, 12-month, randomized, sham-controlled trials; the *G*lobal *E*valuation of impla*N*table d*E*xamethasone in retinal *V*ein occlusion with macular edem*A* (GENEVA) trials [39, 40]. The primary endpoint

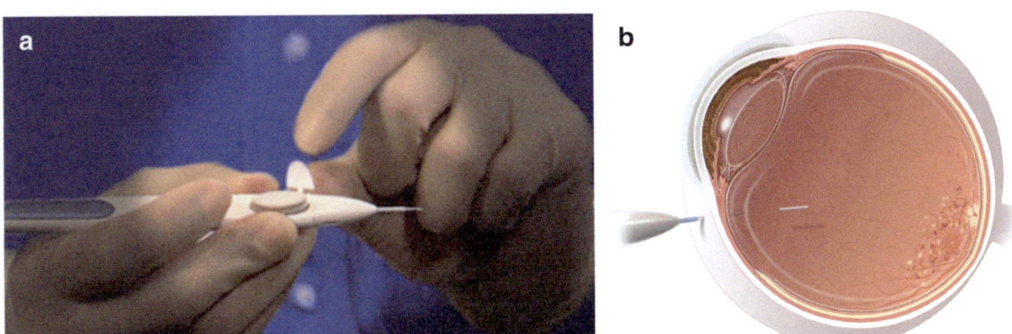

Fig. 3 Ozurdex®. (**a**) The Ozurdex® single-use applicator. (**b**) Ozurdex® after insertion into the vitreous. Reproduced with permission from Future Drugs LTD. [35]

was the time to achieve a ≥15-letter improvement in best-corrected visual acuity (BCVA); secondary efficacy outcomes included the percentage of patients achieving ≥15-letter (3-line) improvement in BCVA, mean change in BCVA, and central retinal thickness. In each study and in the pooled analysis, Ozurdex® achieved its primary endpoint; the time to achieve a ≥15 letter improvement in BCVA cumulative response rate curves were significantly faster with Ozurdex® as compared with a sham procedure ($P < 0.001$). The secondary efficacy measures also supported the efficacy of Ozurdex®, as the percentage of patients achieving ≥15-letters of improvement in BCVA at day 90 was 22 % with Ozurdex® and 13 % with sham ($P < 0.001$) [39]. Benefits were similar following a second treatment 6 months after the first [40]. The most common adverse effect associated with Ozurdex® was increased IOP (percentage with IOP ≥25 mmHg: 16 % vs. <1 % in the sham group; $P < 0.001$) [39]. Phakic eyes treated with a second Ozurdex® implant also had an increased risk of cataract progression (30 % vs. 6 % for sham)—although the rate of cataract surgery was similar to that for sham (1.3 % vs. 1.1 % for sham) [40]. The rate of all other adverse events were similar between Ozurdex®-treated and sham-treated eyes [39, 40].

Marketing approval for the uveitis indication was based on a single, multicenter, masked, 26-week, randomized, sham-controlled study of 153 patients; the c*H*ronic *U*veitis evaluation of the int*R*a-vitreal dexamethas*ON*e implant (HURON) trial [41]. It should be noted that intermediate and posterior uveitis are both rare, so it is appropriate that only a single, small study was conducted for this additional indication. The primary outcome measure was the proportion of eyes with a vitreous haze score of 0 at week 8. The proportion of eyes that achieved this primary endpoint was significantly greater with Ozurdex® treatment (47 %) than with the sham procedure (12 %; $P < 0.001$) and the benefits persisted through week 26. In addition, the percentage of eyes achieving ≥15-letters of improvement in BCVA at day 90 was two- to sixfold greater with Ozurdex® than with sham throughout the follow-up period. Increased IOP (percentage with IOP ≥25 mmHg: 7.1 % vs. 4.2 %) and an increased risk of cataract (15 % vs. 7 % for sham) were more common with Ozurdex® treatment than sham treatment, but these differences were not statistically significant ($P > 0.05$) [41].

4.1 US Approvals

In the US, Ozurdex® was granted a Fast Track Designation by the FDA for the BRVO/CRVO indication and a priority review [36]. It should be noted that, at the time Ozurdex® was submitted for marketing authorization, no approved treatment had been shown to improve vision in eyes with RVO. The FDA concluded that the NDA submitted supported the safety and efficacy of Ozurdex® for this indication. The studies demonstrated that the efficacy of

Ozurdex® was significantly superior to that of a sham injection and that the safety profile was acceptable. They particularly noted that adverse effects other than elevated IOP were similar to sham, and that the increases in IOP were as expected with this drug class [36].

The FDA granted Ozurdex® orphan drug status for the uveitis indication. Approval to market Ozurdex® for intermediate and posterior uveitis was granted on the basis of a supplemental NDA submitted after the approval of Ozurdex® for BRVO/CRVO [37]. A detailed SBA for this indication was not published by the FDA.

4.2 European Union Approvals

Marketing authorizations for Ozurdex® in Europe were obtained through use of the Centralized Procedure [38]. In the European Public Assessment Report issued by the EMA for Ozurdex®, the EMA stated that the recommendation for marketing authorization was granted because the Committee decided that the benefits of Ozurdex® are greater than its risks. The report noted that the Ozurdex® injection appeared to cause only minor trauma to the eye and that the increases in IOP were manageable [38].

5 Notes (Expert Opinion)

The most important steps to ensuring the successful launch of a new drug are very similar in both the US and the EU. Nonetheless, an application that is deemed approvable in the US may not be considered approvable in the EU and vice versa. One reason for this could be that the two regions have different processes for reviewing an application once it has been submitted, and the two mechanisms may focus on different sets of priorities and concerns depending on the candidate drug. This can be avoided by seeking timely advice from both agencies throughout the development process.

In both the US and the EU, a successful application for marketing approval depends on early and frequent consultation with the appropriate contacts at both the FDA and the EMA. These consultations should begin while the candidate drug is still undergoing preclinical testing and continue throughout every clinical trial phase. Meetings with agency contacts will be most productive if the objectives of the meeting are very clear, all appropriate background materials and a specific agenda are sent to the participants in advance, and if the drug sponsor comes to the meeting with a very specific list of questions. The drug sponsor should not ask either agency what to do, but rather present what has already been learned, describe what is proposed as the next step in the development plan (provide specific protocols), and ask if the plan would be sufficient to support a successful application. At all times it is important to provide detailed and prompt responses to any and all concerns and questions raised by the agencies.

Taking advantage of the opportunity to obtain "parallel scientific advice" from both agencies can help to make the development process more efficient and cost-effective by ensuring that all planned investigation will be considered acceptable to support applications in both the US and the EU. Clinical trials are very costly, and discovering that the protocol of a completed clinical trial is considered acceptable in only one market and not the other could be a huge setback to a development plan. In the case study for Ozurdex®, the same clinical studies were deemed acceptable to support marketing approval in both the US and the EU, and this allowed for a more streamlined, cost-effective drug development and approval process than if different studies had been required for each of these major markets.

Technical considerations that can help ensure a successful drug development program include choosing the most clinically relevant animal model(s) for preclinical testing, and designing all clinical trials with great care. Some of the most important aspects of clinical trial design include choosing the most appropriate control group, choosing easily quantifiable and clinically relevant outcome measures (particularly the primary endpoint), and the inclusion of sufficient exploratory and subgroup analyses to help guide decisions about how best to use the drug.

6 Conclusions

The increasing availability of safer and/or more effective medications helps drive ongoing improvements in patient care. The new sustained-delivery implants offer particular promise for the treatment of localized chronic diseases in general and chronic retinal diseases in particular. The ability to bring these innovative new drugs to market is dependent on several factors, including advances in basic science, as well as well-designed drug development plans and successful applications for marketing approval. The keys to the successful launch of a new drug include identifying a promising new drug candidate and then designing a drug development process that takes the requirements for marketing approval into consideration from the very beginning. This will motivate the appropriate consultations with regulatory agencies in both the US and the EU, and ensure that preclinical and clinical trial designs will be appropriate to support a successful application for marketing approval in both regions. Ongoing efforts to harmonize the guidelines, requirements, and document templates across regions are designed to allow the drug development process to be more efficient and cost-effective. The single most important determinant of a successful drug launch—outside of the merits of the drug itself—is taking full advantage of all of the resources and opportunities for communication with both the US FDA and the EMA.

References

1. Black LE, Bendele AM, Bendele RA, Zack PM, Hamilton M (1999) Regulatory decision strategy for entry of a novel biological therapeutic with a clinically unmonitorable toxicity into clinical trials: pre-IND meetings and a case example. Toxicol Pathol 27(1):22–26
2. Food and Drug Administration Website. Drugs @FDA: (http://www.accessdata.fda.gov/scripts/cder/drugsatfda/index.cfm)
3. European Medicines Agency Website. Human medicines: (http://www.ema.europa.eu/ema/index.jsp?curl = pages/regulation/landing/human_medicines_regulatory.jsp&mid = WC0b01ac058001ff89)
4. Kohler M (2011) Regulatory pathways in the European Union. MAbs 3(3):241–242
5. International Conference on Harmonisation Website (http://www.ich.org/)
6. Food and Drug Administration Website. Investigational new drug application (http://www.fda.gov/drugs/developmentapprovalprocess/howdrugsaredevelopedandapproved/approvalapplications/investigationalnewdrugindapplication/default.htm)
7. European Medicines Agency (2009) Document CPMP/ICH/286/95: Note for guidance on non-clinical safety studies for the conduct of human clinical trials and marketing authorization for pharmaceuticals
8. Investigational Medicinal Product Dossier Website (http://www.impd.eu/)
9. International Conference on Harmonisation Website. Safety guidelines (http://www.ich.org/products/guidelines/safety/article/safety-guidelines.html
10. Food and Drug Administration Website. Drug Development and Review Definitions (http://www.fda.gov/Drugs/DevelopmentApprovalProcess/HowDrugsareDevelopedandApproved/ApprovalApplications/InvestigationalNewDrugINDApplication/ucm176522.htm)
11. European Medicines Agency (1998) Document CPMP/ICH/291/95: Note for guidance on general consideration for clinical trials
12. Food and Drug Administration, Center for Drug Evaluation and Research (2009) Guidance for industry: End of phase 2A meetings. Available at: http://www.fda.gov/downloads/Drugs/GuidanceComplianceRegulatoryInformation/Guidances/UCM079690.pdf. Accessed on 18 January 2013
13. Kuppermann BD, Blumenkranz MS, Haller JA et al (2007) Randomized controlled study of an intravitreous dexamethasone drug delivery system in patients with persistent macular edema. Arch Ophthalmol 125(3):309–317
14. Demill DL, Wirostko BM, Nelson LA, Stewart JA, Stewart WC (2013) Average versus highest intraocular pressure analyses in glaucoma clinical trials. Ophthalmic Res 49(1):49–51
15. Miglior S, Bertuzzi F (2013) Relationship between intraocular pressure and glaucoma onset and progression. Curr Opin Pharmacol 13(1):32–35
16. European Medicines Agency (2012) Document EMA/450332/2012. EU Regulatory Workshop—Ophthalmology—Summary and Report: Clinical Development, Scientific Advice and Paediatric Investigation Plans
17. McLeod LD, Coon CD, Martin SA, Fehnel SE, Hays RD (2011) Interpreting patient-reported outcome results: US FDA guidance and emerging methods. Expert Rev Pharmacoecon Outcomes Res 11(2):163–169
18. Vandenbroeck S, De Geest S, Zeyen T, Stalmans I, Dobbels F (2011) Patient-reported outcomes (PRO's) in glaucoma: a systematic review. Eye (Lond) 25(5):555–577
19. Food and Drug Administration Website. New drug application. (http://www.fda.gov/Drugs/ DevelopmentApprovalProcess/HowDrugsareDevelopedandApproved/ApprovalApplications/NewDrugApplicationNDA/default.htm)
20. International Conference on Harmonisation Website. Common technical document (http://www.ich.org/products/ctd.html)
21. Food and Drug Administration Website. Approval process (http://www.fda.gov/Drugs/ResourcesForYou/Consumers/ucm289601.htm#review)
22. Food and Drug Administration Website. Advisory committees (http://www.fda.gov/AdvisoryCommittees/default.htm)
23. Food and Drug Administration Website. Review process overview (http://www.fda.gov/Drugs/ResourcesForYou/Consumers/ucm143534.htm)
24. Congressional Research Service (2001) CRS report for congress. The U.S. drug approval process: a primer
25. Food and Drug Administration Website. Fast Track, Accelerated Approval and Priority Review (http://www.fda.gov/ForConsumers/ByAudience/ForPatientAdvocates/SpeedingAccesstoImportantNewTherapies/ucm128291.htm)
26. Marchand HC, Ros BJ, Fine AM, Kremzner ME (2012) The U.S. Food and drug

administration: drug information resource for formulary recommendations. J Manag Care Pharm 18(9):713–718

27. Food and Drug Administration Website. Orphan drug designation (http://www.fda.gov/ForIndustry/DevelopingProductsforRareDiseasesConditions/default.htm)
28. European Medicines Agency Website. The centralized process (http://www.ema.europa.eu/ema/index.jsp?curl = pages/about_us/general/general_content_000109.jsp&mid = WC0b01ac0580028a47)
29. Coordination Group for Mutual Recognition and Decentralised Procedures—Human (2012) Document CMDh/068/1996/Rev8. Best practice guide for decentralized and mutual recognition procedures. (available at: http://www.hma.eu/fileadmin/dateien/Human_Medicines/CMD_h_/procedural_guidance/Application_for_MA/CMDh_068_1996_Rev8_2012_10-Clean.pdf)
30. European Commission (2007) Document ENTR/F2/ SM. Volume 2A: Procedures for marketing authorization. Chapter 2: mutual recognition
31. European Medicines Agency Website. The CHMP (http://www.ema.europa.eu/ema/index. jsp?curl = pages/about_us/general/general_content_000094.jsp&mid = WC0b01ac0580028c79)
32. European Medicines Agency (2007) Document EMEA/MB/87146/2007. Committee for medicinal products for human use: rules of procedure
33. Chavan PN, Vijayan S, Joshi MM et al (2011) Marketing authorization procedures in Europe: a regulatory perspective. Int J Pharm Pharmaceut Sci Res 1:13–19
34. Ozurdex® Prescribing Information. Allergan, Inc. (2012) Available at: http://www.allergan.com/assets/pdf/ozurdex_pi.pdf
35. Robinson MR, Whitcup SM (2012) Pharmacologic and clinical profile of dexamethasone intravitreal implant. Expert Rev Clin Pharmacol 5(6):629–647
36. Center for Drug Evaluation and Research (2009) Application number 22–315. Summary review: Ozurdex® for Retinal Vein Occlusion
37. Center for Drug Evaluation and Research (2010) Supplemental approval letter: Ozurdex® for Uveitis
38. European Medicines Agency (2011) Document EMA/941595/2011, EMEA/H/C/001140. Ozurdex®: European Public Assessment Report
39. Haller JA, Bandello F, Belfort R Jr et al (2010) Randomized, sham-controlled trial of dexamethasone intravitreal implant in patients with macular edema due to retinal vein occlusion. Ophthalmology 117(6):1134–1146 e1133
40. Haller JA, Bandello F, Belfort R Jr et al (2011) Dexamethasone intravitreal implant in patients with macular edema related to branch or central retinal vein occlusion twelve-month study results. Ophthalmology 118(12):2453–2460
41. Lowder C, Belfort R Jr, Lightman S et al (2011) Dexamethasone intravitreal implant for noninfectious intermediate or posterior uveitis. Arch Ophthalmol 129(5):545–553
42. European Medicines Agency Website. About the EMA (http://www.ema.europa.eu/ema/index.jsp?curl=pages/about_us/general/general_content_000235.jsp&mid)
43. Coordination Group for Mutual Recognition and Decentralised Procedures—Human. Website: About the CMDh (http://www.hma.eu/cmdh.html)

Methods in Pharmacology and Toxicology (2014): 143–203
DOI 10.1007/7653_2013_7

Published online: 29 August 2013

The Ophthalmic Examination as It Pertains to General Ocular Toxicology: Basic and Advanced Techniques and Species-Associated Findings

David A. Wilkie

Abstract

Ocular toxicology pertains to toxicologic effects of drugs administered topically, intraocularly, or systemically. It should also include evaluation of adverse effects of ophthalmic devices such as contact lenses, intraocular lenses, and glaucoma implants. The ophthalmic examination is able to provide detailed in-life information and is used in combination with clinical observations, clinical pathology, and histopathology to assess potential toxicologic effects. The ophthalmologist must be familiar with the wide range of species used in the field of toxicology, be familiar with the anatomic variations associated with these species, be able to determine what is an inherited or a breed-related finding from a study-related effect, be competent with the required ophthalmic equipment, and be capable of examining this wide range of animals.

Key words Laboratory animal, Ophthalmology, Ocular toxicology

1 Introduction

The purpose of this chapter is to discuss laboratory animal ophthalmology as it pertains to industry, not to pocket pets. The industries of interest include contract toxicology laboratories and researchers in an academic environment that may require the expertise of a board-certified veterinary ophthalmologist.

Contract research organizations (CRO) evaluate products for pharmaceutical and agricultural use and are governed by Food and Drug Administration (FDA) and Environmental Protection Agency (EPA) guidelines. In addition they may test cosmetics, contact lenses and associated materials, intraocular devices, and a host of other products that might have an ocular use, contact the eye or be applied topically, or be inhaled, ingested, or injected. The evaluation of potential drug effects and toxicity must integrate the disciplines of pharmacology, toxicology, pathology, and ophthalmology [1]. The CRO study is overseen by a study director and all study-associated personnel, including the consulting ophthalmologist, must be adequately trained and a quality assurance (QA) unit is responsible for monitoring each study to ensure compliance. Toxicology studies conducted for regulatory purposes need to be conducted in compliance with good laboratory practice (GLP). All personnel, including the consulting ophthalmologist, involved in animal studies will be expected to be familiar with GLP and will usually be required to take annual GLP-refresher courses.

Systemic and ocular toxicity studies require evaluation of both systemic toxicity using clinical observations, body weight, and clinical and histologic pathology and ocular toxicity using detailed ophthalmic examinations [1]. The eye, as it pertains to toxicology, can be considered in one of the three ways. With respect to undesirable ophthalmic toxicologic effects the ophthalmologist is concerned with (1) undesirable ocular effects when the eye is the target organ of interest with the drug of interest applied to the eye, (2) undesirable systemic effects associated with an ocularly applied agent, and (3) undesirable ocular effects from an agent applied in a systemic manner (oral, dermal, injection, inhalation) with resulting ocular effects [2–5]. In addition to drug effects, animals may be used to evaluate the effects and side effects of a procedure or a device. With regard to the eye this may include evaluation of a new intraocular device such as an intraocular lens or viscoelastic agent or evaluation of a new surgical procedure.

These studies are designed to evaluate the potential for ocular toxicity or other adverse effects arising from the systemic, topical, or other administration of drugs or compounds, the application of medical devices, or certain surgical procedures. While in some cases the studies are designed to provide proof of concept as regards therapeutic efficacy, in the majority of cases the studies are being conducted specifically to enable an adequate assessment of safety of test materials and devices in consideration of meeting FDA and EPA (or other similar regulating agencies) approval for initiation of human clinical trials (supporting an investigational new drug (IND) and/or investigational device (IDE) application).

The eye, because of its large blood flow by organ weight, is a prime target for various systemic toxicities. In addition to the adnexal structures, vascularized intraocular structures include the retina and uveal tissues (iris, ciliary body, and choroid) [6]. The transparent nature of the eye and the ability to visualize arteries, veins, and neural tissue make the eye an organ where toxicities may be readily detectable. This makes the eye unique in that it is possible to conduct a detailed assessment during the in-life portion of a study [1].

As ophthalmologists, we must be familiar with the normal inter- and intraspecies variations that occur between the species involved in toxicologic studies. We must be able to examine all of these species given the limitations of size, temperament, and restraint. Finally we must be familiar with common naturally occurring abnormalities observed in each of these species and be able to differentiate these from toxicologic effects. A discussion of the anatomy and physiology of the most common animals used in ocular research, including mice, rats, rabbits, guinea pigs, dogs, cats, pigs, and primates, is found in Chap. 2. This chapter emphasizes the routine ophthalmic examination of laboratory animals. It also provides information on more advanced ophthalmic diagnostic tools that are becoming more commonplace in the area of ocular toxicology.

2 Routine Examination

Prior to study initiation, the ophthalmologist should review all ophthalmic procedures, discuss with the study director and/or sponsor any issues or concerns with the study design or the examination procedures, and then follow standard operating procedures (SOPs) when conducting their examinations. It is the position of the American College of Veterinary Ophthalmologists (ACVO) that in order to ensure public safety the status of Diplomate of the ACVO is the minimum qualification for performing these ocular examinations and assessment of findings in a laboratory animal study that is intended to support applications to the FDA (or other similar regulating agencies) for entry into human clinical trials. Evaluation of toxicological effects of pharmaceutical agents involves assessment by a number of personnel, many of which are board-certified specialists, including pathologists, cardiologists, and others in addition to ophthalmologists. Sponsors engaging the services of a CRO must be advised of the participation of veterinary ophthalmologists and the potential limitations that may arise if such studies do not involve veterinary ophthalmologists.

A board-certified veterinary ophthalmologist is uniquely qualified to consult in the development of the experimental design (including the species selected, appropriate diagnostic tests, and frequency of exams) and the assessment of ocular effects of test materials being evaluated. Coordination between the testing agency and the veterinary ophthalmologist is essential throughout the process, to include protocol development, establishing SOPs, and the identification and assessment of ocular findings. If ocular abnormalities are identified, communication between the ophthalmologist and the pathologist will allow correlation of clinical and histopathologic findings.

The components of an ophthalmic examination may vary depending on the species involved and the specific objective of the study. However, if the purpose of such a study is to screen for adverse effects on any ocular tissue including, at a minimum, the adnexal structures (eyelids and conjunctiva), anterior segment (cornea, anterior chamber, iris, and lens), and posterior segment (vitreous and fundus), the following must be included:

1. Pharmacologic pupillary dilation
2. Darkened ambient light conditions
3. Indirect and/or direct ophthalmoscopy
4. Slit lamp biomicroscopy

Additional procedures may be included depending on the objective of the examination. These may include, but are not limited to, corneal staining, corneal esthesiometry, pachymetry, tonometry, fundus photography, fluorescein angiography, optical coherence tomography (OCT), and electrophysiological assessment of the visual system (e.g., electroretinography, multifocal electroretinography, visual evoked potentials (VEP)). Sedation or general anesthesia may or may not be required depending on the species, the procedure being performed, and individual animal.

The routine ophthalmic examination for all animals used in toxicologic studies should begin with the minimum database of both biomicroscopy and indirect ophthalmoscopy. Regardless of the species of interest, these two examination techniques are essential to ensure an accurate and complete examination of both the anterior and posterior segments of the eye. A comparison of techniques by Bellhorn found that of 100 rats with known lens abnormalities diagnosed by biomicroscopy only 65/100 of the lenticular lesions could be found using the direct ophthalmoscopy and only 35/100 were found using indirect ophthalmoscopy [7]. Together these two examinations must, at a minimum, include evaluation of the adnexal structures (eyelids and conjunctiva), anterior segment (cornea, anterior chamber, iris, and lens), and posterior segment (vitreous and fundus).

Ophthalmic examinations should be conducted on an eye that has been pharmacologically dilated and should be performed in a darkened examination room. While some have advocated the use of 10 % phenylephrine to aid in dilation of rodents [8, 9], this is generally not required. Pharmacologic dilation is most commonly performed using tropicamide at a concentration of 0.5 % for rodents and 1 % for larger mammals. The ophthalmologist should be familiar with the length of time required to achieve mydriasis and the duration of the mydriasis for the species being examined. In general, 10–15 min is the minimum time required to achieve acceptable mydriasis and this may be slightly longer in heavily pigmented eyes. The duration of mydriasis is directly related to the amount of intraocular melanin. In albinotic rodents, mydriasis will last no more than 1 h while in a pigmented eye of a dog or a primate the effect will persist for 3–5 h. This information is important so that the ophthalmologist knows when to begin dilation and how many animals should be dilated at one time. The later will depend on how many animals the ophthalmologist can examine in a given time period. For the basic examination, biomicroscopy, and indirect ophthalmoscopy, animals are either manually restrained (rodent, dog, rabbit, pig, guinea pig, cat) or sedated or anesthetized (primates). Rats and mice may be held in a dose-hold and presented to the ophthalmologist with their heads restrained. Some ophthalmologists prefer the eyes to be slightly proptosed in rodents. Dogs and rabbits are most often examined on a table. Rabbits seem to do best if there is a towel on the table as this decreases their movements and may provide some comfort. For rabbits, the ophthalmologist should be seated slightly below the level of the restraint table to allow easy visualization of the rabbits' optic nerve and retinal vasculature which are located in the superior fundus. For dogs, the examiner may be seated or standing. Since primates will be anesthetized or heavily sedated, they may be manually restrained or placed on an examination table. If more extensive examinations such as electrodiagnostic testing or OCT are required sedation or anesthesia may be required regardless of the species.

Additional examination procedures such as direct ophthalmoscopy, corneal staining, tonometry, pachymetry, fluorescein angiography, photographic documentation (anterior or posterior segment), electrodiagnostic testing, ultrasonography, OCT, and other tests may be indicated depending on the study and toxicologic effects of interest. If any of these additional tests are required, the order in which tests are performed and when to perform pupil dilation must be considered. For example, determination of intraocular pressure (IOP) should be performed prior to pupil dilation. In addition, if repeated IOP measurements are required during a study they should be performed at the same time of day to avoid diurnal pressure fluctuation. When possible, examination of the cornea should be performed prior to procedures that may result in corneal changes as a result of corneal contact (pachymetry, tonometry) or the use of topical anesthesia. If sedation is required for the ophthalmic examination then consideration must be given to dosing and feeding schedules, clinical observations, and clinical pathology sampling. Finally, from an animal well-being standpoint, a balance must be struck between multiple procedures performed on the same day as compared with multiple repeated days requiring sedation [1].

Animals will be most commonly be identified by tattoo, ear tag, or microchip. If a tattoo or an ear tag is used, the animal handler will need to have enough light during the examination to read the identification to ensure accurate data collection. This may be provided by a separate light source elsewhere in the examination room or if possible by performing the ophthalmic examinations in a darkened anteroom allowing the handlers to keep the main animal room lights on. When identified by microchip, a computer scanner will allow animal identification to be linked to the computer program for data entry. To ensure accuracy, each animal must be identified to both the ophthalmologist and the data entry person at the time of the examination. The data entry person must verify that the animal being examined and the animal for which the data is being entered correspond.

Depending on the compound being evaluated and the SOP, the ophthalmologist will be expected to wear shoe covers, a lab coat, or surgical scrubs and gloves at a minimum and may be required to wear a Tyvek® suit, surgical cap, mask, and occasionally a respirator. When working with nonhuman primates (NHPs), annual testing for tuberculosis (TB) using a TB intradermal PPD skin test or the new QuantiFERON®-TB blood test will generally be required of all personnel including the ophthalmologist.

The ophthalmologist must be familiar with what is normal for the species being examined and what are the common, spontaneous abnormalities for that species, age of animal, and breed/strain. Albino vs. pigmented eye may be a factor as is the type of retinal vasculature, ranging from anangiotic to merangiotic to holangiotic. The presence or the absence of a tapetum and whether the animal has a fovea should be considered. In addition, the examination techniques to be used, type of biomicroscope and indirect ophthalmoscope, size and diopter of the indirect lens, and number of animals that can be examined in an hour must be understood. The role of the veterinary ophthalmologist is to perform a pretest examination designed to eliminate those animals not suited to the study and to establish a baseline database to compare interim and end-of-study findings. Animals are then subsequently examined one or more times during the study, at the conclusion of the study, and possibly in a recovery phase depending on the study duration and design. Typically studies are divided into acute, subacute, subchronic, and chronic depending on the duration. The ophthalmologist must then interpret findings in light of the species examined, pretest data, compound evaluated, additional study procedures performed (anesthesia, orbital blood collection), and dose group outcome.

Since most laboratory studies involve a significant number of animals, organization and efficiency are essential. In general, most canine, primate, swine, feline, and rabbit studies involve 40–60 animals while rats and mice may involve 250–1,500 animals in a single study. A single ophthalmologist generally requires 2–3 animal handlers, a data entry individual, and in studies over 250 animals 1–2 individuals to go ahead of the animal handlers to dilate the pupils. For efficiency, an animal should be in front of the ophthalmologist at all times. The ophthalmologist's findings are reported verbally to the data entry individual who then either enters it into a computer program or records on a paper record for later entry into a computer database. This data is then verified at the end of the examination and both the ophthalmologist and data entry individual date and initial the accuracy of the report.

When an ophthalmic abnormality is observed, it must be characterized with respect to diagnosis, location, and severity. Depending on the laboratory, some will utilize a standardized scheme for recording of clinical observations such as Provantis® that has a set of preloaded ophthalmic terms for organ location (cornea, lens, iris, etc.), clinical signs/diagnosis (opacity, coloboma, degeneration, hemorrhage, etc.), specific location (cortex, nucleus, tapetal, anterior, posterior, etc.), and severity (slight, moderate, severe). Other CROs may have their own in-house online or hand recording system. The ophthalmologist should be familiar with each laboratory's recording system and terminology to be consistent both within and between studies. When an abnormality is observed, correlation between dose groups is important when evaluating the incidence and severity of lesions so that any association with the test article can be assessed [1]. While it would be best if animals were examined out of dosing order so as to mask the ophthalmologist with respect to dose group being examined, this is often not possible given the way animals are housed and entered into the data collection system.

The ophthalmologist should also have a standardized scoring or grading scheme to assign a severity to any abnormalities seen. In general, a grading scheme of slight, moderate, and severe/marked is most common. When using this grading scheme for the transparent media (cornea, aqueous, lens, and vitreous) a grading of slight would imply a lesion that does not obstruct visualization of the deeper tissues past the lesion, a moderate grade implies a lesion that interferes with but does not fully obstruct the view of the tissues deep to the lesion, and a severe/marked lesion fully obstructs the view of structures deep to the lesion (Table 1). This is analogous to the terms incipient, immature, and mature when applied to a cataract. Lesions may also be characterized with respect to the

Table 1
Biomicroscopy grading criteria for cornea, aqueous, lens, and vitreous opacities

Grade	Definition
0	No observable lesion.
1+	Some loss of transparency. The underlying structures are clearly visible with diffuse illumination.
2+	Moderate loss of transparency. With diffuse illumination the underlying structures are barely visible, but can still be examined and graded.
3+	Severe loss of transparency. With diffuse illumination the underlying structures are not visible when viewed through the lesion and evaluation of them is impaired.

This grading system is based on the modified Hackett–McDonald scoring system
Grade 1—Slight or mild
Grade 2—Moderate
Grade 3—Marked, excessive, or severe

area of involvement with the terms most commonly used being focal, multifocal, and diffuse.

For studies involving topical ophthalmic application of a drug or an ocular/intraocular device a specific more detailed biomicroscopic examination protocol with standardized scoring or grading criteria is frequently used. This is most commonly the modified Hackett–McDonald scoring system (Tables 2 and 3) [10, 11]. Additionally, for studies involving intravitreal injection or intraocular procedures, the Standardization of Uveitis Nomenclature (SUN) grading system can be used or modified to evaluate aqueous flare and cells (Tables 4 and 5) [1, 12, 13]. When counting anterior chamber cells, the type of cell pigmented, white blood cell or red blood cell, should be noted [1]. For grading of intravitreal inflammation and cells, the National Eye Institute system can be used (Table 6) [14, 15].

2.1 Biomicroscopy

Biomicroscopy is used to examine the ocular anterior segment including the eyelids, conjunctiva, third eyelid, tear film, cornea, anterior chamber, iris, lens, and anterior vitreous. Biomicroscopy provides a magnified view of the living eye using a light that can be varied in intensity, width, height, and color. In general for laboratory animals, this is performed using a handheld slit lamp of the ophthalmologist's preference. The slit lamp used for routine examination should be portable, lightweight, and easy to use on a variety of species. The two most common portable slit lamps used for laboratory animals are the Zeiss HSO-10 (Fig. 1) and the Kowa SL-14/15 (Fig. 2). The Zeiss HSO-10 provides a 12× magnification with a 125 mm working distance and is both lightweight and easy to use on all species. The Kowa SL-14/15 has either a 10× or a 16× magnification with a 100 mm working distance. Unlike the Zeiss, the Kowa works from a battery pack and is re-charged in a stand. Both have fixed slit widths (0.15 and 0.75 mm Zeiss; 0.1, 0.2, and 0.8 mm Kowa) and both have a cobalt blue filter for fluorescein. If higher magnification or photographic documentation are required, a table-mounted slit lamp may be used (Fig. 3). Table slit lamps provide higher quality optics, increased magnification, and variable width and height of the slit beam and with additional attachments can allow for photographic documentation, gonioscopy, or specular microscopy. Table slit lamps are however significantly more expensive, less portable, and more difficult to use on a large number of animals or un-sedated animals.

The slit lamp performs two major functions. First, it provides magnification for a more detailed examination of the eye. Secondly it makes use of the slit beam, decreasing the beam of light to a slit allowing an optical cross section of the eye to be obtained (Figs. 4 and 5). This allows precise localization of the depth of a lesion and allows visualization of subtle changes that cannot be seen with full illumination (Figs. 6, 7, 8, 9, and 10). The term for this type of illumination and examination is an optical section and it is the most

Table 2
Criteria used for a modified Hackett–McDonald scoring system [10]

Conjunctival congestion	
0=	Normal. May appear blanched to reddish pink without perilimbal injection (except at 12:00 and 6:00 o'clock positions) with vessels of the palpebral and bulbar conjunctiva easily observed.
1=	A flushed, reddish color predominantly confined to the palpebral conjunctiva with some perilimbal injection but primarily confined to the lower and upper parts of the eye from the 4:00, 7:00, 11:00, and 1:00 o'clock positions.
2=	Bright red color of the palpebral conjunctiva with accompanying perilimbal injection covering at least 75 % of the circumference of the perilimbal region.
3=	Dark, beefy red color with congestion of both the bulbar and the palpebral conjunctiva along with pronounced perilimbal injection and the presence of petechia on the conjunctiva. The petechia generally predominate along the nictitating membrane and the upper palpebral conjunctiva.
Conjunctival swelling (there are five divisions from 0 to 4)	
0=	Normal or no swelling of the conjunctival tissue.
1=	Swelling above normal without eversion of the lids (can be easily ascertained by noting that the upper and lower eyelids are positioned as in the normal eye); swelling generally starts in the lower cul-de-sac near the inner canthus, which needs slit lamp examination.
2=	Swelling with misalignment of the normal approximation of the lower and upper eyelids; primarily confined to the upper eyelid so that in the initial stages the misapproximation of the eyelids begins by partial eversion of the upper eyelid. In this stage, swelling is confined generally to the upper eyelid, although it exists in the lower cul-de-sac (observed best with the slit lamp).
3=	Swelling definite with partial eversion of the upper and lower eyelids essentially equivalent. This can be easily ascertained by looking at the animal head-on and noticing the positioning of the eyelids; if the eye margins do not meet, eversion has occurred.
4=	Eversion of the upper eyelid is pronounced with less pronounced eversion of the lower eyelid. It is difficult to retract the lids and observe the perilimbal region.
Conjunctival discharge—Discharge is defined as a whitish-gray precipitate, which should not be confused with the small amount of clear, inspissated, mucoid material that can be formed in the medial canthus of a substantial number of rabbit eyes. This material can be removed with a cotton swab before the animals are used.	
0=	Normal. No discharge.
1=	Discharge above normal and present on the inner portion of the eye but not on the lids or hairs of the eyelids. One can ignore the small amount that is in the inner and outer canthus if it has not been removed prior to starting the study.
2=	Discharge is abundant, easily observed, and has collected on the lids and around the hairs of the eyelids.
3=	Discharge has been flowing over the eyelids so as to wet the hairs substantially on the skin around the eye.
Aqueous flare—The intensity of the Tyndall phenomenon is scored by comparing the normal Tyndall effect observed when the slit lamp beam passes through the lens with that seen in the anterior chamber. The presence of aqueous flare is presumptive evidence of breakdown of the blood–aqueous barrier.	
0=	The absence of visible light beam in the anterior chamber (no Tyndall effect).

(continued)

Table 2
(continued)

1=	The Tyndall effect is barely discernible. The intensity of the light beam in the anterior chamber is less than the intensity of the slit beam as it passes through the lens.
2=	The Tyndall beam in the anterior chamber is easily discernible and is equal in intensity to the slit beam as it passes through the lens.
3=	The Tyndall beam in the anterior chamber is easily discernible; its intensity is greater than the intensity of the slit beam as it passes through the lens.
Pupillary light reflex—The pupillary diameter of the iris is controlled by the radial and sphincter muscles. Contraction of the radial muscle due to adrenergic stimulation results in mydriasis while contraction of the sphincter muscle due to cholinergic stimulation results in miosis. As an ophthalmic drug can exert potential effects on these neural pathways, it is important to assess the light reflex of an animal as part of the ophthalmic examination. Using full illumination with the slit lamp, the following scale is used.	
0=	Normal pupillary response.
1=	Sluggish pupillary response.
2=	Maximally impaired (i.e., fixed) pupillary response.
Iris involvement—In the following definitions, the primary, secondary, and tertiary vessels are utilized as an aid to determining a subjective ocular score for iris involvement. The assumption is made that the greater the hyperemia of the vessels and the more the secondary and tertiary vessels are involved, the greater the intensity of iris involvement. The scores range from 0 to 4.	
0=	Normal iris without any hyperemia of the iris vessels. Occasionally around the 12:00–1:00 o'clock position near the pupillary border and the 6:00 and 7:00 o'clock position near the pupillary border, there is a small area around 1–3 mm in diameter in which both the secondary and tertiary vessels are slightly hyperemic.
1=	Minimal injection of secondary vessels but not tertiary. Generally, it is uniform, but may be of greater intensity at the 1:00 or 6:00 o'clock position. If it is confined to the 1:00 or 6:00 o'clock position, the tertiary vessels must be substantially hyperemic.
2=	Minimal injection of tertiary vessels and minimal to moderate injection of the secondary vessels.
3=	Moderate injection of the secondary and tertiary vessels with slight swelling of the iris stroma (this gives the iris surface a slightly rugose appearance, which is usually most prominent near the 3:00 and 9:00 o'clock positions).
4=	Marked injection of the secondary and tertiary vessels with marked swelling of the iris stroma. The iris appears rugose; may be accompanied by hemorrhage (hyphema) in the anterior chamber.
Cornea cloudiness—The scoring scheme measures the severity of corneal cloudiness and the area of the cornea involved. Severity of corneal cloudiness is graded as follows:	
0=	Normal cornea. Appears with the slit lamp adjusting to a narrow slit image as having a bright gray line on the epithelial surface and a bright gray line on the endothelial surface with a marble-like gray appearance of the stroma.
1=	Some loss of transparency. Only the anterior half of the stroma is involved as observed with an optical section of the slit lamp. The underlying structures are clearly visible with diffuse illumination, although some cloudiness can be readily apparent with diffuse illumination.

(continued)

Table 2 (continued)

2=	Moderate loss of transparency. In addition to involving the anterior stroma, the cloudiness extends all the way to the endothelium. The stroma has lost its marble-like appearance and is homogeneously white. With diffuse illumination, underlying structures are clearly visible.
3=	Involvement of the entire thickness of the stroma. With the optical section, the endothelial surface is still visible. However, with diffuse illumination, the underlying structures are just barely visible (to the extent that the observer is still able to grade flare and iritis, observe for pupillary response, and note lenticular changes).
4=	Involvement of the entire thickness of the stroma. With the optical section, cannot clearly visualize the endothelium. With diffuse illumination, the underlying structures cannot be seen. Cloudiness removes the capability for judging and grading flare, iritis, lenticular changes, and pupillary response.
Corneal area—The surface area of the cornea relative to the area of cloudiness is divided into five grades from 0 to 4.	
0=	Normal cornea with no area of cloudiness.
1=	1–25 % area of stromal cloudiness.
2=	26–50 % area of stromal cloudiness.
3=	51–75 % area of stromal cloudiness.
4=	76–100 % area of stromal cloudiness.
Pannus—Pannus is vascularization or the penetration of new blood vessels into the corneal stroma. The vessels are derived from the limbal vascular loops. Pannus is divided into three grades.	
0=	No pannus.
1=	Vascularization is present but vessels have not invaded the entire corneal circumference. Where localized vessel invasion has occurred, they have not penetrated beyond 2 mm.
2=	Vessels have invaded 2 mm or more around the entire corneal circumference.
Fluorescein—For fluorescein staining, the area can be judged on a 0 to +4 scale using the same terminology as for corneal cloudiness. The intensity of fluorescein staining can be divided into 0–4 scale.	
0=	Absence of fluorescein staining.
1=	Slight fluorescein staining confined to a small focus. With diffuse illumination the underlying structures are easily visible. (The outline of the pupillary margin is as if there were no fluorescein staining.)
2=	Moderate fluorescein staining confined to a small focus. With diffuse illumination the underlying structures are clearly visible, although there is some loss of detail.
3=	Marked fluorescein staining. Staining may involve a larger portion of the cornea. With diffuse illumination the underlying structures are barely visible but are not completely obliterated.
4=	Extreme fluorescein staining. With diffuse illumination the underlying structures cannot be observed.

(continued)

Table 2
(continued)

Lens—The crystalline lens is readily observed with the aid of the slit lamp biomicroscope, and the location of lenticular opacity can readily be discerned by direct and retro illumination.
The lens is normal (N) or abnormal (A)
If abnormal, the location and severity of lenticular opacities are noted in the comments.

common method of biomicroscopic examination. Using a narrow slit beam, a highly magnified optical section of the eye is obtained. The direction of the slit beam may be varied so that the structures may be viewed using either direct illumination or retroillumination [1]. This will allow the examiner to detect and localize, with respect to depth, abnormalities in the anterior segment of the eye. For example, a corneal lesion can be localized to superficial, stromal, or endothelial; aqueous opacities such as cells (aqueous, vitreous), flare, or hemorrhage are detectable and quantifiable; and lesions of the lens may be localized to anterior, posterior, equatorial, and further to capsular, cortical, or nuclear. Interpretation of the findings on slit lamp biomicroscopy requires extensive knowledge of normal findings as well as background lesions that occur as incidental findings in the species and breed being examined [1].

2.2 Indirect/Direct Ophthalmoscopy

Indirect ophthalmoscopy is the preferred technique of choice for routine screening of the posterior segment in all laboratory animal species. Indirect ophthalmoscopy provides a binocular, inverted, and reversed aerial image with a wide field of view. It requires an indirect headset and a condensing lens. Once perfected, the technique of indirect examination also allows for a more rapid examination of the entire posterior segment as it provides a wider panoramic field of view, allowing the examiner to evaluate more animals, more accurately in a shorter period of time. The indirect headset of choice should be lightweight, comfortable, and easy to manipulate out of the way with one hand and have a small pupil setting. The ease of manipulation will allow the examiner to move efficiently between indirect and biomicroscopic examination techniques. While several excellent choices are available, the Keeler All Pupil® is best suited in the author's opinion (Fig. 11). Alternatively, the Heine indirect ophthalmoscope also offers excellent optics and can be fitted with a portable power supply, but is slightly heavier and more cumbersome for large number of animals (Fig. 12). The indirect condensing lens of choice varies by species examined and by the examiner's choice. In general, a 2.2 Pan Retinal or 30 diopter lens works well for routine screening examination of most

Table 3
Data recording sheet for a modified Hackett–McDonald scoring system

MICROSCOPIC GRADING DATA
(Hackett and McDonald)

Study Number: ______ Study Day: ______ Group: ______

	Animal No.	Conjunctival			Aqueous Flare	Iris		Corneal Cloudiness		Pannus	Time	Fluor. Exam	Time	Lens	Time
		Conges.	Swell	Dis.		Light Reflex	Involve-ment	Sev.	Area						
(Test) Left Eye															
(Control) Right Eye															

Comments: ______

Tech Date/Initials: ______ Ophthalmologist Date/Initials: ______

Conges.=congestion Sev.=Severity
Swell-swelling Fluor, Exam=Fluorescein staining Dis.=Discharge

Table 4
Grading scheme for aqueous cells based on the SUN grading system using a biomicroscope and a 1 mm × 1 mm slit beam

Grade	# cells in the field
0	<1
0.5+	1–5
1+	6–15
2+	16–25
3+	26–50
4+	>50

Cells should be counted at the same location, usually the central anterior chamber [1, 12]

Table 5
Grading scheme for aqueous flare based on the SUN grading system using a biomicroscope [12]

Grade	Description
0	None
1+	Faint
2+	Moderate (iris and lens details clear)
3+	Marked (iris and lens details hazy)
4+	Intense (fibrin or plasmoid aqueous)

Table 6
Grading scheme for vitreous inflammation based on the National Eye Institutes grading system using an indirect ophthalmoscope [14]

Grade	Description
0	None
1+	Posterior pole clearly visible
2+	Posterior pole details slightly hazy
3+	Posterior pole details very hazy
4+	Posterior pole details barely visible
5+	Fundus details not visible

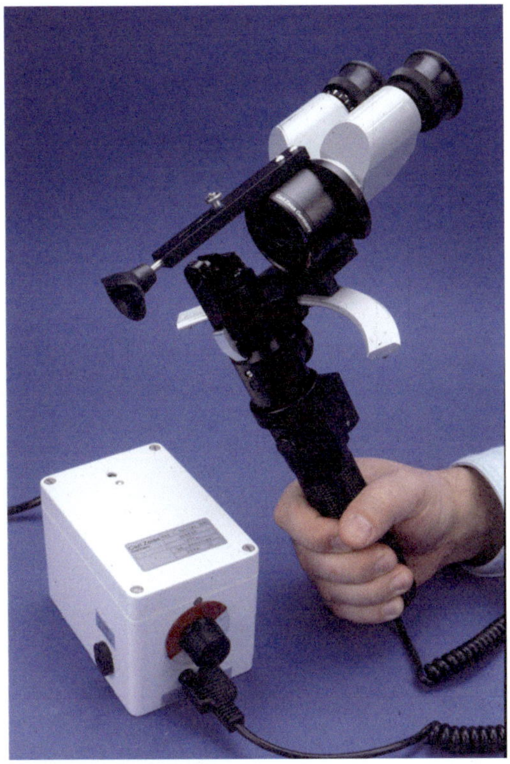

Fig. 1 A Zeiss HSO-10 slit lamp provides excellent optics and portability and is suited for use in all laboratory animal species

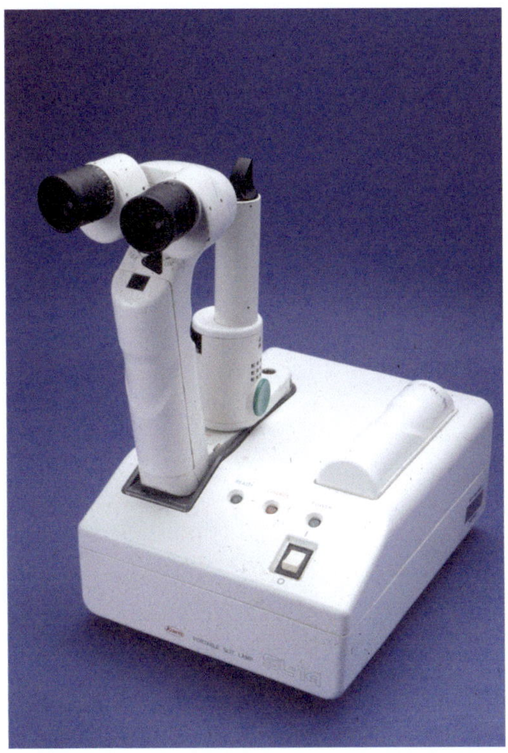

Fig. 2 A Kowa SL-14 or SL-15 handheld slit lamp are rechargeable and portable. As with the Zeiss HSO-10 they are suited for use in all laboratory animal species

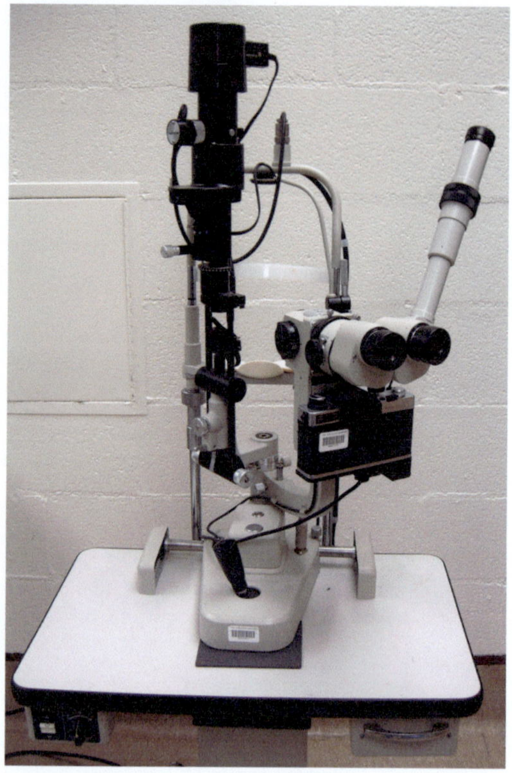

Fig. 3 A Topcon table-mounted slit lamp. This provides excellent optics, higher magnification, and variable slit beam width and height and additionally can be used for other procedures such as photographic documentation and specular microscopy

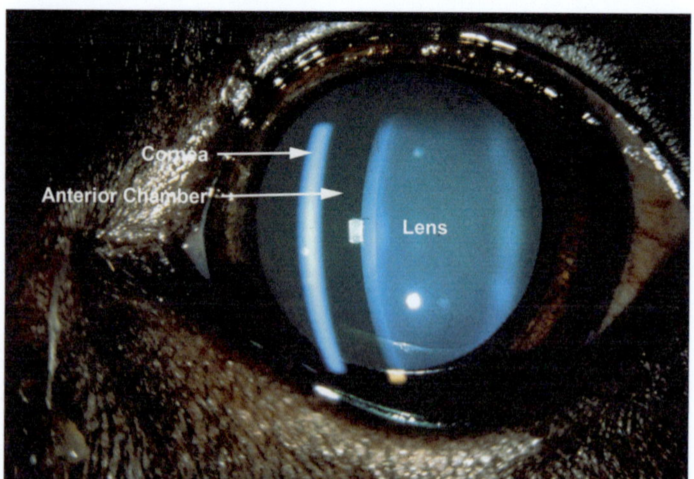

Fig. 4 A normal slit lamp examination using the technique of optical section to examine the anterior segment of a normal beagle

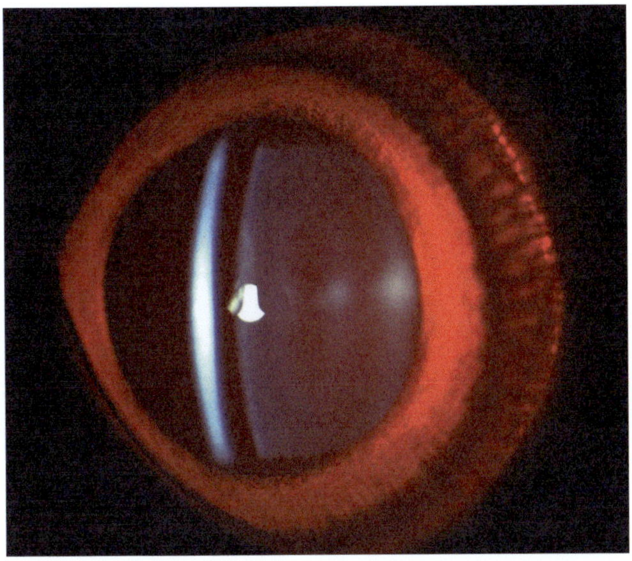

Fig. 5 A normal slit lamp examination using the technique of optical section to examine the anterior segment of a normal New Zealand white rabbit

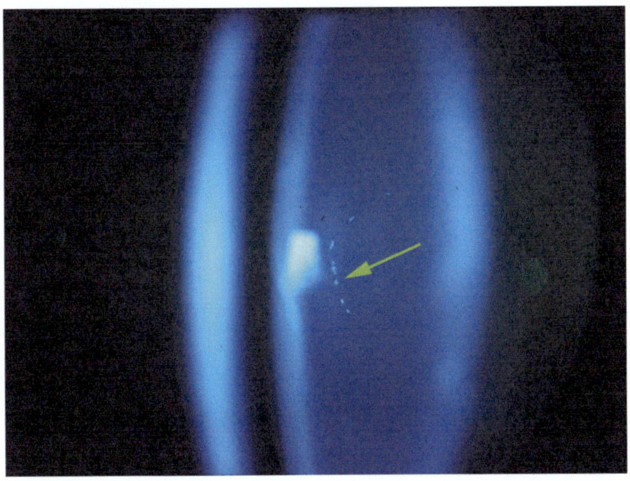

Fig. 6 Multiple anterior cortical suture opacities/cataract are noted (*arrow*) in a beagle in pretest examination

larger species and a 40 or a 60 diopter works best for rats and mice. The addition of a 20 diopter and/or a 15 diopter lens may be advised for higher magnification of the fundus in the canine and to examine the fovea and optic nerve in greater detail in NHPs. Alternately, a direct ophthalmoscope (Fig. 13) can be used to examine the optic nerve head and fovea in NHPs, but given its small field and monocular view, it is less than optimal in the author's opinion. In addition, when performing direct ophthalmoscopy any

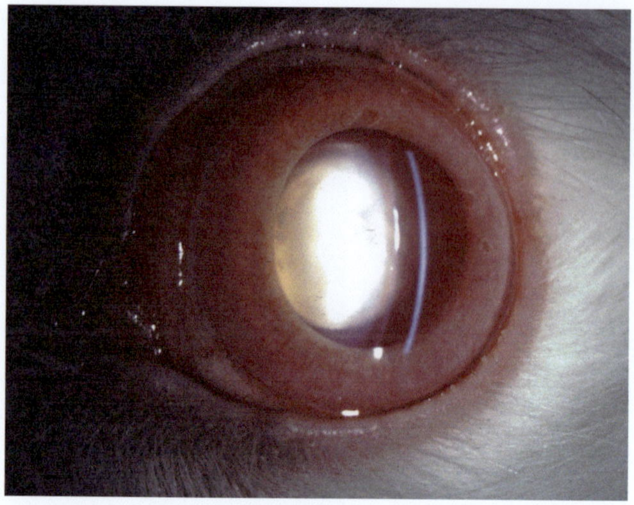

Fig. 7 An immature, nuclear cataract noted in a New Zealand white rabbit in pretest examination

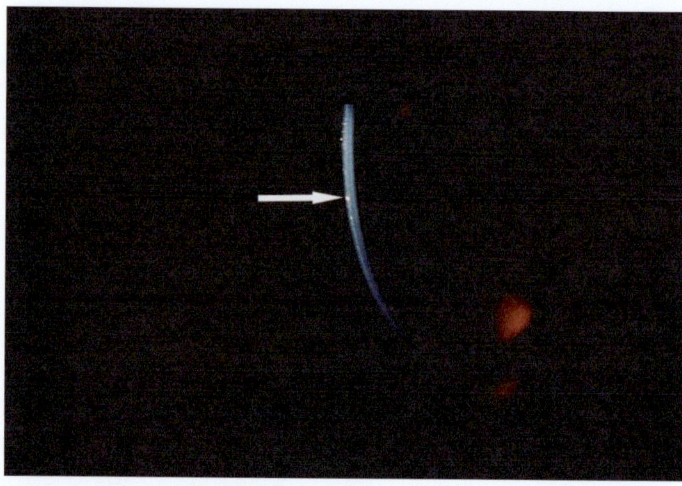

Fig. 8 Multifocal, corneal anterior stromal opacities (*arrow*) observed as a treatment-related effect in high-dose beagles during a chronic study

opacity of the cornea, aqueous, lens, or vitreous will severely impair or prevent visualization of the posterior segment.

Prior to indirect ophthalmoscopy, a short-acting mydriatic agent is required to dilate the pupil. Tropicamide 0.5–1.0 % is the mydriatic of choice. When examining using indirect ophthalmoscopy, the examiner remains at arm's length and places the condensing lens just anterior to the cornea. This technique is used to examine the posterior vitreous, optic nerve, retinal vasculature, retina, and choroid. In addition, opacities of the clear media

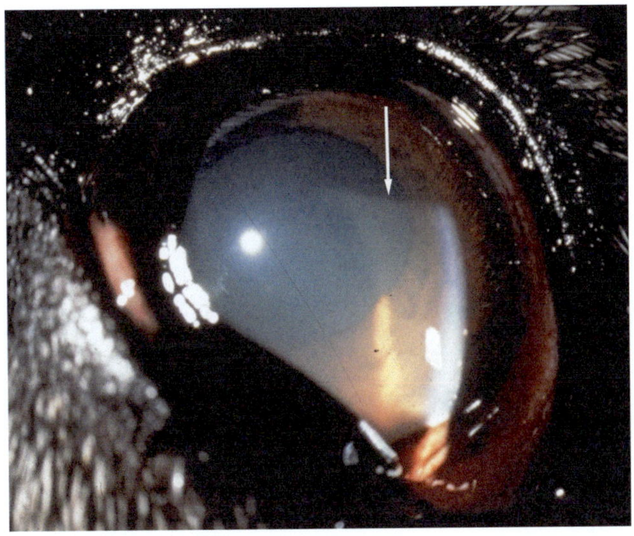

Fig. 9 Aqueous flare is noted in the anterior chamber as a cloudiness (*arrow*) in the normally transparent aqueous humor

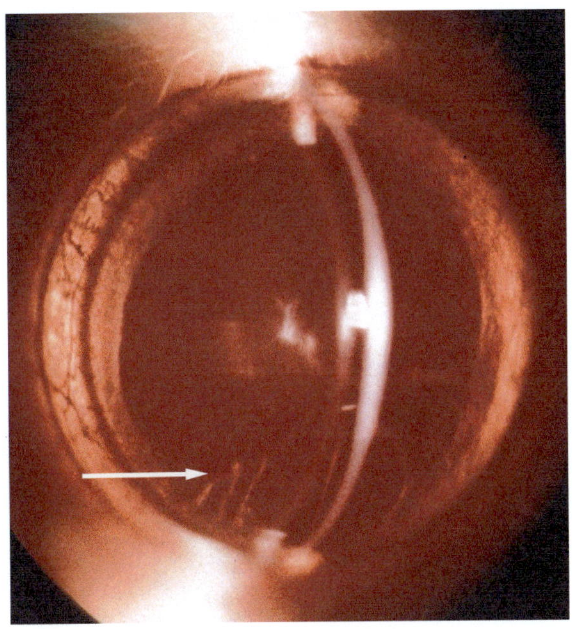

Fig. 10 A Sprague–Dawley rat with several persistent pupillary membranes (*arrow*) noted in pretest examination

(cornea, aqueous, lens, and vitreous) are readily detectable using retroillumination. This technique can be used to grade vitreous inflammation/opacification (Table 6). Given the wide variety of laboratory animals, the examiner must be familiar with the variation of normal anatomy and species variations. The retinal vasculature

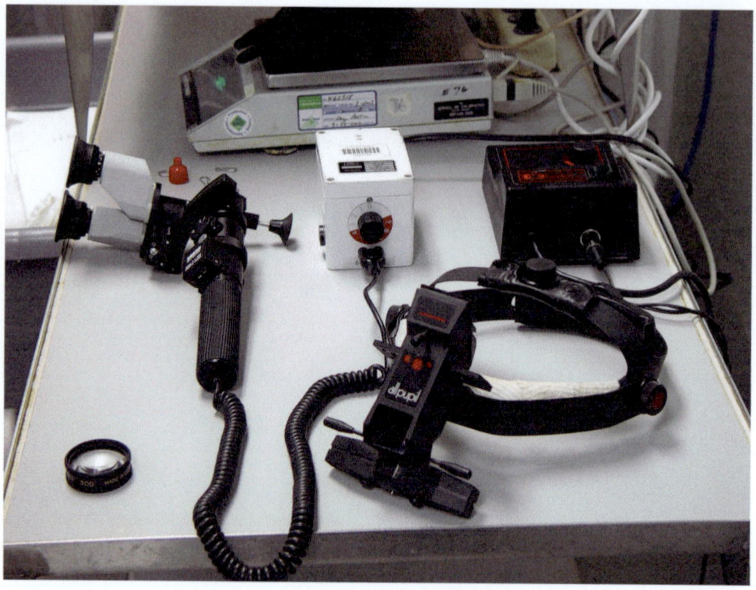

Fig. 11 A Keeler All-Pupil® indirect ophthalmoscope, 30D condensing lens, and a Zeiss HSO-10 slit lamp used for ophthalmic examination of laboratory animals

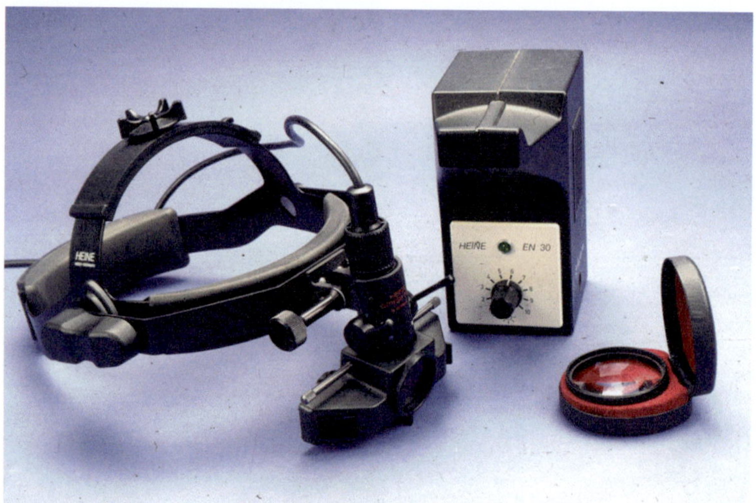

Fig. 12 A Heine® indirect ophthalmoscope with a power source and a 30 diopter indirect condensing lens

will vary with the species anangiotic (guinea pig), merangiotic (rabbit), and holangiotic (rodent, canine, swine, primate). The pigmentation of the retinal pigment epithelium (RPE) and the choroid vary between albinotic, sub-albinotic, and pigmented animals of the same species (mouse, rat, rabbit). Some species such as the canine will have a tapetum located in the superior choroid, but

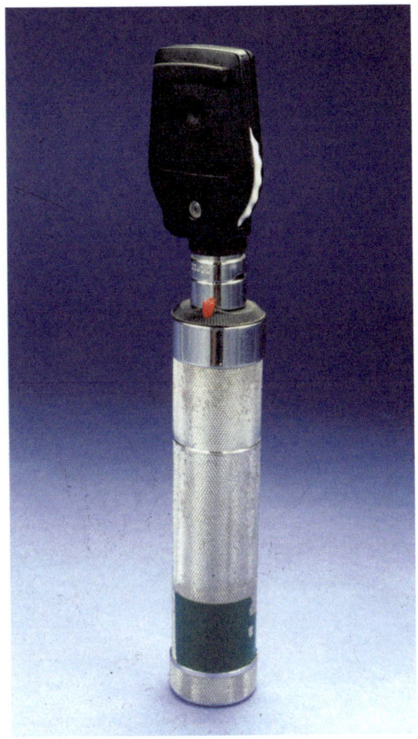

Fig. 13 A Welch-Allyn direct ophthalmoscope

this can be lacking in color dilute or lemon beagles. Finally, NHPs are foveated and this region must be examined carefully for abnormalities.

Additional techniques to evaluate the retina may include fluorescein angiography, OCT, confocal scanning laser ophthalmoscopy, fundus photography, and electrodiagnostic testing. When these tests are used correctly and in combination they can provide additional en face, cross-sectional, and functional information of the retina that may be then correlated with histopathology.

2.3 Pretest Examination

Prior to study initiation, a pretest ophthalmic examination should be performed on all study animals. This is done for two reasons. The first is to eliminate from the study animals with current significant or potentially progressive ophthalmic abnormalities. The second is to establish a baseline of ocular findings to compare to as the study progresses and subsequent ophthalmic examinations are performed. Examples of pretest abnormalities that should automatically result in an animal's elimination from the study would include all ocular findings with a severity score of moderate or higher and all abnormalities that currently prevent or may prevent if progressive complete examination of intraocular structures. Examples of ocular findings that may be progressive during the course of the study and

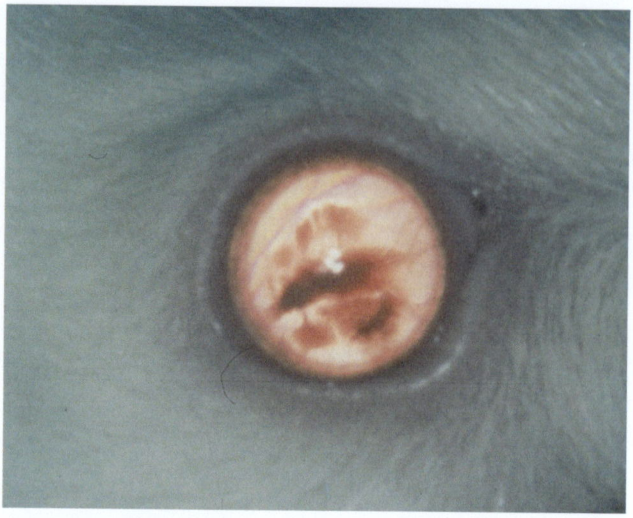

Fig. 14 A Sprague–Dawley rat with significant intravitreal extravasated blood associated with a persistent hyaloid. This was noted in pretest examination and the animal was eliminated from the study

would result in elimination would include cataract, intraocular hemorrhage, uveitis, and any other findings that may result in progressive opacification and interfere with a complete ophthalmic examination on subsequent examinations.

Common background abnormalities will vary by species, but may include ocular trauma associated with shipping, congenital embryonic remnants such as persistent pupillary membrane (PPM) and persistent hyaloid artery (PHA), extravasation of blood in association with a PHA, corneal opacity/dystrophy, coloboma (iris, lens, choroid), cataract, micropapilla, optic nerve hypoplasia, and retinal dysplasia [1, 7–9, 11, 16–28]. PPM and PHA are commonly observed in rodents (Figs. 10 and 14) and less frequently in the beagle (Figs. 15 and 16). In general, they are noted and graded. However, if they result in significant opacity of the cornea, lens, or vitreous at pretest examination elimination of the affected animal from study should be considered. If a persistent hyaloid has a significant component of extravasated blood, elimination from study is advised (Fig. 14).

Whenever possible, animals with ocular abnormalities are eliminated from inclusion in the study. This is especially true if the lesion may be progressive during the study. However, some abnormalities are so common as to preclude elimination. The most common example of this would be corneal dystrophy in the rat and mouse [23, 29–38]. The prevalence of corneal dystrophy varies by stain, age, and sex of the rat. In the Sprague–Dawley, males are more commonly affected than females and prevalence will increase with age and may vary from 20 to 50 % (Fig. 17). In the Wistar, corneal

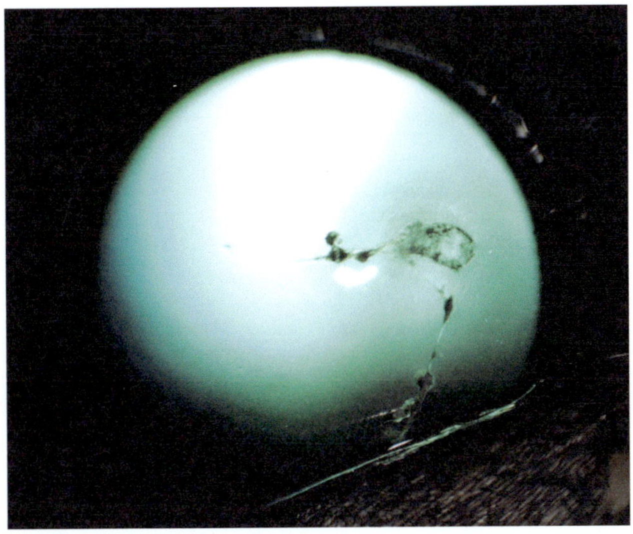

Fig. 15 A persistent pupillary membrane with attachment to the corneal endothelium is observed using retroillumination in a beagle

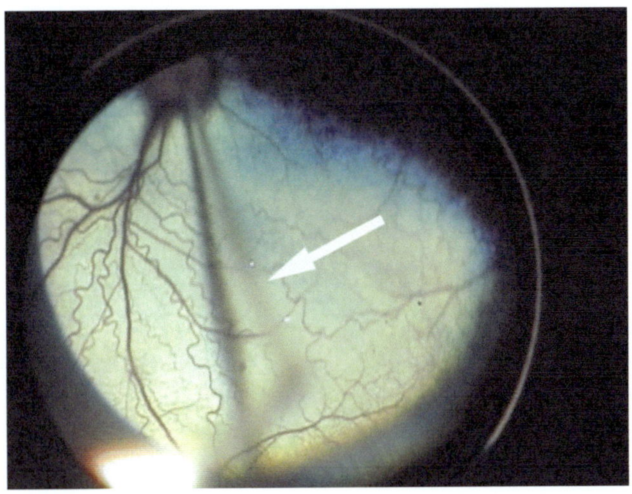

Fig. 16 A persistent hyaloid remnant (*arrow*) extends from the optic nerve to the posterior lens in a beagle

dystrophy has been reported to affect >65 % (Fig. 18) and in the Fisher 344 (Fig. 19), the prevalence is generally 100 %. As a result of such a high prevalence, affected animals cannot be eliminated from inclusion in study. However, animals affected with corneal dystrophy with a severity grade of greater than slight or with secondary keratitis should be eliminated at pretest. Corneal dystrophy lesions are also observed in other species including the beagle (Fig. 20) and Dutch Belted rabbit (Fig. 21). It should also be noted that lesions such as corneal dystrophy can be exacerbated in both

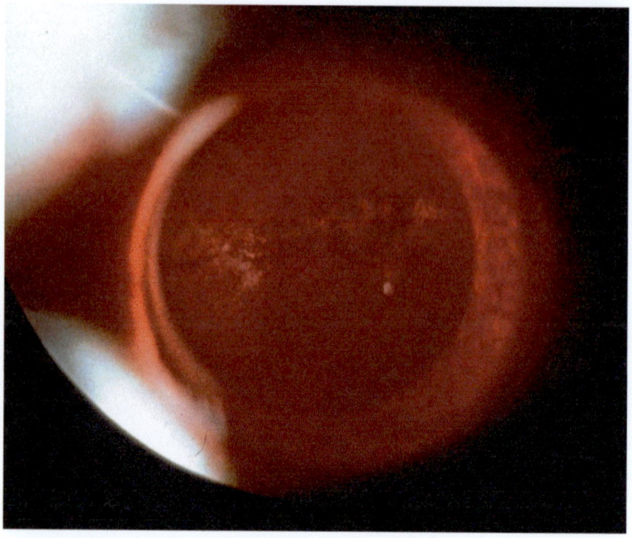

Fig. 17 Corneal dystrophy in a Sprague–Dawley rat

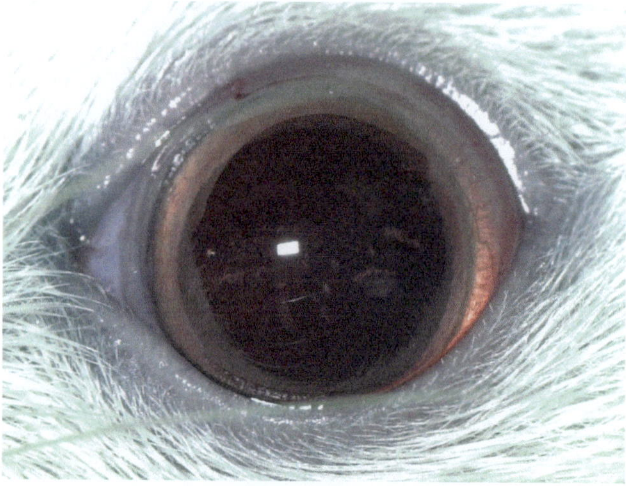

Fig. 18 Corneal dystrophy in a Wistar rat

prevalence and severity by corneal exposure caused by desiccation, sedation/anesthesia, orbital bleeding, environmental irritants, and the test article itself.

2.4 Species-Specific Ophthalmic Findings

The ophthalmologist must be familiar with what is normal for the species in question and what are the common spontaneous abnormalities for that species, age of animal, and breed/strain [39]. Common laboratory species of interest may include mice, rats, guinea pigs, cats, rabbits, dogs, Gottingen mini-pigs, and NHPs (cynomolgus, rhesus). For the common laboratory species

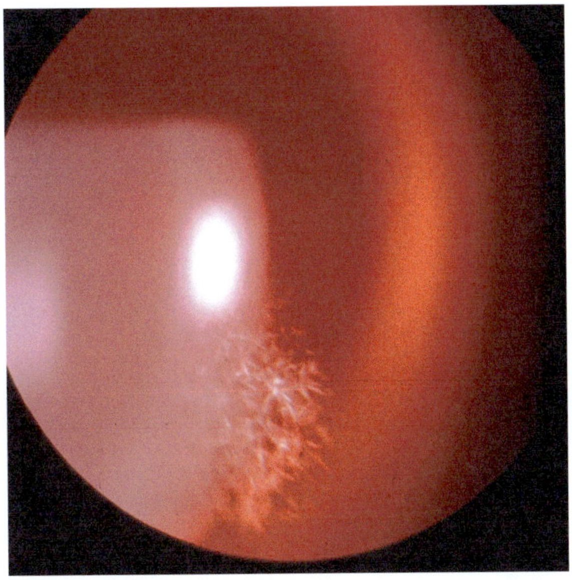

Fig. 19 Corneal dystrophy in a Fisher 344 rat

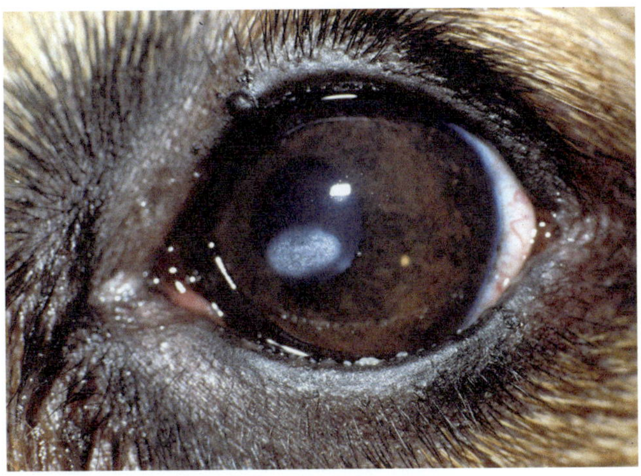

Fig. 20 Corneal dystrophy in a Marshall Farms beagle

examined, the type of retinal vasculature includes anangiotic (guinea pig), merangiotic (rabbit), and holangiotic (rodent, feline, canine, swine, primate) (Figs. 22, 23, 24, 25, 26, 27, 28, and 29). An albinotic vs. pigmented eye may be a factor in clinical findings as well as response to mydriasis or test article effect. The presence of a nictitating membrane (third eyelid), number, location, and type of lacrimal/orbital glands, location and number or lacrimal puncta, presence or absence of a tapetum, myelination of the optic nerve, anatomy and physiology of aqueous outflow, and whether the animal has a fovea should all be understood and considered [39].

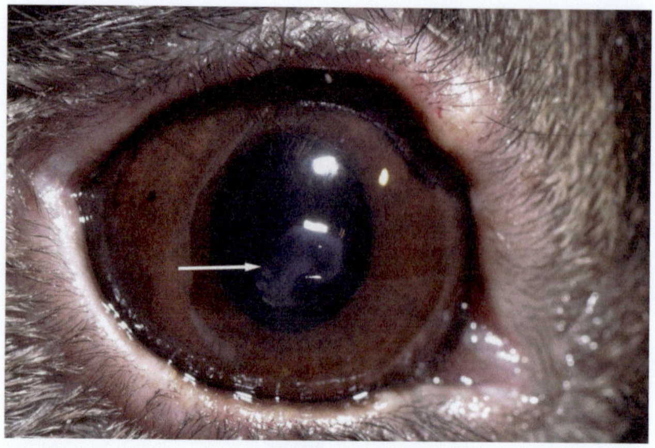

Fig. 21 Corneal dystrophy in a Dutch Belted rabbit (*arrow*). This was not present in pretest examination, but appeared during the study

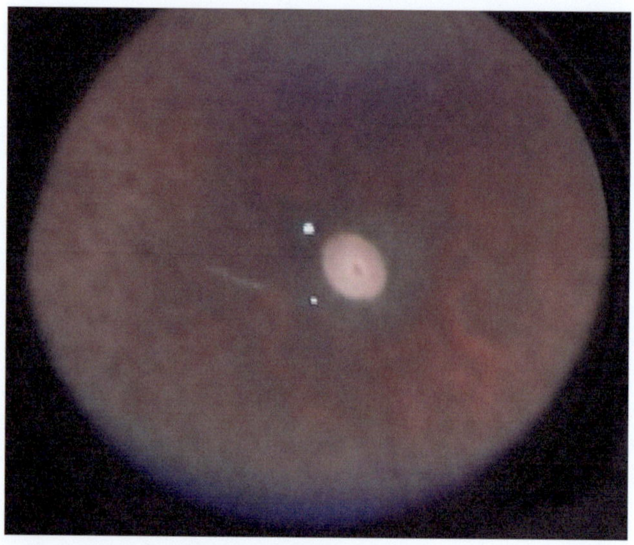

Fig. 22 Normal anangiotic fundus of the guinea pig

For intraocular procedures or intraocular dosing the specific size of the globe and the size and volume of all intraocular structures and the aqueous and vitreous must be understood in order to avoid inadvertent trauma during the procedure [39]. For topical ophthalmic dosing, the volume capacity of the conjunctival cul-de-sac and volume of the pre-corneal tear film must be known.

In addition, the examination and restraint techniques, need for sedation, type of biomicroscope and indirect ophthalmoscope, diopter power of the indirect lens, and number of animals that can be examined in the time period that the mydriatic effect will persist must be understood. The role of the veterinary

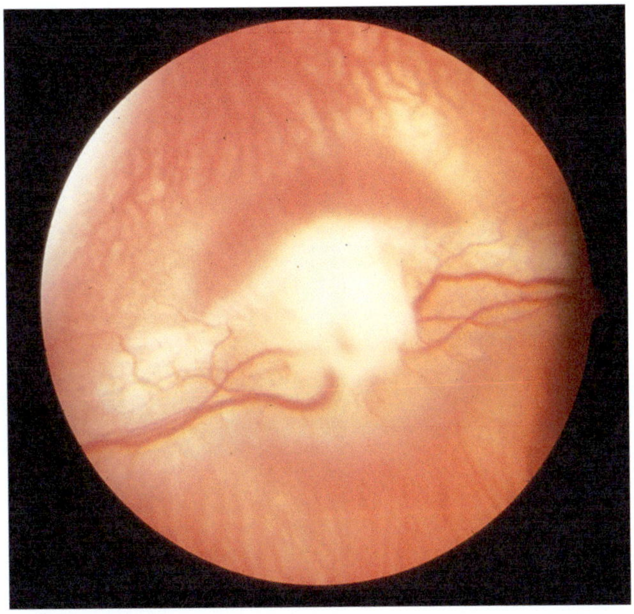

Fig. 23 Normal merangiotic fundus of an albinotic New Zealand white rabbit

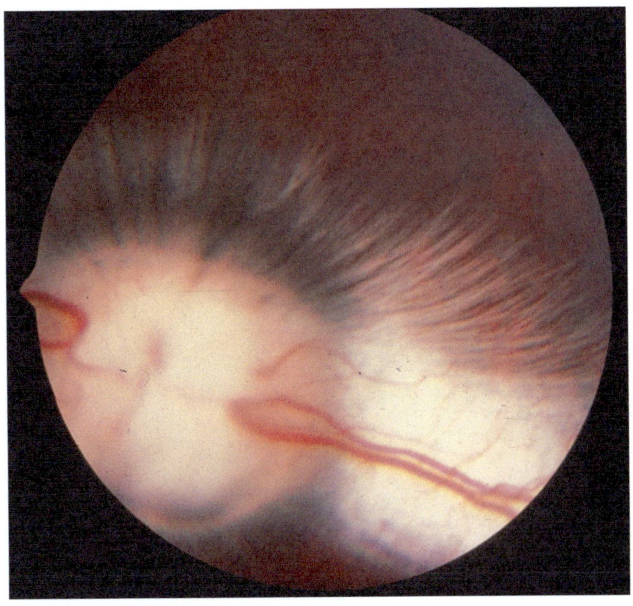

Fig. 24 Normal merangiotic fundus of a pigmented Dutch Belted rabbit. Note the prominent myelinated medullary rays and optic cup

ophthalmologist is to perform a pretest examination designed to eliminate those animals not suited to the study and to establish a baseline database to compare to. Animals are then subsequently examined one or more times during and at the conclusion of the

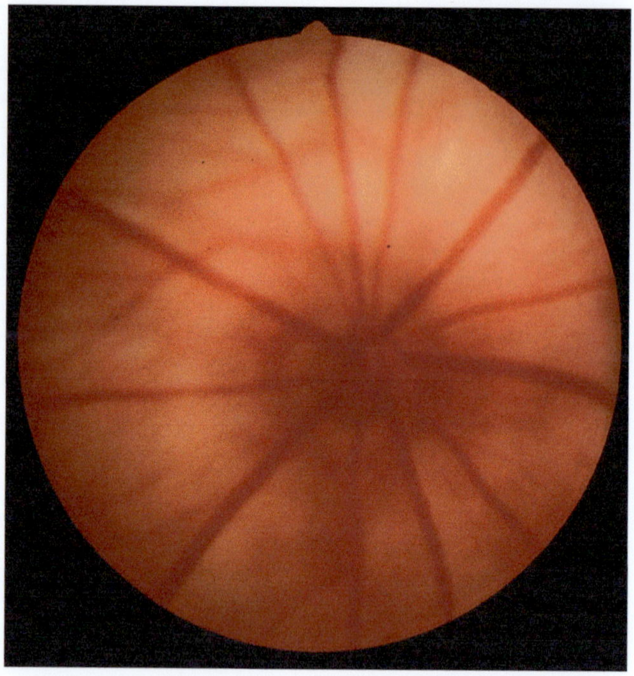

Fig. 25 Normal holangiotic fundus of an albinotic Sprague–Dawley rat

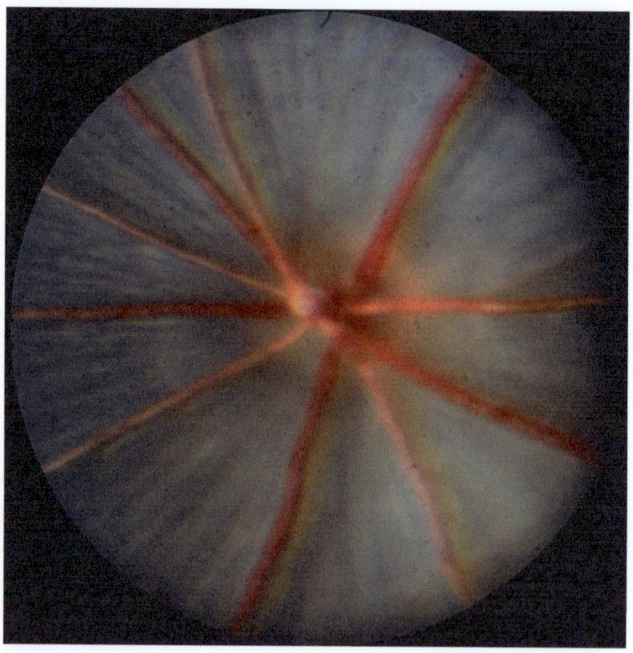

Fig. 26 Normal holangiotic fundus of a pigmented Long–Evans rat

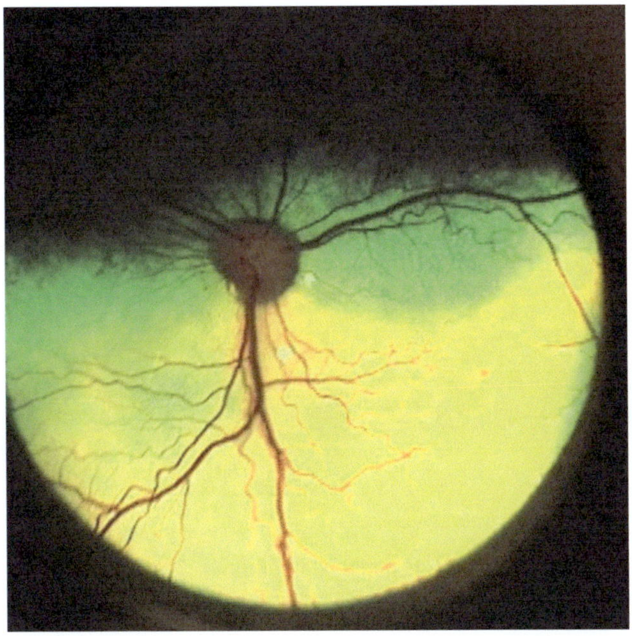

Fig. 27 Normal holangiotic fundus of a beagle. Note the yellow-green tapetum which appears ventral as the indirect image is inverted and reversed

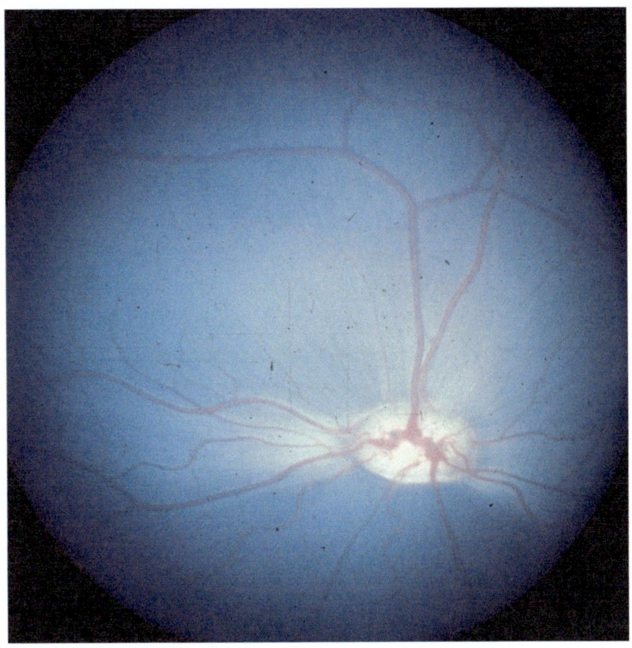

Fig. 28 Normal holangiotic fundus of a Gottingen pig. Observe the lack of a tapetum

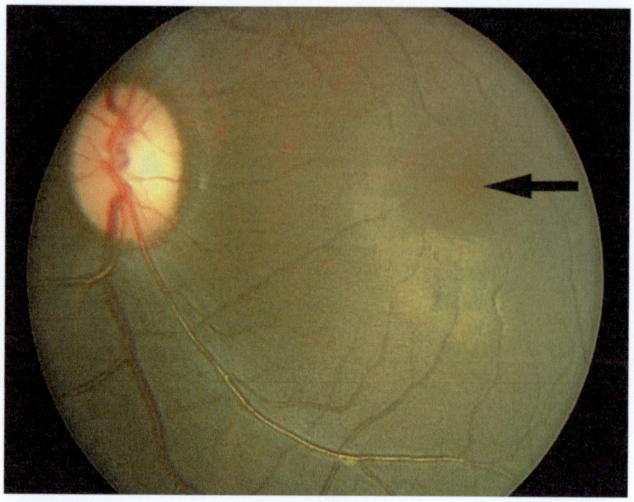

Fig. 29 Normal holangiotic fundus of a cynomolgus monkey. The fovea is denoted by the *arrow*

study depending on the study duration. Typically studies are divided into acute, subacute, subchronic, and chronic depending on the duration. The ophthalmologist must then interpret findings in light of the species examined, pretest data, compound evaluated, and dose group outcome.

2.4.1 Beagle

The beagle is a canine like any other and most veterinary ophthalmologists are both familiar and comfortable with the examination and abnormalities of this breed [16–18, 23]. The breed-related abnormalities will vary according to the supplier and are often seen with a prevalence that waxes and wanes according to the current sires and dams. For example in the author's experience, micropapilla is more common in a specific supplier's beagles, but rare in beagles from other suppliers. Keep in mind that these are tightly controlled breeding programs to yield a beagle with specific characteristics and their ocular lesions while similar in kind may differ in prevalence from the pet beagles seen in a clinical setting. In the author's experience, prolapse of the gland of the nictitans (Fig. 30), retinal dysplasia (folds) (Figs. 31 and 32), optic nerve micropapilla/hypoplasia (Fig. 33), and incipient posterior cortical or anterior suture cataract (Figs. 6, 34, and 35) are the most common breed-related findings in the laboratory beagle [17, 18, 21, 40]. These are similar to the previously reported prevalence of ophthalmic findings in 8–10-month-old beagles (Table 7) [17]. Corneal dystrophy is also observed in the laboratory beagle [19, 20]. It should be noted that corneal dystrophy, cataracts, and retinal degeneration may also be noted as a treatment-related finding (Figs. 36, 37, and 38).

The beagle has a holangiotic retina and, unlike most laboratory animal species, has a tapetum located in the superior choroid

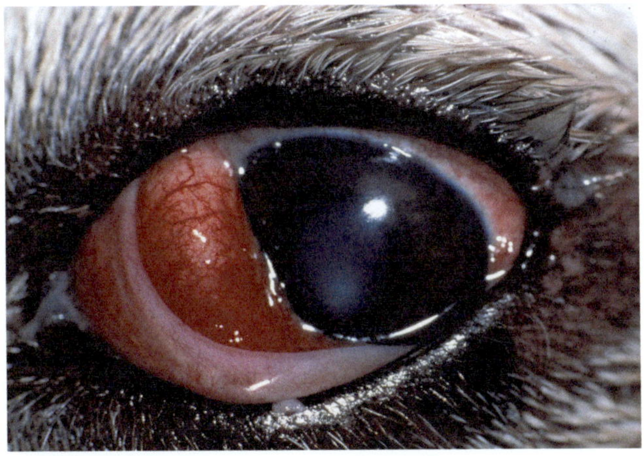

Fig. 30 Prolapse of the gland of the nictitans with associated mucoid epiphora, conjunctival hyperemia, and a focal corneal opacity

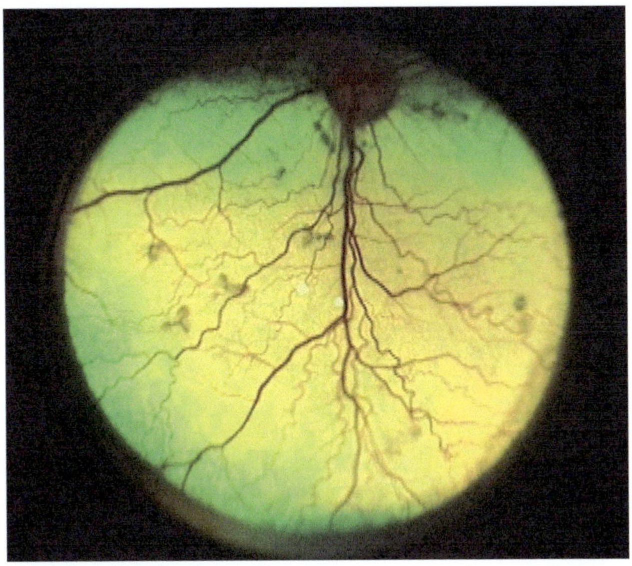

Fig. 31 Multiple, focal retinal folds are observed in the tapetal fundus. They appear as linear hyporeflective areas obscuring the underlying tapetum

(Fig. 27). The tapetum is cellular in nature and is located between the large choroidal vessels and the choriocapillaris in the dorsal aspect of the fundus. The tapetal color is variable with blue, green, orange, and yellow the most common variations. There are also atapetal beagles, usually color dilute, which are reported to have tapetal cells that are deficient in tapetal rodlets [41]. The tapetum can have a role in ocular toxicity [42] and in such instances atapetal beagles can be used. The tapetum of the dog contains a high concentration of zinc and as such zinc chelators may result in

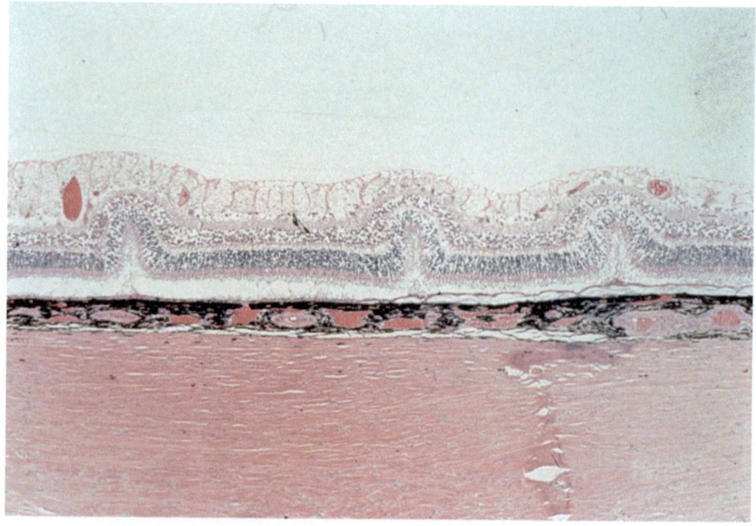

Fig. 32 Histopathology of retinal folds. H&E 100×

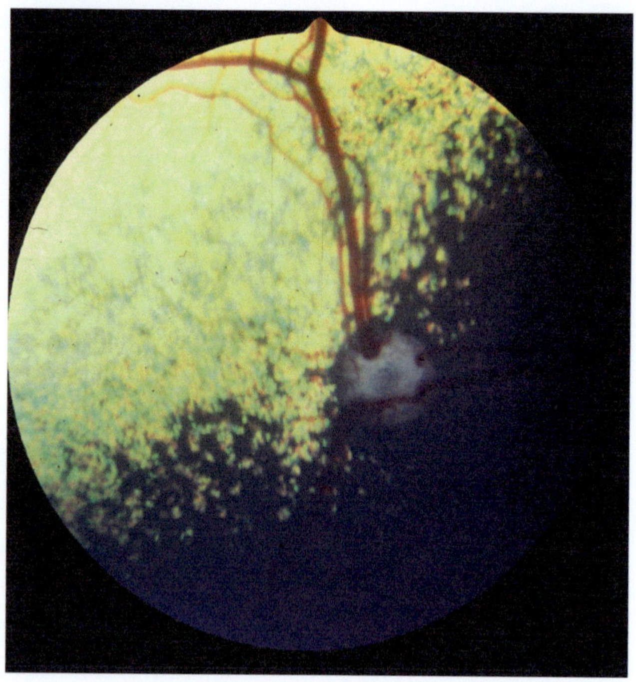

Fig. 33 Optic nerve micropapilla is present as a congenital lesion in a beagle

tapetal necrosis and secondary retinopathy [43]. Additional drug-associated lens and retinal changes have also been described in the beagle (Figs. 37 and 38) [44, 45].

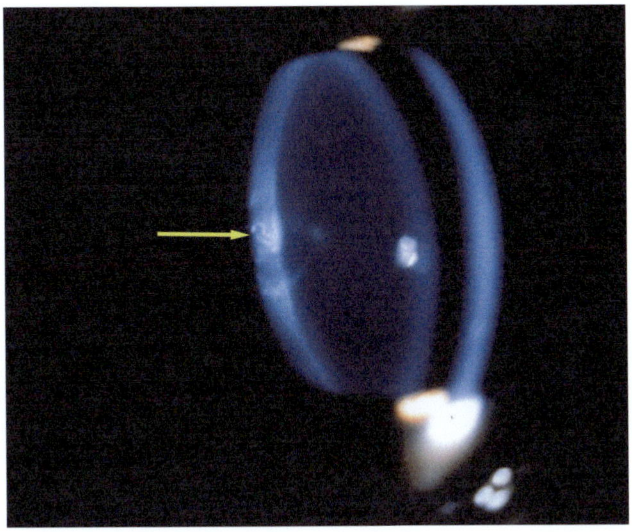

Fig. 34 An axial incipient, posterior cortical cataract is noted in pretest examination

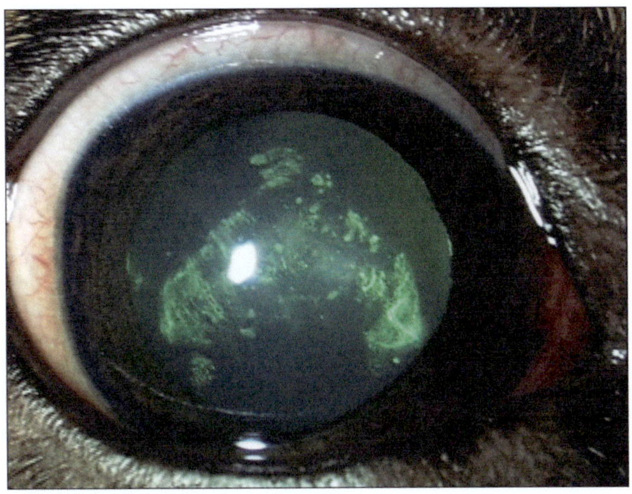

Fig. 35 An immature posterior cataract is noted in pretest examination

2.4.2 Rat/Mouse

In general, spontaneous ocular lesions in rodents may include microophthalmos, buphthalmos, corneal dystrophy, keratitis, persistent hyaloid (PH) (with or without hemorrhage), PPM, peripheral anterior synechiae, cataract (often nuclear), retinal hemorrhage, coloboma, saccular aneurysm of retinal vessels, and choroidal and optic nerve coloboma as the most common species-associated findings in laboratory rats and mice (Figs. 39 and 40) [9, 23, 27, 29, 35, 46–51].

Table 7
Summary of findings in 8–10-month-old laboratory beagles [17]

Finding	# dogs (479 examined)	# dogs (479 examined)
Prolapsed gland	4	0.83
Corneal opacity	7	1.46
Persistent pupillary membrane	1	0.21
Lens cortical vacuoles/opacity	23	4.8
Fetal nucleus opacity	7	1.46
Prominent nucleus	2	0.42
Peripheral capsular opacity	1	0.21
Prominent posterior lens sutures	25	5.23
Posterior capsular opacity	27	5.64
Persistent hyaloid remnant	15	3.13
Tapetal scar/pigment	13	2.71
Micropapilla	22	4.59

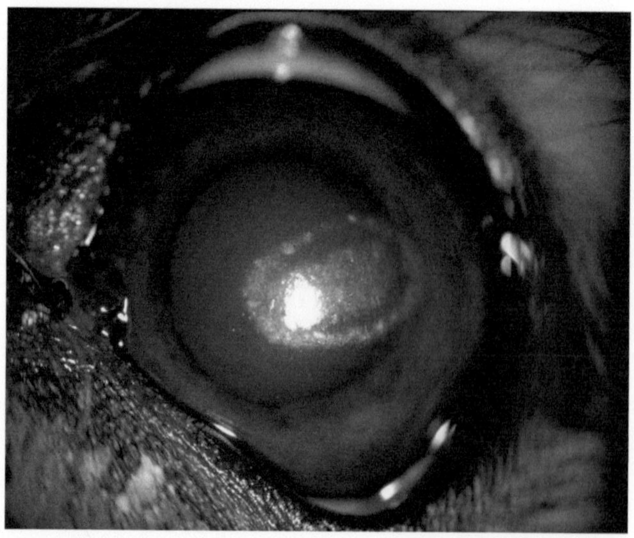

Fig. 36 Corneal opacity with a dystrophy-like appearance secondary to a treatment-related effect

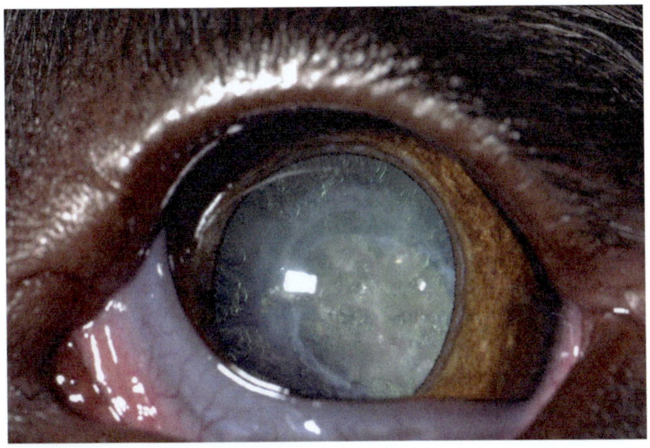

Fig. 37 Acute-onset, immature anterior and posterior cortical cataract with vacuolization secondary to a treatment-related effect

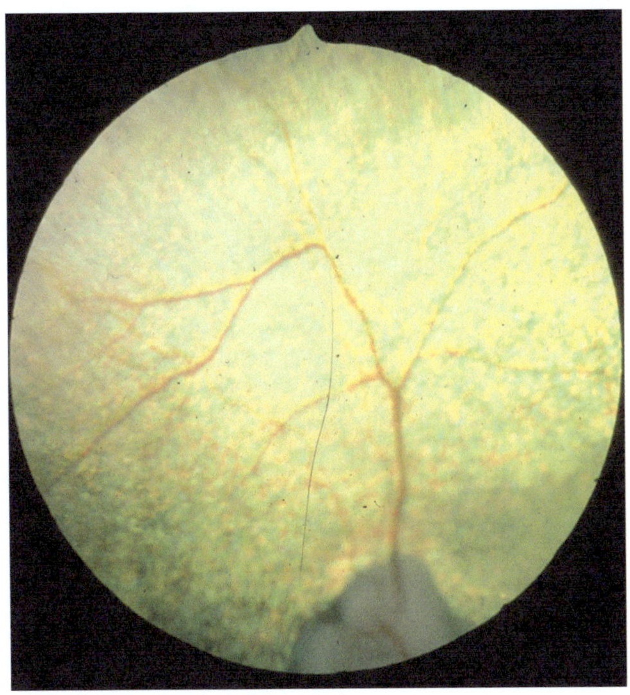

Fig. 38 Retinal degeneration characterized by vascular attenuation, tapetal hyper-reflectivity, and optic nerve pallor secondary to a treatment-related effect

In general, young animals are more likely to have PH or PPM (Figs. 10, 14, and 41). In one report the prevalence of hyaloid remnants may be as high as 60 % at 6 weeks of age, but decrease to less than 17 % by 1 year of age [26, 52, 53]. In mice, the prevalence of a PH has been reported to range between 28 and 32 % with a

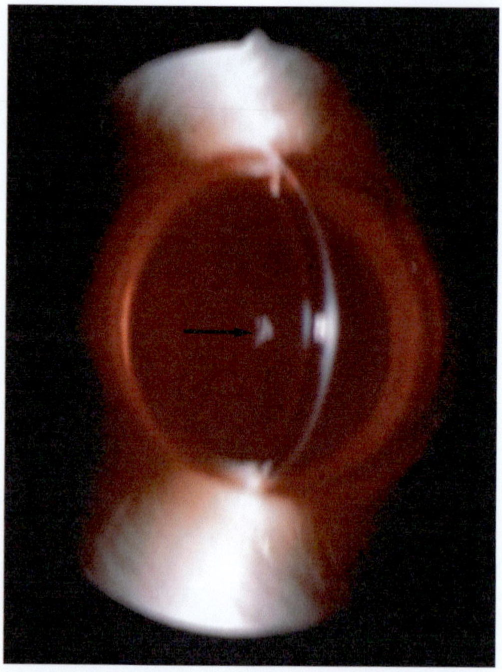

Fig. 39 A focal, incipient cataract (*arrow*) is noted in pretest examination

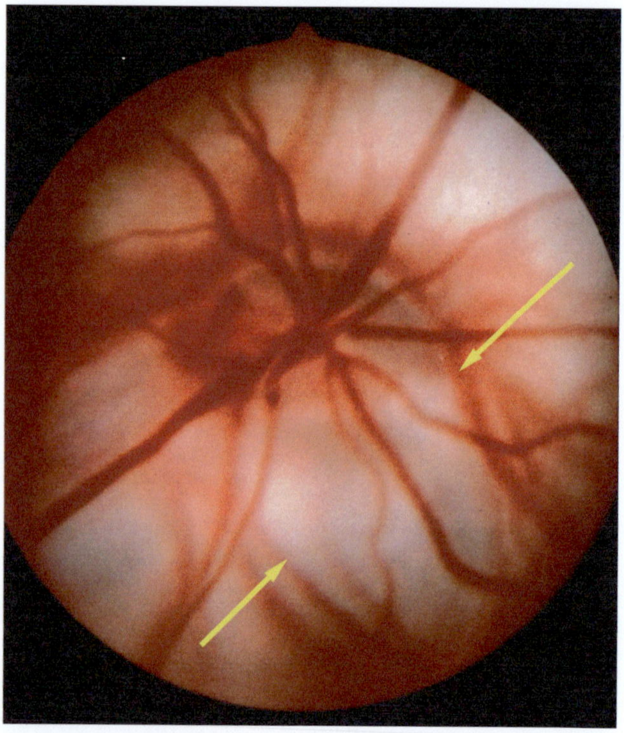

Fig. 40 A coloboma involving the optic nerve and adjacent structures is noted in pretest examination (*arrows*)

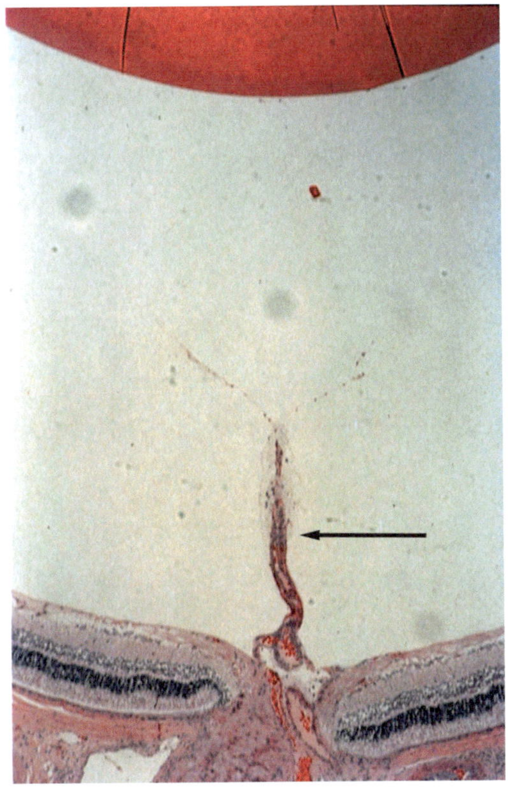

Fig. 41 Histologic section of the posterior globe in a rat demonstrating a persistent hyaloid remnant (*arrow*)

higher prevalence in females [48]. On a pretest examination, animals with PPM/PH and associated hemorrhage (vitreous, aqueous) should typically be eliminated from the study if possible (Fig. 14). Anterior synechia, microophthalmos, and anterior cleavage anomalies are also occasionally seen as congenital ocular anomalies in rats and mice.

The term corneal dystrophy implies a bilateral, noninflammatory inherited, degenerative disorder and is a specific term. Unfortunately, the terms corneal opacity or corneal crystals are also used and are less specific and more general terms. The term calcific band keratopathy has also been applied to the lesions observed in rodents [43]. Clinically, the lesions of corneal dystrophy most commonly appear as fine granular or linear opacities in the nasal and axial palpebral fissure (Figs. 17–19). They are most frequently bilateral. Histologically, corneal dystrophy in rodents is typically a basement membrane, anterior stromal corneal defect resulting in deposits of mineral and phospholipid in and adjacent to the epithelial basement membrane (Fig. 42) [34, 43]. Corneal dystrophy, while common in a pretest examination, will be observed to increase in prevalence and severity with age. Corneal dystrophy is common in rats and less

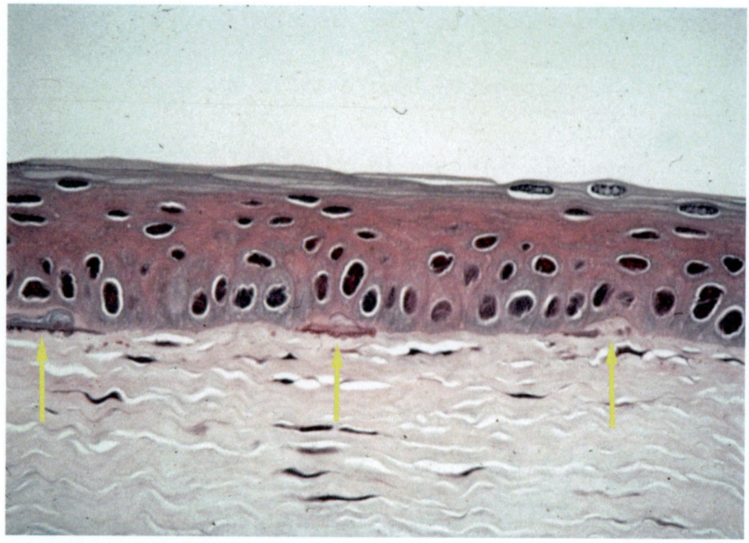

Fig. 42 Histologic section of the anterior cornea of a Sprague–Dawley rat with corneal dystrophy. The areas of basement membrane thickening, disorganization, and mineralization are indicated by the *arrows*. H&E 100×

common in mice, and varies in prevalence, appearance, and severity by strain of rat/mouse, sex, age, and shipment and supplier. It is more prevalent in males and increases in prevalence and in some species severity with age [23]. The prevalence will vary from 5 to 100 % [30–36]. It has been variously termed corneal dystrophy, calcific keratopathy, corneal opacity, corneal calcification, and spontaneous corneal degeneration. It has also been reproduced experimentally in rats by corneal desiccation which can occur secondary to dehydration, a decrease in blink rate, sedation, or anesthesia. As it increases in severity with age it can be associated with secondary keratitis (typically nasal), especially in the Fischer 344 rat (Fig. 43). In addition, keratitis can occur secondary to anesthesia, corneal exposure, keratoconjunctivitis sicca, sialodacryoadenitis (SDA), environment (dust, irritants), and conjunctivitis.

Cataracts may be seen during pretest screening and are most often nuclear (Fig. 39). They can be unilateral or bilateral and if possible, these animals are eliminated from the study. Posterior cortical cataracts are also seen, often associated with a PH with or without hemorrhage. Cataracts may also be spontaneous, associated with age, secondary to retinal degeneration, or associated with trauma, anesthesia, or other external factors (Fig. 44) [29, 54–56]. Acquired cataracts may also be treatment related and the result of a toxicologic effect. The examiner should always ascertain if orbital bleeding was performed during the study in question, especially if the cataracts are unilateral and typically in the same eye within the study animals. Reversible lens opacities may be

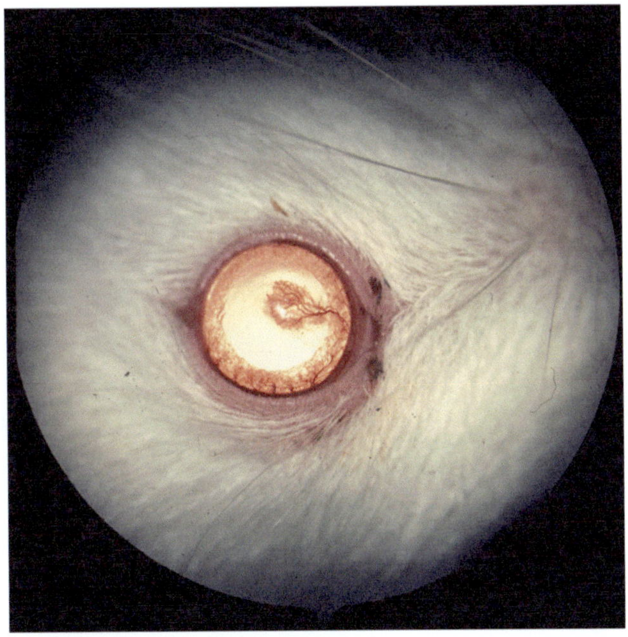

Fig. 43 Nasal corneal vascularization and keratitis in a Fisher 344 rat secondary to corneal dystrophy

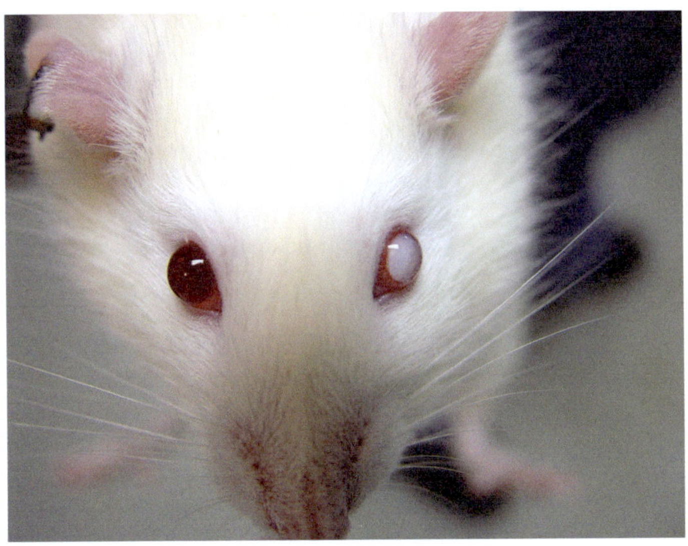

Fig. 44 A unilateral, mature cataract is seen secondary to the trauma of orbital bleeding

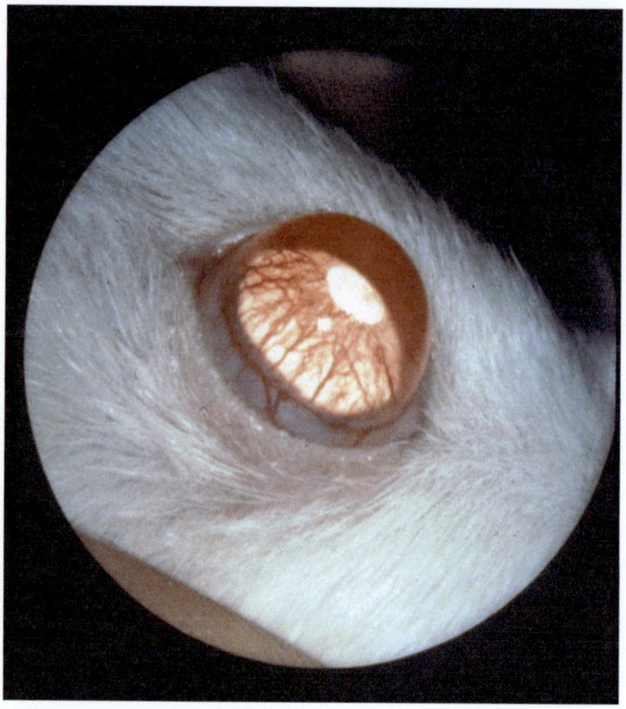

Fig. 45 Slit lamp examination of a rat with buphthalmos noted in pretest examination

induced in the rat by temperature (cold), dehydration, anoxia, and specific drugs (opiates, opioids, phenothiazine) [53, 57, 58].

Buphthalmos and glaucoma have been observed and are typically congenital (Fig. 45) [49]. Unfortunately, the intraocular pressure is generally not determined in affected animals as this is most often noted in young rats in a pretest examination and they are usually eliminated from study without further diagnostics or follow-up.

Retinal dysplasia may be noted in rats and can be unilateral or bilateral [27]. Retinal degeneration may occur spontaneously, be associated with aging, occur as a result of orbital bleeding techniques, occur secondary to phototoxicity, or be inherited [27, 47, 59–66]. It is reported that the prevalence of senile retinal degeneration in the 2-year-old Wistar rat may be as high as 10 % [60]. In addition, retinal degeneration can be a toxicologic effect [53]. Care should be taken to evaluate retinal "blanching" in combination with the temperament and restraint required to examine a particular animal. Excessive restraint will result in apparent retinal degeneration.

As rats age, the prevalence of corneal, lenticular, and retinal abnormalities will increase and in a 2-year chronic study abnormalities may be found in >50 % of the animals examined [29, 38].

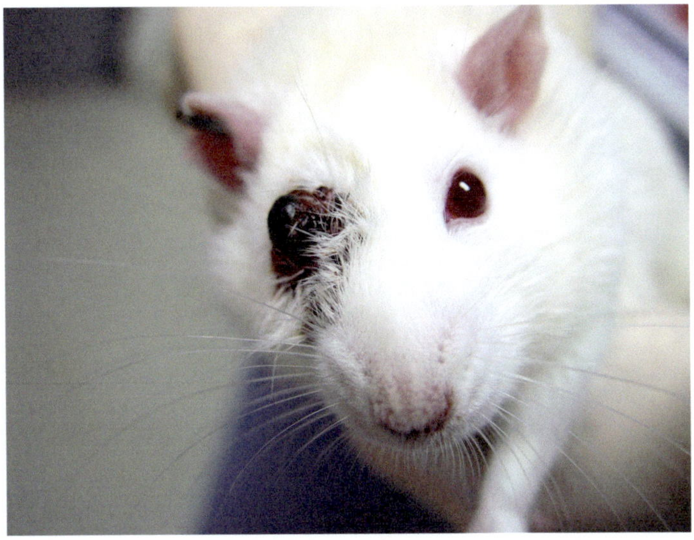

Fig. 46 Marked exophthalmos and exposure keratitis are observed secondary to the trauma of orbital bleeding

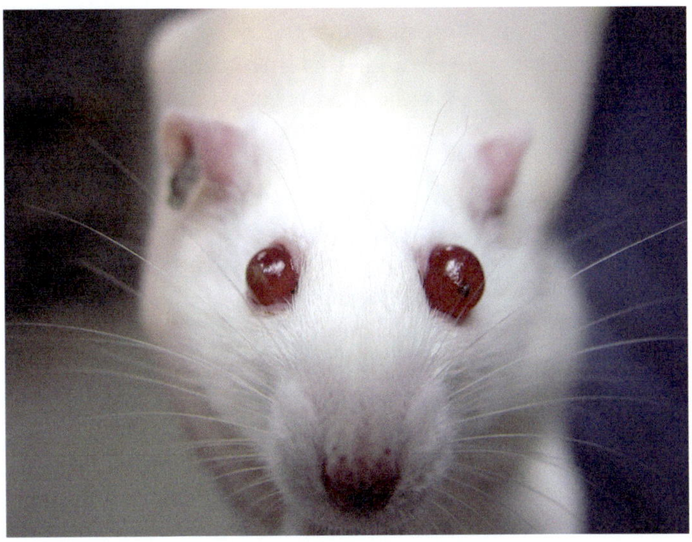

Fig. 47 Bilateral exophthalmos secondary to orbital bleeding

There is also often a sex predilection with corneal and possibly lens abnormalities seen more often in males than females.

The technique of orbital bleeding may be used to collect venous blood from the retrobulbar sinus of rodents during a study [8, 9]. Most often one side is preferred, usually the right. The side effects of orbital bleeding can be severe and include exophthalmos, corneal rupture, exposure keratitis, retinal degeneration, hyphema, cataract, and phthisis bulbi (Figs. 44, 46, 47, and 48). The frequency of these

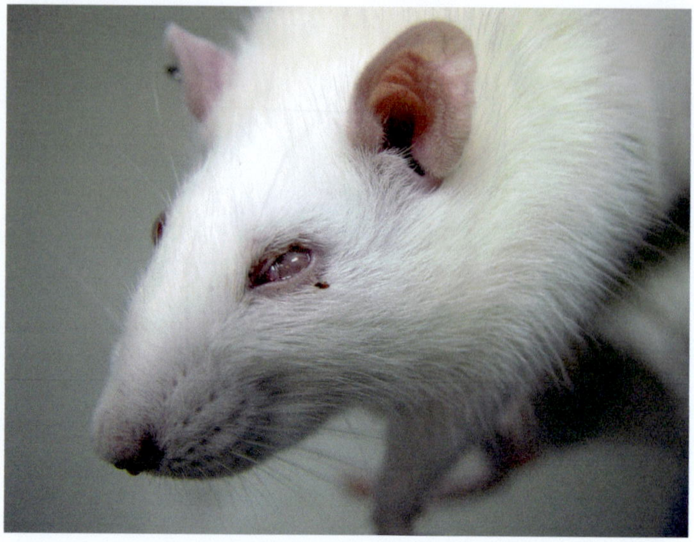

Fig. 48 Unilateral phthisis bulbi secondary to orbital bleeding

complications likely relates directly to the skill of the individual performing the procedure. However, complications are frequent enough that the technique should be discouraged, especially in studies that require ophthalmic examination.

If a rodent study requires general anesthesia the ophthalmologist can expect exacerbation of corneal dystrophy and in some instances cataract formation. Xylazine has been incriminated as being cataractogenic in one study [58].

Chromodacryorrhea appears as a red-brown periorbital discharge (Fig. 49) [8, 9, 47]. Ocular irritation, respiratory infection, stress, and SDA (coronavirus) can all result in chromodacryorrhea [67]. Irritation can occur from something as simple as a diet formulation change in an effort to get a test article into the feed.

Sprague–Dawley

Corneal dystrophy is common affecting 20–50 % of animals in the author's clinical experience. This is higher than what is reported in the literature most likely due to the failure to use biomicroscopy in several published reports. Corneal dystrophy appears more prevalent in males than females and increases in prevalence with age [23, 35, 36, 46]. In the Sprague–Dawley, the lesions of corneal dystrophy involve the axial cornea and appear as fine granules or crystals in the subepithelial stroma (Fig. 17). A basement membrane dystrophy and calcium deposits are noted histologically and ultrastructurally (Fig. 42). The severity is generally mild, keratitis is uncommon, and prevalence increases with age. Rats as young as a few weeks of age can be affected.

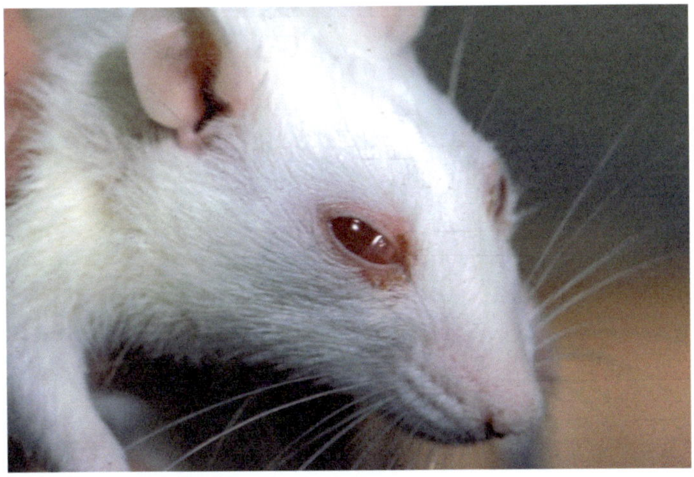

Fig. 49 Conjunctivitis and chromodacryorhea in a Sprague–Dawley rat

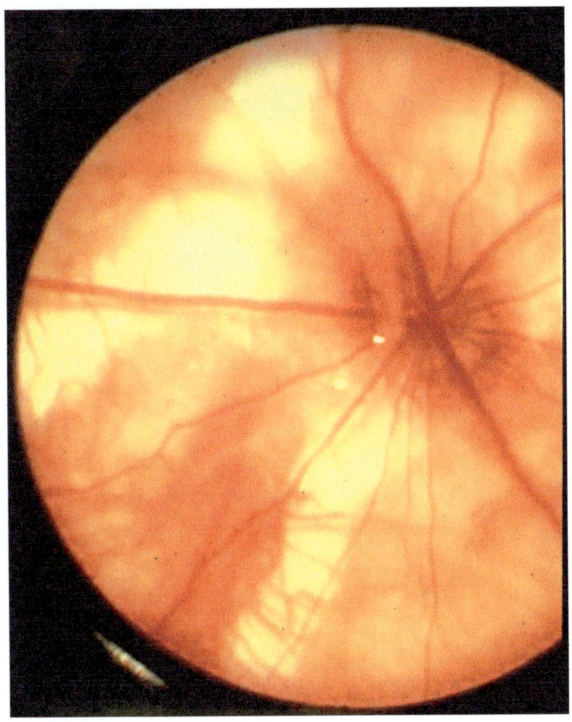

Fig. 50 Linear retinopathy in a Sprague–Dawley rat

Lens opacities in the Sprague–Dawley aged 101–134 weeks have been reported to be 18–21 % [54, 55]. A chorioretinal abnormality, termed linear retinopathy, retinochoroidal degeneration/atrophy, retinal dysplasia, or choroidal coloboma, is described in 7–10-week-old Sprague–Dawley rats (Fig. 50) [23, 27, 29, 35, 68]. Histologically the lesion is characterized by thinning of the outer

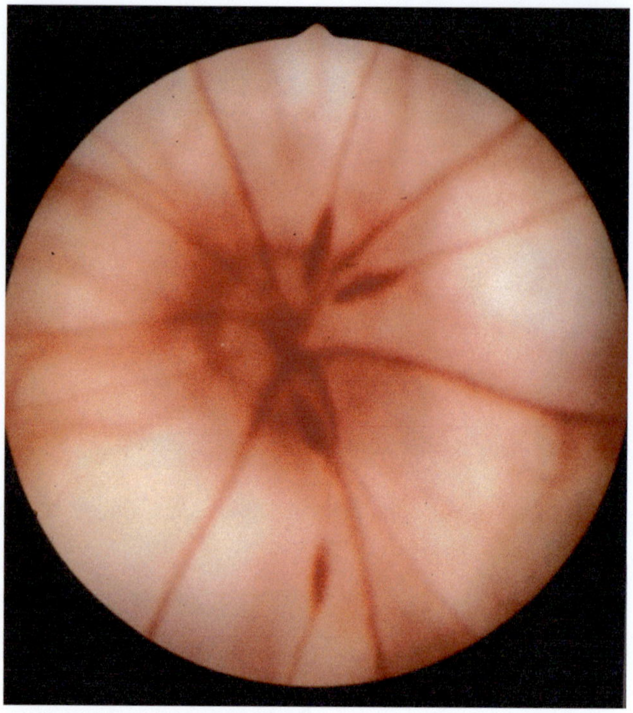

Fig. 51 Saccular aneurysms in a Sprague–Dawley rat

retina and choroid [53]. Posterior segment vascular anomalies have been described in the Sprague–Dawley and may include a preretinal vascular loop and saccular aneurysms (Fig. 51) [51]. In one study this was observed in 12 % of rats examined [27].

Fisher 344

I have never examined a Fisher 344 that did not have corneal dystrophy (Fig. 19); in my clinical experience the prevalence is 100 %. It should be noted that papers citing prevalence below this often fail to examine using biomicroscopy [33, 34]. When compared to the Sprague–Dawley the lesions in the Fischer 344 are more numerous and larger and may have a linear pattern in the axial cornea. As the Fischer 344 rat ages, the corneal dystrophy severity score is expected to increase and keratitis, corneal vascularization, and corneal ulceration may occur in association with corneal dystrophy. In addition to corneal dystrophy, in one report affected rats were also found to have basement membrane changes in other organs [34]. Corneal changes are characterized histologically by thickened, fragmented, and mineralized corneal basement membranes. These lesions have also been described to be associated with limbal inflammatory reaction which may be the precursor to the keratitis and vascularization. It should be noted that as corneal dystrophy in the Fisher 344 worsens clinically the opacities increase in size and density. The overlying epithelium will become elevated, as the dystrophy becomes a space-occupying lesion. Histologically, the epithelium overlying a severe area of dystrophy will be thin and possibly keratinizing indicating irritation. It is this space-occupying, foreign-body effect combined with the disruption of the corneal epithelial basement membrane that results in corneal vascularization and keratitis. It has been the author's experience that in some instances dystrophy will even result in the loss of the overlying corneal epithelium exposing the underlying basement membrane and possibly the corneal stroma. Severity may be more severe in males.

Wistar

Corneal dystrophy has been reported to affect >65 % of Wistar rats and to be composed of extracellular calcium and phosphorous at the level of the corneal epithelial basement membrane (Fig. 18). In one clinical study, 40/43 males and 26/29 females were affected with an interpalpebral corneal opacity [32, 36, 37]. Histologically, the lesions are located at the level of the basement membrane and consist of calcium and phosphorus [32]. Clinically, when compared to the Sprague–Dawley rat the axial corneal lesions in the Wistar are larger, linear, and more opaque.

Another biomicroscopy study found lenticular water clefts in 5 and 13 % of 1-year-old female and male Wistar rats and in 30 and 48 % of 2-year-old female and male Wistar rats. The same study found cortical/nuclear lens opacities in approximately 20 % of 2-year-old male/female Wistars and posterior capsular opacities in up to 37 and 67 % of 2-year-old female and male Wistars [38].

A retinal dystrophy/degeneration has been reported in the Wistar rat [69]. It is reported that the prevalence of senile retinal degeneration in the 2-year-old Wistar rat may be as high as 10 % [60].

2.4.3 Rabbit

Rabbits have long been used in ophthalmic and toxicologic research for topical irritancy testing (Draize, modified Hackett–McDonald) [10, 70], contact lens evaluation, ocular pharmacology, intraocular device biocompatibility, and intravitreal injection protocols as well as in systemic toxicity studies. The most common rabbits examined in toxicologic studies are New Zealand white (NZW) and American Dutch Belted. Most rabbits are found to be normal on routine ophthalmic examination. The eye of the rabbit may be albinotic or pigmented and has a single nasolacrimal punctum, a merangiotic fundus, and deep physiologic optic disc cup with a heavily myelinated optic nerve termed a medullary ray [71].

Congenital and spontaneous sporadic findings include optic nerve coloboma, corneal dystrophy, cataract, glaucoma, epiphora, pseudopterygium, and dacryocytitis (Figs. 7, 52, 53, and 54). Corneal dystrophy has been reported in American Dutch Belted and NZW rabbit (Fig. 21) [25, 72] and can also occur as a result of diet.

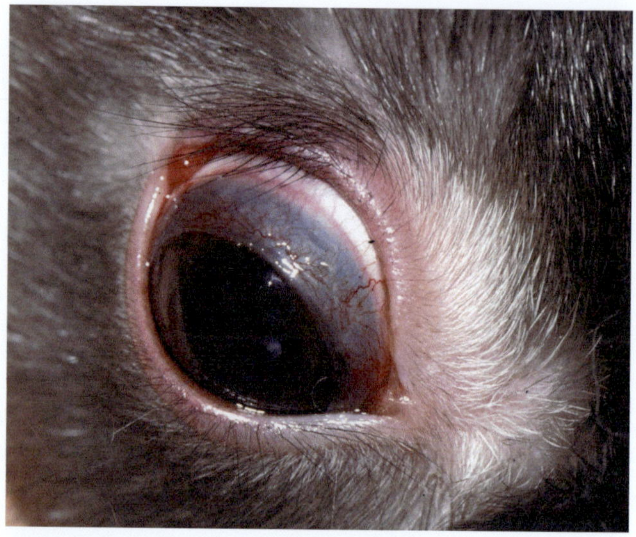

Fig. 52 Conjunctival overgrowth in a Dutch Belted rabbit

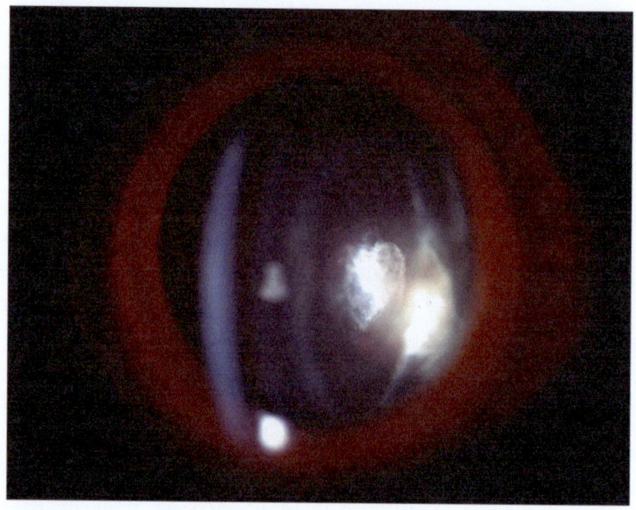

Fig. 53 Slit lamp of a posterior cortical immature cataract in a New Zealand white rabbit

In corneal dystrophy of the Dutch Belted rabbit there is a thickening of the corneal basement membrane and a thinning and disorganization of the overlying corneal epithelium [25]. In the Watanabe rabbit, altered lipid metabolism may be associated with corneal lipidosis especially when fed a high-fat diet (Fig. 55) [43, 73]. Inherited glaucoma and associated buphthalmia are seen in the NZW rabbit and occur as the result of goniodysgenesis with the mode of inheritance being autosomal recessive (bu/bu gene) [74–76]. IOP increases beginning at 1–3 months of age with resulting buphthalmia [77].

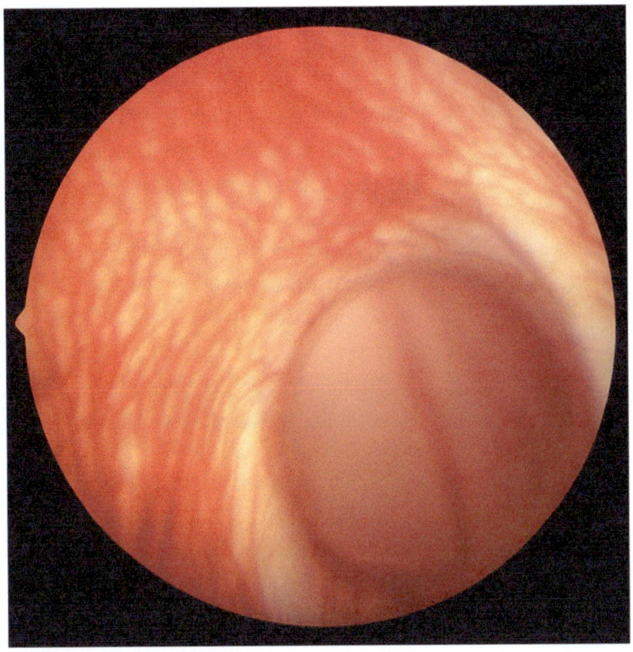

Fig. 54 A coloboma involving the optic nerve and adjacent structures is noted in pretest examination

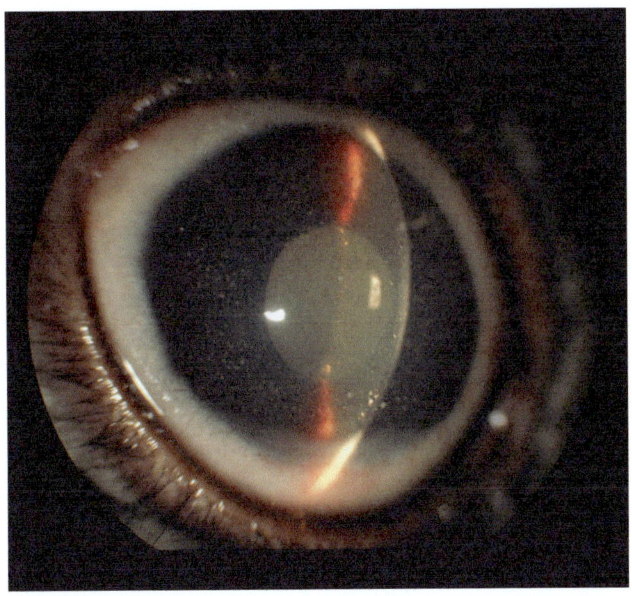

Fig. 55 Slit lamp examination of a Watanabe rabbit with lipid aqueous flare and corneal lipidosis

2.4.4 Nonhuman Primate

The use of NHPs in toxicologic research seems to have become more common over the past 10 years with cynomolgus and rhesus monkeys the most commonly examined. The ocular anatomy of the NHP is similar to that of man with a canal of Schlemm for aqueous outflow, well-developed accommodative abilities, a central retinal artery, and a fovea resulting in a visual acuity and color vision similar to humans (Fig. 29) [9, 78, 79]. As with other species, there can be variations in pigment distribution and amount in the fundus and the examiner needs to be familiar with normal variations [80].

For safety purposes, NHPs are generally examined under a short-acting general anesthetic such as ketamine with the mydriatic administered following sedation. The examiner will generally be required to wear gloves (usually double glove), a Tyvec® jump suit, surgical bouffant, and a mask. Safety goggles are advised until the animals are anesthetized and you are examining the eyes.

Traumatic lesions are most common and may include eyelid lacerations and corneal scars. In addition, traumatic cataract and retinal scars have been noted. Focal iris nevi are not considered abnormal and are observed not infrequently. In one study of 2,100 wild-caught cynomolgus monkeys 167 animals (7.95 %) had 185 findings, the majority of which involved the posterior segment [24]. The lesions of the posterior segment are predominately chorioretinal scars [28]. Glaucoma has been described in several species of NHPs [81] as has macular degeneration [82, 83] and cataract [84, 85].

3 Additional Ophthalmic Diagnostic Procedures

There are numerous noninvasive ophthalmic diagnostic techniques that, depending on the tissue of interest, can provide both structural and functional information of both the anterior and posterior segments of the eye. Some of the more common techniques are discussed below and a more detailed discussion of these and additional techniques as they apply to toxicologic, ophthalmic research and clinical application has recently been published [86, 87].

3.1 Tonometry

Tonometry is used to measure and obtain an indirect measurement of the IOP. There are several methods that are considered portable and they include indentation, applanation, and rebound tonometry. Of these, indentation tonometry, utilizing the Schiotz tonometer, would be considered inaccurate and unreliable and so it should not be used for laboratory studies. As all tonometers are originally designed for the human cornea, readings in animals may be slightly inaccurate, but provided the same tonometer is used throughout a study, the changes in IOP will still remain valid [88–97].

The IOP in most laboratory animals will range between 12 and 25 mmHg and there should be ≤ 5 mmHg difference between the two eyes. The IOP can be affected by restraint techniques, animal

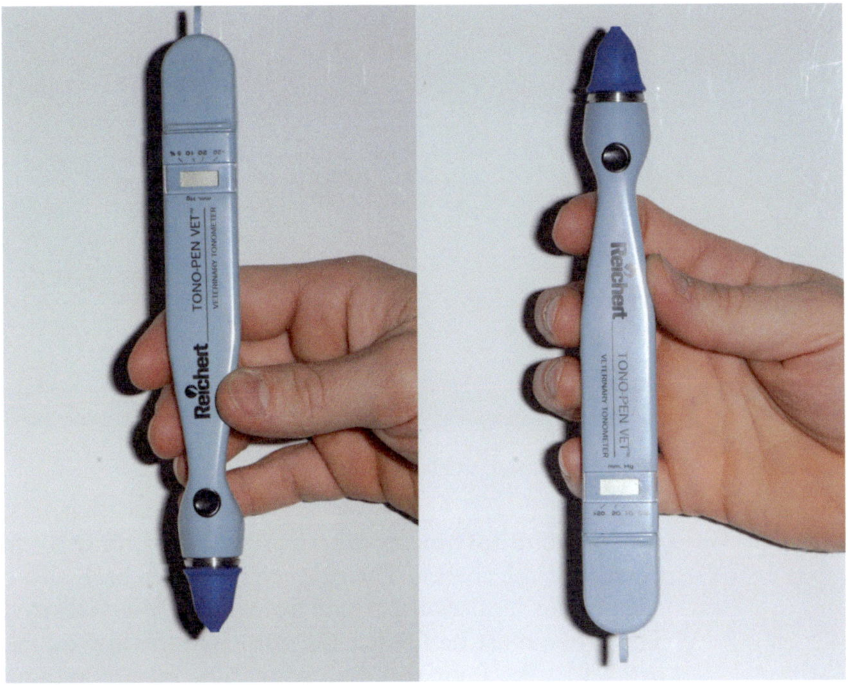

Fig. 56 A Tonopen Vet® being calibrated prior to use

stress, diurnal or circadian rhythm [92, 98], eye position, sedation or anesthesia, corneal thickness, and several other variables. If possible, the IOP should be obtained for all animals at the same general time of day throughout the study and by the same examiner, using the same tonometer, same handling personnel, and same technique each time. Determination of IOP should be performed prior to pharmacologic dilation. When IOP is a critical aspect of a study, it is also advisable for the animals to be acclimatized to both the procedure and restraint techniques prior to study initiation.

Applanation tonometry is most commonly performed using the Tonpen XL®, Tonopen Vet®, Tonopen Avia®, or pneumotonograph. It requires topical anesthesia of which 0.5 % proparacaine is the most common topical ophthalmic anesthetic of choice. This technique measures the force required to applanate or flatten a given area of cornea and then converts this into an IOP value in mmHg. These tonometers have the advantage of being able to be self-calibrated for a GLP study (Fig. 56) and the pneumotonograph can also provide a hard paper copy for record keeping. The Tonpen XL and Tonopen Vet® obtain four independent readings, average them, and indicate both the IOP and the % error indicating the variability between the four readings obtained. The Tonopen Avia® obtains ten independent readings, averages them, and reports the IOP and reports the variability in readings as a % confidence. For the Tonopen XL® the % error should be <5 % and for the Tonopen Avia® the % confidence should be >95 %.

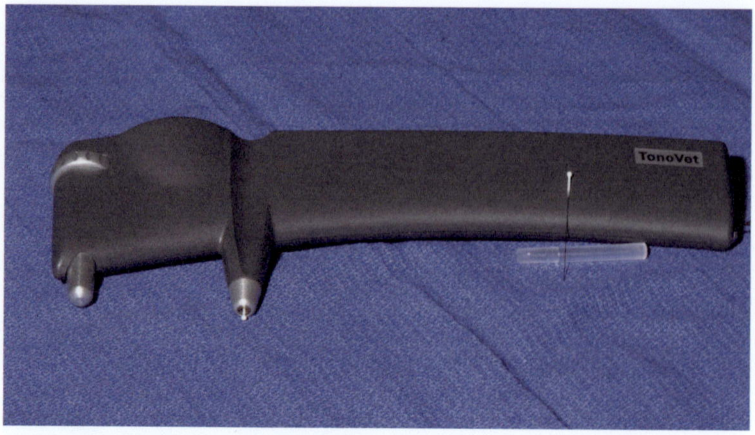

Fig. 57 A Tonovet® rebound tonometer

Rebound tonometry determines IOP by firing a small plastic tip against the cornea. The tip then rebounds back into the device creating an induction current from which the IOP is calculated. The probe must be fired at the cornea in the horizontal position, parallel to the floor to be accurate. The most common rebound tonometer for laboratory animals is the Tonovet® (Fig. 57). Unfortunately the Tonovet® is most specifically calibrated for the dog and horse, but it has been used reliably in other species [95–97, 99–103]. It has the advantage of not requiring topical anesthesia and seems to obtain the IOP more easily than the Tonpen® in many laboratory animals including the dog, rabbit, and rat. Its disadvantage is that it cannot be self-calibrated prior to use. Like the Tonopen® the Tonovet® also averages six readings and gives an indication of % error using a bar at the left of the IOP value. There should be no error bar or the bar should be at the left ventral aspect of the screen for a reading to be acceptable.

Regardless of the tonometer used, typically a minimum of 2–3 final averaged readings per eye should be obtained and recorded. As both the Tonpen® and Tonovet® give only digital readouts, the IOP must be either hand recorded or entered into a computer database as no permanent record is created by the device.

3.2 Pachymetry

Pachymetry is the evaluation of corneal thickness. It is most commonly performed by use of a contact ultrasound specifically designed for this purpose, but the corneal thickness measurement can also be obtained by high-resolution ultrasound or OCT. Pachymetry allows evaluation of subtle changes in corneal thickness prior to the appearance of clinically detectable corneal edema on biomicroscopy. The corneal thickness varies between species, but also varies by region of the cornea (axial vs. peripheral). As a result of the regional variation readings must be obtained from the same region of the cornea, usually axially, at each time point.

3.3 Fluorescein Staining

Sodium fluorescein to evaluate the cornea is routinely used in studies involving topical ophthalmic drug administration and contact lens evaluation and other studies that use the modified Hackett–McDonald scoring system [10]. Fluorescein is a water-soluble dye that is retained by the hydrophilic corneal stroma, but not by the corneal epithelium. It is used to evaluate for corneal epithelial defects and can also be used in evaluation of the pre-corneal tear film. Fluorescein is available in individual impregnated strips that are moistened at the time of use using sterile saline. The moistened strip is gently applied to the dorsal sclera taking care not to contact the cornea. The excess fluorescein is then gently irrigated from the eye using a gravity-fed stream of saline rather than a forced high-velocity stream. The eye is then examined by the ophthalmologist using a biomicroscope and the cobalt blue filter to excite the fluorescein should any remain following irrigation.

3.4 Photographic Documentation

Ophthalmic photography may be used to demonstrate a lack of change in an area like the fundus, to document abnormalities, or to monitor progression of a lesion. Serial photographs taken at various time points during a study will allow comparison to accurately establish whether an abnormality is static or progressive. As photography adds additional time, cost, and animal stress, it is not routinely performed in all studies. Rather it is in a study protocol as an option to be used to document a lesion when observed or for studies where abnormalities are more likely to occur, such as with an intraocular implant, or for intravitreal injection studies.

Photography can be divided into external and intraocular. External photography can be performed using a standard SLR digital camera with a macro lens or with a digital Kowa Genesis-D fundus camera with the diopter settings adjusted to allow external and anterior segment imaging (Fig. 58). Photography of the posterior segment requires some type of fundus camera and the digital Kowa Genesis-D camera is suitable for most routine laboratory animal photography. The Kowa Genesis-D can also be adapted for indirect ophthalmic photography, rodent fundus photography, and fluorescein angiography [61]. In addition, alternate methods for fundus photography in small rodents have been described [104–108]. The advantages of fundus photography are the ability to have a permanent stored record to compare potential study-related findings and if indicated to obtain an independent review by another ophthalmologist [86].

When obtaining photographs, the magnification and illumination settings should be standardized for all images. In addition, the eyes (left vs. right) should be photographed in the same order and all photographs should be accompanied by an animal identification photograph and a photographic log should be maintained as part of SOP.

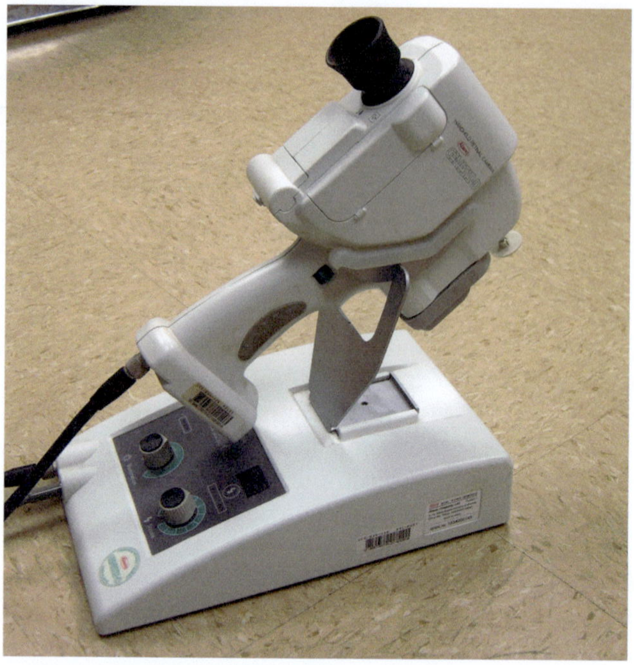

Fig. 58 A Kowa Genesis-D® fundus camera

3.5 Fluorescein Angiography

Fluorescein angiography is used to evaluate the vascular integrity of the intraocular arteriolar and venous vasculature. While it is most commonly used for examination of the retinal and choroidal vessels, it can be applied to iris vasculature as well. It is most frequently used in toxicology studies to evaluate a compounds effect on neovascularization. It has been applied to various laboratory animals with 10 % fluorescein most commonly used, but with the use of indocyanine green also described [61, 82, 108–117].

The technique of fluorescein angiography requires sedation or anesthesia and pupil dilation [115]. The excitable compound, fluorescein, is injected intravenously and a series of timed images of the tissue of interest (chorioretinal, iris) are obtained. Complications associated with fluorescein injection may include extravasation and tissue irritation, vomiting, and anyphylaxis. An excitation filter (490 nm) and a barrier filter (520–520 nm) must be used on a fundus camera that is capable of taking multiple, rapid sequenced images. The Kowa Genesis-Df is designed for fluorescein angiography and is portable. Prior to injection a baseline color image is obtained and then sequential black and white images are taken every 20 s. As the fluorescein fills the chorioretinal vasculature various phases of vascular filling are described. They include the prearteriolar, retinal arteriolar, capillary, early venous, late venous, and recirculation. Abnormalities noted on fluorescein angiography may include vascular anomalies (aneurysms, neovascularization), blocked fluorescence, leakage of fluorescein, hypofluorescence, and hyperfluorescence.

3.6 Electroretinography/Visual Evoked Potential

Depending on the toxicologic study and the specific aspect of the visual system that may be affected, there are various electrophysiologic tests that are available to evaluate the retina and visual pathways. Electroretinography (ERG) is the measurement of the electrical potential generated by the retina when stimulated by light. The standard ERG is a full-field stimulation that provides information about the retina as a whole and is a mass response of the retinal pigment epithelium, photoreceptors, and inner retinal layer [87]. For localized retinal evaluation the multifocal electroretinogram (mfERG) and for evaluation of macular ganglion cells the pattern reversal electroretinogram (PERG) are indicated [87]. To evaluate the entire visual pathway from the retina to the visual cortex, a VEP is the technique of choice [87]. Of these tests, the full-field ERG is most common for preclinical toxicologic testing. The ERG provides a noninvasive means of repeatedly assessing retinal function that in combination with indirect ophthalmoscopy and histology provides integrated assessment of retinal anatomy and function.

The ERG should be conducted in a standardized manner following pupil dilation and there are standardized protocols developed for human and canine ERGs that can serve as a study design guide [118, 119]. The conditions for obtaining a full-field ERG must be consistent with respect to room illumination, dark adaptation, flash intensity and frequency, and sedation or anesthetic used and their dosage. Discussion of these details and protocols is provided elsewhere and is beyond the scope of this chapter [87, 118, 119].

3.7 Optical Coherence Tomography

OCT is a high-resolution, noninvasive imaging technique that can provide a real-time cross-sectional imaging of ocular structures, most commonly retina and optic nerve, at an axial resolution of 2–10 μm [1, 120–122]. It can also be used to image the anterior segment of the eye. Like many advanced imaging techniques it requires sedation or anesthesia, pupil dilation, and specialized equipment. When imaged by OCT, all individual retinal layers can be seen and their thickness measured to allow a quantitative and repeated evaluation of all retinal layers over time. The optic disc can be measured with respect to the cup area, disc area, cup diameter, disc diameter, and rim area [121]. Evaluation of the anterior segment by OCT provides structural information of the cornea, anterior chamber, iris, and iridocorneal angle without the need for corneal contact as is required for ultrasound biomicroscopy (UBM) [121]. It also provides greater axial resolution than that provided by UBM [121]. The use of OCT in laboratory animals has been well described in a variety of species and its use is increasing in animal models of human disease and preclinical trials [122–136].

A recent advancement, spectral-domain OCT (SD-OCT), uses a significantly faster, nonmechanical technology than traditional OCT or time-domain OCT (TD-OCT) [122, 124, 137]. SD-OCT simultaneously measures multiple wavelengths of reflected light across a spectrum, hence the name spectral-domain. SD-OCT is 100 times faster than TD-OCT and acquires 40,000 A-scans per second. The increased speed and number of scans translate into higher resolution.

3.8 Specular Microscopy

Specular microscopy provides in vivo, noninvasive imaging of the corneal endothelial cells [86, 138]. It can be performed using a contact or non-contact method. Once visualized, the corneal endothelial cells can be evaluated with regard to cell morphology and can be quantified as to the number of cells per mm [2]. Normal corneal endothelial cells are regular in arrangement and hexagonal in shape. Cells are evaluated for cell density, pleomorphism, and polymegethism. As cell counts vary by age of the animal and region of the cornea these variables must be standardized using animals of the same age and examining the axial cornea. Animals must be sedated or anesthetized to obtain an accurate image and automated systems are available that simplify the technique. Guidelines for specular microscopy in human FDA clinical trials have been established and these can be used as a guideline for preclinical study design [138].

3.9 Confocal Microscopy

In vivo confocal microscopy is a noninvasive method for the microscopic imaging of the living tissues that allows optical sectioning of almost any material with increased axial and lateral spatial resolution and better image contrast [86, 139, 140]. It allows in vivo, noninvasive, real-time images of the eye at magnifications (630×) which allow resolution of anatomical detail at the cellular level [139]. Three-dimensional confocal microscopy of the eye has also been described [141, 142]. Confocal microscopy has been used to image the cornea of various laboratory species including rabbits, rats, and mice [143]. Its use has also been described in dogs, cat, birds, guinea pigs, and horses [144–148]. Confocal microscopy can provide detailed imaging of the corneal architecture at the cellular level of each corneal epithelial cell layer, the epithelial basement membrane, corneal stroma including nerve fibers and keratocytes, Descemet's membrane, and endothelium [86]. While confocal microscopy is most commonly used in the clinical arena [149–153], its use may be indicated to evaluate the cornea and corneal thickness in contact lens studies, to evaluate the stromal keratocytes or corneal endothelium for toxicity, or to monitor wound healing [86, 144].

3.10 Confocal Scanning Laser Ophthalmoscopy

Confocal scanning laser ophthalmoscopy (cSLO) is an ophthalmic imaging technology that uses laser light instead of a bright flash of white light to illuminate the retina en face [154]. The advantages of using cSLO over traditional fundus photography include improved image quality, small depth of focus, suppression of scattered light, patient comfort through less bright light, 3D imaging capability,

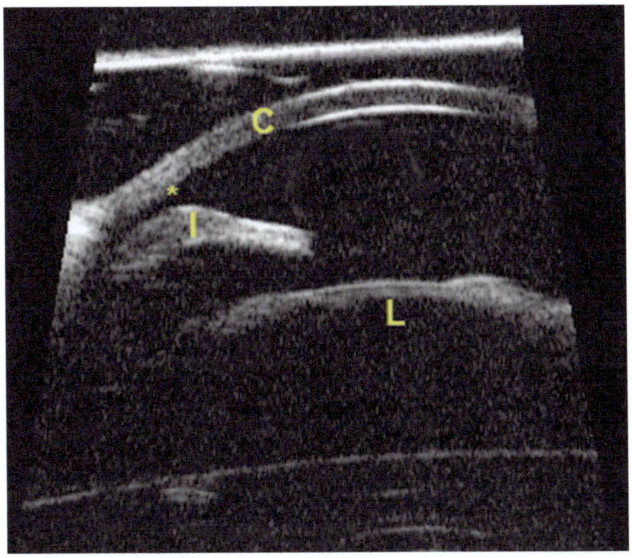

Fig. 59 Ultrasound biomicroscopy of the anterior segment of a canine eye using a 35 mHz transducer. C = cornea, I = iris, L = lens, * = iridocorneal angle

video capability, and effective imaging of patients who do not dilate well. cSLO has been used in several laboratory animal models [124]. When cSLO is combined with SD-OCT the combination provides both en face and cross-sectional imaging of the retina [124].

3.11 Ultrasound and Ultrasound Biomicroscopy

Traditional ocular ultrasound uses frequencies ranging from 7.5 to 20 mHz and is used to image the entire globe and orbit. UBM utilizes higher frequencies (35–50 mHz) to image the anterior segment of the eye, specifically the cornea, iridocorneal angle, iris, ciliary body, and lens (Fig. 59) [86, 155–157]. It can be used to determine corneal thickness, document, and monitor changes in the iridocorneal angle, ciliary cleft, angle opening distance, and anterior chamber depth in response to various pharmacologic agents and in studies of accommodation [86, 158].

References

1. Munger RJ, Collins M (2013) Assessing ocular toxicity potential: basic theory and techniques. In: Weir AB, Collins M (eds) Molecular and integrative toxicology: assessing ocular toxicology in laboratroy animals. Humana, New York, pp 23–52
2. Novack GD (1994) Ocular toxicology. Curr Opin Ophthalmol 5:110–114
3. Novack GD (1995) Ocular toxicology. Curr Opin Ophthalmol 6:108–112
4. Novack GD (1997) Ocular toxicology. Curr Opin Ophthalmol 8:88–92
5. Santaella RM, Fraunfelder FW (2007) Ocular adverse effects associated with systemic medications: recognition and management. Drugs 67:75–93
6. Bill A (1975) Blood circulation and fluid dynamics in the eye. Physiol Rev 55:383–417
7. Bellhorn R (1991) Laboratory animal ophthalmology. In: Gelatt KN (ed) Veterinary ophthalmology, 2nd edn. Lea & Febiger, Philadelphia, PA, pp 656–679
8. Williams DL (2007) Laboratory animal ophthalmology. In: Gelatt KN (ed) Veterinary

ophthalmology, 4th edn. Blackwell Publishing, Ames, IA, pp 1336–1369

9. Williams DL (2013) Laboratory animal ophthalmology. In: Gelatt KN, Gilger BC, Kern TJ (eds) Veterinary ophthalmology, 5th edn. Wiley, Ames, IA, pp 1692–1724
10. Hackett RB, McDonald TO (1996) Ophthalmic toxicology and assessing ocular irritation. In: Marzulli FN, Maibach HI (eds) Dermatotoxicology, 5th edn. Hemisphere Publishing Corp, Washington, DC, pp 749–815
11. Munger RJ (2002) Veterinary ophthalmology in laboratory animal studies. Vet Ophthalmol 5:167–175
12. Jabs DA, Nussenblatt RB, Rosenbaum JT (2005) Standardization of uveitis nomenclature for reporting clinical data. Results of the first international workshop. Am J Ophthalmol 140:509–516
13. Khairallah M (2010) Are the Standardization of the Uveitis Nomenclature (SUN) Working Group criteria for codifying the site of inflammation appropriate for all uveitis problems? Limitations of the SUN Working Group classification. Ocul Immunol Inflamm 18:2–4
14. Nussenblatt RB, Palestine AG, Chan CC et al (1985) Standardization of vitreal inflammatory activity in intermediate and posterior uveitis. Ophthalmology 92:467–471
15. Zierhut M, Deuter C, Murray PI (2007) Classification of uveitis—current guidelines. Eur Ophthal Rev, 77–78
16. Bellhorn RW (1973) Survey of ocular findings in 16- to 24-week-old beagles. J Am Vet Med Assoc 162:139–141
17. Bellhorn RW (1974) A survey of ocular findings in eight- to ten-month-old Beagles. J Am Vet Med Assoc 164:1114–1116
18. Heywood R, Hepworth PL, Van Abbe NJ (1976) Age changes in the eyes of the Beagle dog. J Small Anim Pract 17:171–177
19. Morrin LA, Waring GO 3rd, Spangler W (1982) Oval lipid corneal opacities in beagles: ultrastructure of normal beagle cornea. Am J Vet Res 43:443–453
20. Spangler WL, Waring GO, Morrin LA (1982) Oval lipid corneal opacities in beagles. Vet Pathol 19:150–159
21. Schiavo DM, Field WE (1974) Unilateral focal retinal dysplasia in beagle dogs. Vet Med Small Anim Clin: VM, SAC 69:33–34
22. Schiavo DM, Field WE (1974) The incidence of ocular defects in a closed colony of Beagle dogs. Lab Anim Sci 24:51
23. Taradach C, Greaves P (1984) Spontaneous eye lesions in laboratory animals: incidence in relation to age. Crit Rev Toxicol 12:121–147
24. Kuhlman SM (1992) Prevalence of ophthalmic lesions in wild-caught cynomolgus monkeys. Prog Vet Comp Ophthalmol 2:20–28
25. Moore CP (1987) Anterior corneal dystrophy of American Dutch belted rabbits: biomicroscopic and histopathologic findings. Vet Pathol 24:28–33
26. Poulsom R (1985) Persistent hyaloid vasculature and vitreal hemorrhage in albino rats: a morphological and histological study. Exp Eye Res 40:155–160
27. Hubert MF, Gillet JP, Durand-Cavagna G (1994) Spontaneous retinal changes in Sprague Dawley rats. Lab Anim Sci 44:561–567
28. Schmidt RE (1971) Ophthalmic lesions in non-human primates. Vet Pathol 8:28–36
29. Taradach C, Regnier B, Perraud J (1981) Eye lesions in Sprague–Dawley rats: type and incidence in relation to age. Lab Anim 15:285–287
30. Verhagen C, Rowshani T, Willekens B et al (1995) Spontaneous development of corneal crystalline deposits in MRL/Mp mice. Invest Ophthalmol Vis Sci 36:454–461
31. Van Winkle TJ, Balk MW (1986) Spontaneous corneal opacities in laboratory mice. Lab Anim Sci 36:248–255
32. Wojcinski ZW, Houston B, Gragtmans B et al (1999) A spontaneous corneal change in juvenile Wistar rats. J Comp Pathol 120:281–294
33. Losco PE, Troup CM (1988) Corneal dystrophy in Fischer 344 rats. Lab Anim Sci 38:702–710
34. Bruner RH, Keller WF, Stitzel KA et al (1992) Spontaneous corneal dystrophy and generalized basement membrane changes in Fischer-344 rats. Toxicol Pathol 20:357–366
35. Kuno H, Usui T, Eydelloth RS et al (1991) Spontaneous ophthalmic lesions in young Sprague–Dawley rats. J Vet Med Sci/Jpn Soc Vet Sci 53:607–614
36. Bellhorn RW, Korte GE, Abrutyn D (1988) Spontaneous corneal degeneration in the rat. Lab Anim Sci 38:46–50
37. Eiben R (2001) Frequency of spontaneous opacities in the cornea and lens observed in chronic toxicity studies in Wistar rats: experience with a standardized terminology glossary. Res Commun Pharm Toxicol 6:238–245
38. Wegner A, Kaegler K, Stinn W (2002) Frequency and nature of spontaneous age-related eye lesions observed in 2-year inhalation toxicity study in rats. Ophthalmic Res 34:281–287
39. Vezina M (2013) Comparative ocular anatomy in commonly used laboratory animals. In: Weir AB, Collins M (eds) Molecular

and integrative toxicology: assessing ocular toxicology in laboratroy animals. Humana, New York, pp 1–21

40. Bellhorn RW (1973) A survey of ocular findings in 16- to 24-week-old beagles. JAVMA 162:139–141
41. Bellhorn RW, Bellhorn MB, Swarm RL et al (1975) Hereditary tapetal abnormality in the beagle. Ophthal Res 7:250–260
42. Schiavo DM (1972) Retinopathy from administration of an imidazo quinazoline to beagles. Toxicol Appl Pharmacol 23:782–783
43. Schafer KA, Render JA (2013) Toxicologic pathology of the eye: Preparation and anterior segment. In: Weir AB, Collins M (eds) Molecular and integrative toxicology: assessing ocular toxicology in laboratory animals. Humana, New York, pp 159–217
44. Heywood R (1974) Drug-induced retinopathies in the Beagle dog. Br Vet J 130:564–569
45. Heywood R (1971) Drug-induced lenticular lesions in the dog. Br Vet J 127:301–303
46. Heywood R (1973) Some clinical observations on the eyes of Sprague–Dawley rats. Lab Anim 7:19
47. Williams DL (2002) Ocular disease in rats: a review. Vet Ophthalmol 5:183–191
48. Park SA, Jeong SM, Yi NY et al (2006) Study on the ophthalmic diseases in ICR mice and BALB/c mice. Exp Anim/Jpn Assoc Lab Anim Sci 55:83–90
49. Young C, Festing MF, Barnett KC (1974) Buphthalmos (congenital glaucoma) in the rat. Lab Anim 8:21–31
50. Lee P (1989) Ophthalmic findings in laboratory animals. Anim Eye Res 8:1–12
51. Matsui K, Kuno H (1987) Spontaneous ocular fundus abnormalities in the rat. Anim Eye Res 6:25–41
52. Suckow MA, Weisbroth SH, Franklin CL (2006) The laboratory rat, 2nd edn. Elsevier, Boston, MA
53. Schafer KA, Render JA (2013) Toxicologic pathology of the eye: lens and posterior segment. In: Weir AB, Collins M (eds) Molecular and integrative toxicology: assessing ocular toxicology in laboratory animals. Humana, New York, pp 219–257
54. Balazs T, Ohtake S, Noble JF (1970) Spontaneous lenticular changes in the rat. Lab Anim Care 20:215–219
55. Balazs T, Rubin L (1971) A note on the lens in aging Sprague–Dawley rats. Lab Anim Sci 21:267–268
56. Zigler JS Jr, Hess HH (1985) Cataracts in the Royal College of Surgeons rat: evidence for initiation by lipid peroxidation products. Exp Eye Res 41:67–76
57. Grant WM (1986) Toxicology of the eye, 3rd edn. Charles C. Thomas, Springfield
58. Calderone L, Grimes P, Shalev M (1986) Acute reversible cataract induced by xylazine and by ketamine-xylazine anesthesia in rats and mice. Exp Eye Res 42:331–337
59. Bellhorn RW, Burns MS, Benjamin JV (1980) Retinal vessel abnormalities of phototoxic retinopathy in rats. Investig Ophthalmol Vis Sci 19:584–595
60. Tucker MJ (1997) Special sense organs and associated tissues. In: Tucker MJ (ed) Diseases of the Wistar rat. Taylor and Francis, London, pp 237–245
61. Hawes NL, Smith RS, Chang B et al (1999) Mouse fundus photography and angiography: a catalogue of normal and mutant phenotypes. Mol Vis 5:22
62. Von Sallmann L, Grimes P (1972) Spontaneous retinal degeneration in mature Osborne-Mendel rats. Arch Ophthalmol 88:404–411
63. Lai YL, Jacoby RO, Jonas AM (1978) Age-related and light-associated retinal changes in Fischer rats. Investig Ophthalmol Vis Sci 17:634–638
64. Lai YL, Jacoby RO, Yao PC (1979) Animal model: peripheral retinal degeneration in rats. Am J Pathol 97:449–452
65. DiLoreto D Jr, Ison JR, Bowen GP et al (1995) A functional analysis of the age-related degeneration in the Fischer 344 rat. Curr Eye Res 14:303–310
66. DiLoreto D Jr, Cox C, Grover DA et al (1994) The influences of age, retinal topography, and gender on retinal degeneration in the Fischer 344 rat. Brain Res 647:181–191
67. Weisbroth SH, Peress N (1977) Ophthalmic lesions and dacryoadenitis: a naturally occurring aspect of sialodacryoadenitis virus infection of the laboratory rat. Lab Anim Sci 27:466–473
68. Schardein JL, Lucas JA, Fitzgerald JE (1975) Retinal dystrophy in Sprague–Dawley rats. Lab Anim Sci 25:323–326
69. Lin WL, Essner E (1988) Retinal dystrophy in Wistar-Furth rats. Exp Eye Res 46:1–12
70. Draize JH (1944) Method for the study of irritation and toxicity of substances applied topically to the skin and mucous membranes. J Pharmacol Exp Ther 82:377–384
71. Williams DL (2013) The rabbit. In: Gelatt KN, Gilger BC, Kern TJ (eds) Veterinary ophthalmology, 5th edn. Wiley, Ames, IA, pp 1725–1749

72. Port CD, Dodd DC (1983) Two cases of corneal epithelial dystrophy in rabbits. Lab Anim Sci 33:587–588
73. Garibaldi BA, Goad ME (1988) Lipid keratopathy in the Watanabe (WHHL) rabbit. Vet Pathol 25:173–174
74. Bunt-Milam AH, Dennis MB Jr, Bensinger RE (1987) Optic nerve head axonal transport in rabbits with hereditary glaucoma. Exp Eye Res 44:537–551
75. Knepper PA, Goossens W, McLone DG (1997) Ultrastructural studies of primary congenital glaucoma in rabbits. J Pediatr Ophthalmol Strabismus 34:365–371
76. Fox RR, Crary DD, Babino EJ Jr et al (1969) Buphthalmia in the rabbit. Pleiotropic effects of the (bu) gene and a possible explanation of mode of gene action. J Hered 60:206–212
77. Burrows AM, Smith TD, Atkinson CS et al (1995) Development of ocular hypertension in congenitally buphthalmic rabbits. Lab Anim Sci 45:443–444
78. Fukui M (1983) Observations on the ocular fundus of primates, anthropoids and prosimians. Anim Eye Res 2:10–15
79. Suzuki MT, Narita H, Cho F (1983) Ophthalmoscopic observations of the ocular fundus in colony-born cynomolgus monkeys aged from 0 days to 19 years. Anim Eye Res 2:21–25
80. Dawson WW, Jeffery G, Dawson JC et al (2004) Fundus pigment distribution in rhesus monkeys. Vet Ophthalmol 7:391–396
81. Dawson WW, Brooks DE, Hope GM et al (1993) Primary open angle glaucomas in the rhesus monkey. Br J Ophthalmol 77:302–310
82. Dawson WW, Ulshafer RJ, Engel HM et al (1989) Macular disease in related rhesus monkeys. Doc Ophthalmol Adv Ophthalmol 71:253–263
83. Suzuki MT, Ogawa H, Cho F (1989) Visual function in cynomolgus monkeys with macular degeneration. Anim Eye Res 8:33–38
84. Beltran WA, Vanore M, Ollivet F et al (2007) Ocular findings in two colonies of gray mouse lemurs (Microcebus murinus). Vet Ophthalmol 10:43–49
85. Souri E (1973) Eye diseases in two families of animals. Vet Med Small Anim Clin: VM, SAC 68:1011–1014
86. Nork TM, Rasmussen CA, Christian BJ et al (2013) Emerging imaging technologies for assessing ocular toxicity in laboratory animals. In: Weir AB, Collins M (eds) Molecular and integrative toxicology: assessing ocular toxicology in laboratroy animals. Humana, New York, pp 53–121
87. Ver Hoeve JN, Munger RJ, Gourley IM et al (2013) Emerging electrophysiological technologies for assessing ocular toxicity in laboratory animals. In: Weir AB, Collins M (eds) Molecular and integrative toxicology: assessing ocular toxicology in laboratroy animals. Humana, New York, pp 123–157
88. Lim KS, Wickremasinghe SS, Cordeiro MF et al (2005) Accuracy of intraocular pressure measurements in New zealand white rabbits. Investig Ophthalmol Vis Sci 46:2419–2423
89. Acosta AC, Espana EM, Nose I et al (2007) Estimation of intraocular pressure in rabbits with commonly used tonometers. Ophthal Surg Lasers Imaging 38:43–49
90. Abrams LS, Vitale S, Jampel HD (1996) Comparison of three tonometers for measuring intraocular pressure in rabbits. Investig Ophthalmol Vis Sci 37:940–944
91. Leiva M, Naranjo C, Pena MT (2006) Comparison of the rebound tonometer (ICare) to the applanation tonometer (Tonopen XL) in normotensive dogs. Vet Ophthalmol 9:17–21
92. Pereira FQ, Bercht BS, Soares MG et al (2011) Comparison of a rebound and an applanation tonometer for measuring intraocular pressure in normal rabbits. Vet Ophthalmol 14:321–326
93. Suzuki MT, Narita H, Park SW (1993) What are the optimal tonometers for different animals species: cynomologous monkey. Anim Eye Res 12:41–46
94. Moore CG, Milne ST, Morrison JC (1993) Noninvasive measurement of rat intraocular pressure with the Tono-Pen. Investig Ophthalmol Vis Sci 34:363–369
95. Kontiola AI, Goldblum D, Mittag T et al (2001) The induction/impact tonometer: a new instrument to measure intraocular pressure in the rat. Exp Eye Res 73:781–785
96. Goldblum D, Kontiola AI, Mittag T et al (2002) Non-invasive determination of intraocular pressure in the rat eye. Comparison of an electronic tonometer (TonoPen), and a rebound (impact probe) tonometer. Graefe's Arch Clin Exp Ophthalmol 240:942–946
97. Danias J, Kontiola AI, Filippopoulos T et al (2003) Method for the noninvasive measurement of intraocular pressure in mice. Investig Ophthalmol Vis Sci 44:1138–1141
98. Rowland JM, Potter DE, Reiter RJ (1981) Circadian rhythm in intraocular pressure: a rabbit model. Curr Eye Res 1:169–173
99. Wang X, Dong J, Wu Q (2013) Twenty-four-hour measurement of IOP in rabbits using rebound tonometer. Vet Ophthalmol. doi:10.1111/vop.12020

100. Johnson TV, Fan S, Toris CB (2008) Rebound tonometry in conscious, conditioned mice avoids the acute and profound effects of anesthesia on intraocular pressure. J Ocul Pharmacol Ther 24:175–185
101. Lobler M, Rehmer A, Guthoff R et al (2011) Suitability and calibration of a rebound tonometer to measure IOP in rabbit and pig eyes. Vet Ophthalmol 14:66–68
102. McLellan GJ, Kemmerling JP, Kiland JA (2013) Validation of the TonoVet(R) rebound tonometer in normal and glaucomatous cats. Vet Ophthalmol 16:111–118
103. Rusanen E, Florin M, Hassig M et al (2010) Evaluation of a rebound tonometer (Tonovet) in clinically normal cat eyes. Vet Ophthalmol 13:31–36
104. Paques M, Guyomard JL, Simonutti M et al (2007) Panretinal, high-resolution color photography of the mouse fundus. Investig Ophthalmol Vis Sci 48:2769–2774
105. Guyomard JL, Rosolen SG, Paques M et al (2008) A low-cost and simple imaging technique of the anterior and posterior segments: eye fundus, ciliary bodies, iridocorneal angle. Investig Ophthalmol Vis Sci 49:5168–5174
106. Link D, Strohmaier C, Seifert BU et al (2011) Novel non-contact retina camera for the rat and its application to dynamic retinal vessel analysis. Biomed Opt Express 2:3094–3108
107. Hernandez V, Albini T, Lee W et al (2012) A portable, contact animal fundus imaging system based on Rol's GRIN lenses. Vet Ophthalmol 15:141–144
108. DiLoreto D Jr, Grover DA, del Cerro C et al (1994) A new procedure for fundus photography and fluorescein angiography in small laboratory animal eyes. Curr Eye Res 13:157–161
109. Satoh T, Yamaguchi K (2000) Ocular fundus abnormalities detected by fluorescein and indocyanine green angiography in the Royal College of Surgeons dystrophic rat. Exp Anim 49:275–280
110. Herren JI, Kunzelman KS, Vocelka C et al (1998) Angiographic and histological evaluation of porcine retinal vascular damage and protection with perfluorocarbons after massive air embolism. Stroke 29:2396–2403
111. Gelatt KN, Henderson JD, Steffen GR (1976) Fluorescein angiography of the normal and diseased ocular fundi of the laboratory dog. J Am Vet Med Assoc 169:9
112. Ninomiya H, Kuno H, Inagaki S (2005) Vascular changes associated with chorioretinal and optic nerve colobomas in rats (Crj: CD (SD), IGS). Vet Ophthalmol 8:319–323
113. Kommonen B, Koskinen L (1984) Fluorescein angiography of the canine ocular fundus in ketamine-xylazine anesthesia. Acta Vet Scand 25:346–351
114. Narfstrom K (1985) Progressive retinal atrophy in the Abyssinian cat. Clinical characteristics. Invest Ophthalmol Vis Sci 26:193–200
115. Gasthuys F, Pollet L, Simoens P et al (1990) Anaesthesia for fluorescein angiography of the ocular fundus in the miniature pig. Vet Res Commun 14:393–402
116. Hyvarinen L, Flower RW (1980) Indocyanine green fluorescence angiography. Acta Ophthalmol 58:528–538
117. Flower RW (1973) Injection technique for indocyanine green and sodium fluorescein dye angiography of the eye. Investig Ophthalmol 12:881–895
118. Ekesten B, Komaromy AM, Ofri R, et al. (2013) Guidelines for clinical electroretinography in the dog: 2012 update. Doc Ophthalmol 2013 Jun 1 Epub
119. Marmor MF, Fulton AB, Holder GE et al (2009) ISCEV standard for full-field clinical electroretinography (2008 update). Doc Ophthalmol 118:69–77
120. Fujimoto JG, Pitris C, Boppart SA et al (2000) Optical coherence tomography: an emerging technology for biomedical imaging and optical biopsy. Neoplasia 2:9–25
121. Gabriele ML, Wollstein G, Ishikawa H et al (2011) Optical coherence tomography: history, current status, and laboratory work. Investig Ophthalmol Vis Sci 52:2425–2436
122. McLellan GJ, Rasmussen CA (2012) Optical coherence tomography for the evaluation of retinal and optic nerve morphology in animal subjects: practical considerations. Vet Ophthalmol 15(Suppl 2):13–28
123. Fischer MD, Huber G, Beck SC et al (2009) Noninvasive, in vivo assessment of mouse retinal structure using optical coherence tomography. PLoS One 4:e7507
124. Huber G, Beck SC, Grimm C et al (2009) Spectral domain optical coherence tomography in mouse models of retinal degeneration. Investig Ophthalmol Vis Sci 50:5888–5895
125. Kim KH, Puoris'haag M, Maguluri GN et al (2008) Monitoring mouse retinal degeneration with high-resolution spectral-domain optical coherence tomography. J Vis 8:17.1–17.11
126. Li Q, Timmers AM, Hunter K et al (2001) Noninvasive imaging by optical coherence tomography to monitor retinal degeneration in the mouse. Investig Ophthalmol Vis Sci 42:2981–2989

127. Gabriele ML, Ishikawa H, Schuman JS et al (2010) Reproducibility of spectral-domain optical coherence tomography total retinal thickness measurements in mice. Investig Ophthalmol Vis Sci 51:6519–6523
128. Nagata A, Higashide T, Ohkubo S et al (2009) In vivo quantitative evaluation of the rat retinal nerve fiber layer with optical coherence tomography. Investig Ophthalmol Vis Sci 50:2809–2815
129. Gloesmann M, Hermann B, Schubert C et al (2003) Histologic correlation of pig retina radial stratification with ultrahigh-resolution optical coherence tomography. Investig Ophthalmol Vis Sci 44:1696–1703
130. Gekeler F, Gmeiner H, Volker M et al (2007) Assessment of the posterior segment of the cat eye by optical coherence tomography (OCT). Vet Ophthalmol 10:173–178
131. Huang Y, Cideciyan AV, Papastergiou GI et al (1998) Relation of optical coherence tomography to microanatomy in normal and rd chickens. Investig Ophthalmol Vis Sci 39:2405–2416
132. Cong L, Sun D, Zhang Z et al (2008) A novel rabbit model for studying RPE transplantation. Investig Ophthalmol Vis Sci 49:4115–4125
133. Reiser BJ, Ignacio TS, Wang Y et al (2005) In vitro measurement of rabbit corneal epithelial thickness using ultrahigh resolution optical coherence tomography. Vet Ophthalmol 8:85–88
134. Hosseini K, Kholodnykh AI, Petrova IY et al (2004) Monitoring of rabbit cornea response to dehydration stress by optical coherence tomography. Investig Ophthalmol Vis Sci 45:2555–2562
135. Schuman JS, Pedut-Kloizman T, Pakter H et al (2007) Optical coherence tomography and histologic measurements of nerve fiber layer thickness in normal and glaucomatous monkey eyes. Investig Ophthalmol Vis Sci 48:3645–3654
136. Alario AF, Pirie CG (2013) Intra and interuser reliability of central corneal thickness measurements obtained in healthy feline eyes using a portable spectral-domain optical coherence tomography device. Vet Ophthalmol. doi:10.1111/vop.12029
137. Fleckenstein M, Charbel Issa P, Helb HM et al (2008) High-resolution spectral domain-OCT imaging in geographic atrophy associated with age-related macular degeneration. Investig Ophthalmol Vis Sci 49:4137–4144
138. McCarey BE, Edelhauser HF, Lynn MJ (2008) Review of corneal endothelial specular microscopy for FDA clinical trials of refractive procedures, surgical devices, and new intraocular drugs and solutions. Cornea 27:1–16
139. Cavanagh HD, Jester JV, Essepian J et al (1990) Confocal microscopy of the living eye. CLAO J 16:65–73
140. Nubile M, Mastropasqua L (2009) In vivo confocal microscopy of the ocular surface: where are we now? Br J Ophthalmol 93:850–852
141. Masters BR, Bohnke M (2002) Three-dimensional confocal microscopy of the living human eye. Annu Rev Biomed Eng 4:69–91
142. Masters BR, Bohnke M (1999) Video-rate, scanning slit confocal microscopy of living human cornea in vivo: three-dimensional confocal microscopy of the eye. Methods Enzymol 307:536–563
143. Labbe A, Liang H, Martin C et al (2006) Comparative anatomy of laboratory animal corneas with a new-generation high-resolution in vivo confocal microscope. Curr Eye Res 31:501–509
144. Kafarnik C, Fritsche J, Reese S (2007) In vivo confocal microscopy in the normal corneas of cats, dogs and birds. Vet Ophthalmol 10:222–230
145. Cafaro TA, Ortiz SG, Maldonado C et al (2009) The cornea of Guinea pig: structural and functional studies. Vet Ophthalmol 12:234–241
146. Kafarnik C, Fritsche J, Reese S (2008) Corneal innervation in mesocephalic and brachycephalic dogs and cats: assessment using in vivo confocal microscopy. Vet Ophthalmol 11:363–367
147. Ledbetter EC, Scarlett JM (2009) In vivo confocal microscopy of the normal equine cornea and limbus. Vet Ophthalmol 12 (Suppl 1):57–64
148. Ledbetter EC, Irby NL, Kim SG (2011) In vivo confocal microscopy of equine fungal keratitis. Vet Ophthalmol 14:1–9
149. Babu K, Murthy KR (2007) Combined fungal and acanthamoeba keratitis: diagnosis by in vivo confocal microscopy. Eye 21:271–272
150. Winchester K, Mathers WD, Sutphin JE et al (1995) Diagnosis of Acanthamoeba keratitis in vivo with confocal microscopy. Cornea 14:10–17
151. Grise-Dulac A, Brasnu E, Goldchmidt P et al (2010) In vivo confocal microscopy: a new tool for the diagnosis of Acanthamoeba keratitis. Journal francais d'ophtalmologie 33:383–390
152. Alomar T, Matthew M, Donald F et al (2009) In vivo confocal microscopy in the diagnosis and management of acanthamoeba keratitis

showing new cystic forms. Clin Exp Ophthalmol 37:737–739

153. Winchester K, Mathers WD, Sutphin JE (1997) Diagnosis of Aspergillus keratitis in vivo with confocal microscopy. Cornea 16:27–31
154. Rosolen SG, Saint-MacAry G, Gautier V et al (2001) Ocular fundus images with confocal scanning laser ophthalmoscopy in the dog, monkey and minipig. Vet Ophthalmol 4:41–45
155. Gilger BC, Reeves KA, Salmon JH (2005) Ocular parameters related to drug delivery in the canine and equine eye: aqueous and vitreous humor volume and scleral surface area and thickness. Vet Ophthalmol 8:265–269
156. Aubin ML, Powell CC, Gionfriddo JR et al (2003) Ultrasound biomicroscopy of the feline anterior segment. Vet Ophthalmol 6:15–17
157. Crumley W, Gionfriddo JR, Radecki SV (2009) Relationship of the iridocorneal angle, as measured using ultrasound biomicroscopy, with post-operative increases in intraocular pressure post-phacoemulsification in dogs. Vet Ophthalmol 12:22–27
158. Lutjen-Drecoll E, Kaufman PL, Wasielewski R et al (2010) Morphology and accommodative function of the vitreous zonule in human and monkey eyes. Investig Ophthalmol Vis Sci 51:1554–1564

Methods in Pharmacology and Toxicology (2014): 205–242
DOI 10.1007/7653_2013_8

Published online: 23 August 2013

Study Design and Methodologies for Evaluation of Anti-glaucoma Drugs

Paul E. Miller

Abstract

A large number of factors are important in conducting anti-glaucoma drug efficacy studies. It is essential to have an understanding of aqueous humor dynamics and how the tonometer, tonometrist, and animal may affect IOP estimates. Additional critical considerations in the design of an anti-glaucoma drug efficacy studies include the following: (1) selecting the most appropriate species, (2) identifying the rate of nonresponders within the study population, (3) determining whether normotensive or glaucomatous animals should be used, and deciding (4) what secondary endpoints (if any) to include, and (5) whether one eye or both should be dosed. Anti-glaucoma drug efficacy studies have an acclimation phase in which the animal becomes conditioned to the procedures, a predose phase in which baseline data is collected, a dosing phase in which the drug is administered and IOP and possibly other endpoints are monitored, and a recovery phase in which IOP returns to predose values as the drug is washed out before another predose phase is started.

Key words Glaucoma, Anti-glaucoma drugs, Intraocular pressure, Tonometry, Aqueous humor dynamics, Animal models

1 Introduction

Glaucoma is a group of diseases which result in a characteristic pattern of damage to the optic nerve and subsequently vision loss [1, 2]. In animals with spontaneous glaucoma this injury is believed to be almost always initiated by an abnormal increase in intraocular pressure (IOP) [2]. In humans, however, the relationship between glaucomatous optic neuropathy and IOP appears to be more complex and other risk factors are thought to play significant roles such as the ease with which the lamina cribrosa (the sieve-like portion of the sclera through which the axons of the retinal ganglion cells [RGCs] exit the eye) becomes distorted and vascular alterations in the perfusion of the optic nerve (Fig. 1) [2, 3]. Hence, some humans may exhibit mild increases in IOP with no signs of glaucomatous damage or vision loss (so-called *ocular hypertension*), presumably due to a lamina cribrosa that offers greater resistance to distortion and compression of the optic nerve fibers (RGC axons) passing through it, or due to an increased ability to maintain

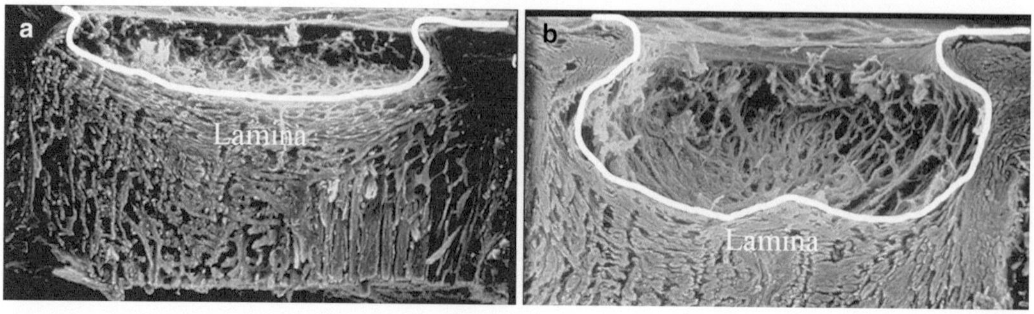

Fig. 1 Scanning electron micrographs of trypsin-digested optic nerve heads from normal (*left*) and advanced glaucoma (*right*) human eyes. The lamina cribrosa is distorted (cupped) in the glaucomatous eye, resulting in damage to the optic nerve fibers which pass through this region. From Downs JC, Roberts MD, Sigel IA (2011) Glaucomatous cupping of the lamina cribrosa: A review of the evidence for active progressive remodeling as a mechanism. Exp Eye Res 93(2):133–140

perfusion of the optic nerve despite increased IOP. Alternatively, up to 1/3 of humans may show glaucomatous damages and vision loss despite having IOPs that are considered to be within the normal range for the population as a whole (so-called *normotensive glaucoma*), presumably due to a more flexible lamina cribrosa or more tenuous perfusion of the optic nerve [4]. Other factors involved in RGC cell death may include deprivation of neuronal growth factors due to impaired axoplasmic flow, peroxynitrile toxicity from increased nitric oxide synthase activity, immune-mediated nerve damage and oxidative stress [3]. Additionally, dying RGCs may release mediators that can lead to vicious cycle of programmed cell death (apoptosis) of previously healthy adjacent RGCs [3]. Because IOP is the only clinical risk factor that can be therapeutically manipulated to date, the overwhelming majority of anti-glaucoma drug studies involve drugs which alter IOP. As our understanding of the pathogenic mechanisms behind glaucomatous optic neuropathy improves, however, numerous other drug targets aimed at preventing RGC cell death or stimulating the regeneration of RGCs will emerge.

1.1 Forms of Glaucoma

Glaucoma occurs in two main forms: primary and secondary [2]. *Secondary glaucoma*, which is infrequently a target of anti-glaucoma drug studies, results when there is another structural abnormality in the eye that leads to impaired outflow from the eye. Examples include obstruction of the outflow pathways by inflammatory debris, red blood cells, or tumor cells; displacement of the lens, occlusion of the pupil, and many others. *Primary glaucoma* occurs when the abnormality lies in the iridocorneal angle or trabecular meshwork. In both forms of glaucoma the iridocorneal angle can be further classified as “open” or “closed” angle by use of a specialized goniolens.

Primary open angle glaucoma (POAG) in humans is the target disorder for most anti-glaucoma drugs [2]. It is a chronic life-long disorder in which IOP slowly increases due to impaired outflow via the trabecular meshwork [2]. It affects 70 million people worldwide [5] and its prevalence increases with age. The prevalence also varies with race, affecting 6 % of whites, 16 % of blacks, and 3 % of Asians over 70 years of age [6]. This high prevalence makes glaucoma the second leading cause of world blindness after cataracts [7]. In part because the IOP increase in POAG is slow, insidious, and painless, glaucoma is undiagnosed in 50 % of patients in developed countries and in nine of ten affected people worldwide [5]. Lowering IOP has been demonstrated to be an effective therapy and typically allows some vision to be maintained in most patients [8, 9]. However, although generally effective [9], current anti-glaucoma drugs often need to be used in combination or as an adjunct to surgery to sufficiently control IOP and typically do not directly target the source of the impairment to outflow in the trabecular meshwork. In the aggregate these clinical features create strong incentives to develop new anti-glaucoma drugs.

1.2 Aqueous Humor and Its Outflow

Aqueous humor is responsible for the supply of nutrients and the removal of metabolic wastes from the avascular tissues of the eye [10]. It also plays a critical role in maintaining the optical clarity of the eye [10]. The production and drainage of aqueous humor are influenced not only by the anatomy of the anterior segment but also by a large number of endogenous compounds, including neurotransmitters, hormones, prostaglandins, proteins, lipids, and proteoglycans [10]. Indeed, so many factors influence the production and drainage of aqueous humor that it is difficult to identify a single pathway, and therefore a single drug, that is capable of dramatically lowering IOP in every patient.

Aqueous humor is produced in the ciliary body by both active secretion (which requires energy and accounts for 80–90 % of aqueous humor production) and passive diffusion/ultrafiltration [10]. Aqueous exits the eye via the conventional (trabecular) and unconventional (uveoscleral) outflow pathways [10]. In the conventional pathway aqueous humor passes from the posterior chamber, through the pupil, into the anterior chamber, into the iridocorneal angle, and into the sponge-like trabecular meshwork (Fig. 2). After filtering between the beams of the trabecular meshwork, aqueous crosses through the endothelial cell membranes of the meshwork to enter a series of radially oriented, blood-free collecting vessels, and ultimately into the episcleral veins or scleral venous plexus and ultimately the general circulation. Contraction of smooth muscle fibers of the ciliary muscle that insert into the trabecular meshwork are capable of increasing drainage of aqueous from the eye by enlarging the spaces in the trabecular meshwork. In the unconventional route aqueous humor passes through the root of the iris and the interstitial spaces of the ciliary muscle to reach the supraciliary space (between the ciliary body and the sclera) or the suprachoroidal space (between the choroid and

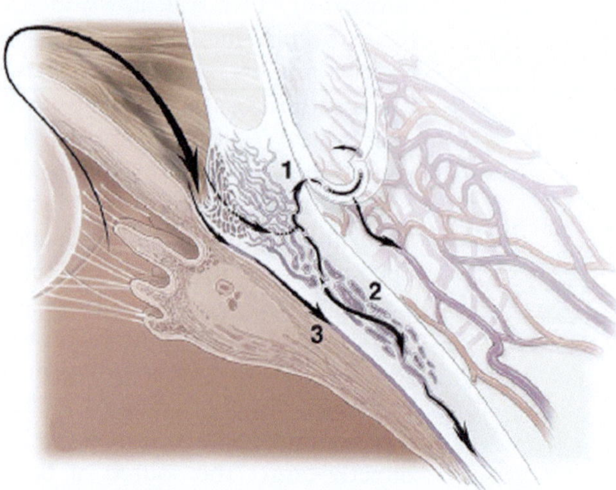

Fig. 2 Outflow pathways of the canine eye, other species are comparable. Aqueous humor is made by the ciliary processes, flows into the posterior chamber and through the pupil into the anterior chamber. From the anterior chamber it may flow into trabecular meshwork and into the angular aqueous plexus and be directed interiorly into more superficial episcleral venues (1) or posterior into the scleral venous plexus and the vortex venous system (2) and eventually into the general circulation. Alternatively, (3) aqueous may pass through the ciliary muscle interstitial to the suprachoroidal space and diffuse through the sclera (uveoscleral outflow) and enter the orbit. From Tsai S, Miller PE, Strule C et al (2012) Topical application of 0.005 % latanoprost increases episcleral venous pressure in normal dogs. Vet Ophthalmol 15 (suppl 1):71–78

the sclera) [10]. From these locations it passes through the sclera into the orbit. In most species the majority of aqueous humor (approximately 50 % in horses, 85 % in dogs, and 97 % in cats) leaves the eye via the traditional outflow route [1].

The relationship between the various components of aqueous humor production and outflow has been described by the following equation [11]:

$$\text{Flow in} = \text{Flow out}$$

$$\text{Rate of formation} = \textit{Pressure gradient across entire outflow pathway} \times \text{Ease with which fluid can exit} + \text{uveosceral outflow}$$

$$F = (P_i - P_e) \times C + U$$

$F =$ rate of aqueous formation in μl/min

$P_i =$ IOP in mmHg

$P_e =$ episcleral venous pressure in mmHg

$C =$ facility of aqueous outflow in μl/min/mmHg

$U =$ Uveoscleral outflow (assumes is pressure independent)

This equation is subject to a number of assumptions and is somewhat simplified, but it conveys the overall relationships between the various components of aqueous humor dynamics and the pathways by which anti-glaucoma drugs alter IOP. Methods have been developed for directly measuring or estimating the various components described above and these form the foundation for determining the mechanism of action of an IOP lowering drug.

2 Measuring IOP

The only method for directly measuring IOP is manometry in which the anterior chamber is cannulated with a fine needle which is connected to fluid filled tubing and ultimately a calibrated pressure transducer. This is an invasive, generally one-time procedure and in living animals introduces numerous artifacts including inflammation (which may occlude the needle and confound results), making it unsuitable for clinical use in which IOP needs to be sequentially followed or in studies that are more than a few hours in duration. Manometry is most frequently used in species in which noninvasive tonometry is difficult, such as rats and mice, or to evaluate how well a given tonometer performs in a specific species [12, 13].

Noninvasive tonometers, however, do not actually measure IOP but instead measure the "tone" of the eye-wall (usually the cornea) and use a mechanical property of that tissue to estimate actual IOP. There are a number of potential inherent errors in these measurements, and most of these instruments are calibrated for the human eye which generally results in an underestimation of true IOP in animals. However, as long as this underestimation is linear over the range of IOP being measured (as determined by comparison with a manometer) the device is still useful in determining the effect of a given test article on IOP (Fig. 3). This linearity makes it generally unnecessary to convert tonometric IOP estimates to "true" IOP values (as determined with a manometer) using equations which describe the relationship between the two instruments. It is also important that normative values be established by tonometer, species, and tonometrist as they may vary considerably [13, 14]. In other words, IOP values with one tonometer in one species by a given tonometrist are not necessarily directly comparable to those acquired with a different tonometer in a different species by a different tonometrist.

There are two principle forms of tonometry in use today: *Applanation* and *Rebound*. Applanation tonometry (as exemplified by the Tono-Pen, Pneumatonometer, Perkins and Goldmann tonometers) is based on the principle that the force required to flatten (applanate) any portion of the surface of a sphere is directly proportional to the pressure inside the sphere multiplied by the area being flattened [15]. This assumes, however, that the sphere's

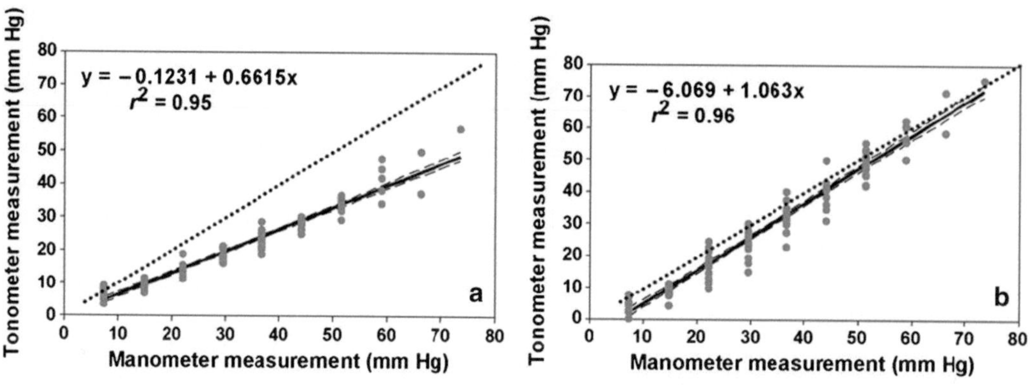

Fig. 3 Comparison of the Tono-Pen XL applanation tonometer (**a**) and TonoVet rebound tonometer (**b**) to a manometer in normal dog eyes. Both tonometers demonstrate a linear relationship to true IOP making them suitable for use in glaucoma efficacy studies in this species. The rebound tonometer, however, more closely approximates true IOP than does the Tono-Pen which tends to underestimate actual IOP. From Goring C, Coonan RTI, States FC et al (2006) Comparison of the use of new handheld tonometers and established applanation tonometers in dogs. Am J Vet Res 67:134–144

surface is perfectly spherical, flexible, infinitely thin, and dry—features that the cornea only roughly approximates. By carefully selecting the area being applanated it is possible to have the corneal surface's resistance to bending roughly cancel out the effect of tear film surface tension on the tonometer tip. For all applanation tonometers, even veterinary versions, however, the area of applanation has been selected based on the characteristics of the human cornea, and across species there are substantial variations in corneal thickness, tear film viscosity, and the proportion of the cornea being applanated. For example, the mean corneal thickness (and hence part of the ease with which the cornea is applanated) varies from 366 ± 15.5, 452 ± 24.9 and 538 ± 36.1 for rabbit, cynomolgus monkey, and dog respectively [16]. Additionally, IOP measurements with applanation tonometers may be altered by drugs which substantially alter the tear film viscosity (ointments or gels), ocular surface drying by topical or general anesthesia, or by preceding diagnostic procedures such as gonioscopy in which the goniolens is coupled to the eye with a viscous gel [17].

Mechanically the pressure-sensitive working end of the Tono-Pen is metal rod that projects slightly above a surrounding insensitive annulus whose purpose is to overcome the cornea's resistance to bending [18]. The sensitive metal rod is covered by an inexpensive ($0.21 to $0.33 each) disposable latex rubber tip that is easily changed between animals. The Tono-Pen has been available since the 1980s and there are several variations on this basic principle; the original Tono-Pen, Tono-Pen II, Tono-Pen XL, Tono-Pen Vet, Tono-Pen Avia, and Tono-Pen Avia Vet. It is essentially a miniaturized, hand-held strain gauge that creates an electrical signal as the sensitive tip and surrounding insensitive annulus flattens the cornea. The voltage change is amplified, digitized, and analyzed by an on-board microprocessor using discriminatory algorithms. Three to six accepted waveforms (indicated by an audible click) are averaged and the mean IOP in mm Hg is shown on a liquid crystal display. The coefficient of variance is also indicated as 5, 10, 20, or >20 % [18]. Only results with ≤10 % should be regarded as valid. The models differ primarily in battery size and whether individual readings (in addition to the average) are displayed. The veterinary version (Tono-Pen Vet) differs from the human version (Tono-Pen XL) essentially only in color. Gravity is used to calibrate all versions of the Tono-Pen, but there is no easy way for the user to externally verify that the internal calibration program is correctly functioning. In general, the Tono-Pen tonometer tends to underestimate true IOP in most species including rabbits, dogs, and monkeys [19–21].

The pneumotonometer uses a central column of air under a silastic membrane as the sensing device [19]. Changes in air pressure in the column resulting from applanation are recorded on a moving paper strip and on a LCD screen. Several variations exist and some require prolonged (5 s) contact with the eye, making them difficult to use in animals that are not fully acclimated to the process. The contact area with the cornea is larger than that of the Tono-Pen or TonoVet (5 mm versus 1.0 mm for the Tono-Pen and even less for the TonoVet), resulting in somewhat greater ocular surface trauma during tonometry. Its calibration, however, is easy to verify as it is calibrated daily against a water column that is supplied with the instrument. Sterilization of the tonometer tip between animals or prevention of cross-contamination of vehicle control and test article is difficult with this instrument as the silastic membrane is relatively expensive ($50 to $60 each) and cumbersome to change. In practice tips are usually cleaned between animals by gently touching them to a gauze square soaked in 70 % isopropyl alcohol. Cross-contamination with test article is minimized by measuring IOP in ascending group order.

In general the pneumatonometer tends to underestimate IOP in dogs [22] and does not give linear estimates of IOP in rabbits at IOPs between 0 and 30 mmHg [19]. It is, however, quite close to a manometer in rhesus monkeys at IOPs between 5 and 35 mmHg [23].

The Perkins tonometer is a portable tonometer that is based on the Goldmann applanation tonometer that is widely used in humans [24–26]. Instead of using a probe or pneumatically driven disc to applanate the cornea, the cornea is applanated by the examiner manually adjusting a variable tension spring until the edges of two green semicircles are precisely aligned in a viewfinder [24–26]. Although in manometric studies the Perkins has been suggested to more closely approximate true IOP than the Tono-Pen and pneumatonometer in cats, dogs, and rabbits [24–26]; it is more cumbersome to use and has a much longer learning curve than the other applanation or rebound tonometers. It still underestimates true IOP in rabbits [25, 26]. It also requires much greater cooperation on the part of the animal to get accurate readings. In manometric studies its IOP estimates are comparable to those obtained with the rebound tonometer, although the latter is much easier to use. In practice the mean IOPs obtained with the Perkins in conscious cats and dogs are not statistically significantly different from those obtained with the Tono-Pen [23]. As the sensitive tip is reused cross-contamination between groups is possible.

Rebound or induction/impact tonometry was introduced 2004 as an offshoot of efforts to develop accurate methods of measuring IOP in rats and mice for glaucoma research [27]. The fundamental premise of this instrument is that a precisely characterized disposable tonometer probe resembling a sewing pin is electromagnetically propelled (induced) to come into contact with (impact) and then rebound from the corneal surface. The motion parameters of the probe have been determined to vary with IOP and this experimentally derived calibration data has been used to create species-specific internal algorithms. The internal calibration curve for the TonoLab has been optimized for mice and rats [27] whereas the related TonoVet has three independent internal calibration curves (cat/dog = d, horse = h and other = p) [13]. The probe is so light (0.027 g) that it can be used to estimate IOP without the instillation of topical ocular anesthesia. This allows one to avoid this potentially confounding variable in topical anti-glaucoma drug studies [28]. Six individual measurements are obtained, internally averaged, and the IOP estimate is displayed accompanied by a letter indicating the species-specific calibration curve that was used. The rebound tonometer can also display a variety of error messages reflecting poor standard deviation of the measurements, problems with the probe motion, and misalignment contact with the central cornea. The tip is relatively inexpensive ($1.66 each) and faster to change than the pneumatonometer, but not as fast as the Tono-Pen. In practice the probe is so small that in the author's experience less than 0.0002 g of tear (and even less test article) may adhere to it after use. Of the commercially available tonometers the TonoVet in the "d" setting comes the closest to estimating true IOP in monkeys/dogs/cats but, like the Tono-Pen and pneumatonometer, the "d" setting underestimates IOP in rabbits [13, 25, 29, 30]. Measurements with the TonoVet also tend to exhibit less variability than Tono-Pen which may be useful in detecting statistically significant differences between groups.

3 Continuous IOP Measurements

The ability to continuously measure IOP would allow IOP measurement in unrestrained animals and a more thorough characterization of the diurnal variations in IOP [31, 32]. It also would help determine whether the test article has an effect on the frequent transient, but potentially important, IOP spikes that occur over the course of a day. Clinical management of glaucoma patients typically relies upon single IOP measurements acquired during clinic hours, although the majority of glaucoma patients reach their peak IOP levels outside of clinic hours or during brief spikes [33]. The latter spikes may be some of the most damaging to the eye and are typically missed during less frequent sampling.

McLaren published a technique in rabbits in which a commercially available battery powered pressure transducer and transmitter (Model PA-C40, Data Sciences International) was implanted subcutaneously and a fluid-filled catheter was threaded subcutaneously from the transducer into the vitreous cavity [31]. This device has been used to demonstrate the efficacy of several IOP lowering drugs in rabbits over the course of days to months [32, 34]. It also demonstrated that the effects of many common procedures such as animal handling, tonometry, and water drinking were often of a magnitude comparable to that of a pharmacologic agent, and as such they can create an unacceptable level of "noise" in IOP measurements which make it more difficult to determine the efficacy of a candidate drug [32]. The sensing probe is generally well tolerated in the vitreous cavity, although cataracts and vitreous opacities commonly develop in chronically implanted animals. A similar implantable device also has been described for monkeys [35], and a less invasive prototype has been described for rabbits utilizing a 30 g needle in the vitreous cavity [36]. Recently, a telemetric contact lens sensor (SENSIMED Triggerfish®) has been used in humans to frequently measure IOP over a 24 h period [33, 37]. This device has demonstrated that IOP is very dynamic and that measurements at just a few time points may not fully reflect the physiologic changes in IOP [33, 37]. The device does not, however, measure IOP per se but instead measures relative changes in IOP in arbitrary units which cannot be easily translated into absolute IOP values [33, 37].

4 Other Technical Considerations in Measuring IOP

Accurate and repeatable IOP measurements are critical to the success of anti-glaucoma drug studies. Failure to eliminate all of the following potentially confounding variables can render an efficacy study meaningless.

4.1 Tonometer-Associated Factors

In addition to the above, each tonometer has an inherent variability which is typically ±2 mmHg. As with many instruments, individual tonometers of the same model may also give somewhat different measurements [38]. Although it is often considered more reliable to collect and average three IOP estimates at each interval, this approach does not always make the data more accurate, especially with certain tonometers which already collect multiple measurements to generate the single displayed reading. For example, the potential errors in IOP estimates with the Tono-Pen and many other tonometers are not normally distributed, but instead these errors almost always result in overestimation of true IOP [39]. This means that averaging three readings is likely to increase the error in those IOP estimates.

4.2 Tonometrist-Associated Factors

Just as there are inter-instrument variations in IOP measurements there are inter-tonometrist differences as well. These can be several mm Hg or more, and may be due not only to differences in individual technique but also to variations in the animal's acclimation to one individual over another. Therefore the ideal situation is to have one experienced individual collect all measurements. It is also important that the tonometrist (or the assistant) avoids compressing the jugular veins or eyelids, ensures that the instrument cleanly contacts the cornea, and is aware of confounding factors that may affect the accuracy of an individual reading (globe retraction, excessive eye movements, panting, contacting paraxial cornea or the cornea at an angle, nonparallel to the ground positioning of the TonoVet, etc.). As the animal's acclimation to tonometry can rapidly fade, it is important on long-duration studies to continue to periodically collect measurements from the animals so as to maintain acclimation even if this data is not to be used for data interpretation purposes. For example, acclimation is likely to be lost, and IOP values become more variable, if measurements are collected once every 4 weeks in a typical 3 or 6 month efficacy study. Most species do best with collection two to three times a week, although this varies by tonometrist, species, the extent of the time the animal has been acclimated to the procedure, and to some extent the device being used.

Eyelid Manipulation. Manipulation of the eyelids can result in marked alterations in IOP. In one study retracting the eyelids of a dog laterally or in a dorsoventral direction resulted in IOP estimates that were increased by 16.5 mmHg and 6.4 mmHg respectively [40]. The low scleral rigidity of rabbits suggests that this effect would be even greater in rabbits.

Compression of the External Jugular Veins. Compression of the external jugular veins frequently occurs in dogs during restraint for IOP measurements and may also occur in some primate studies in which the animal is wearing a rigid neck collar to facilitate capture or identification. In one study in dogs compression of both jugular veins increased IOP estimates by 3.0 mmHg [40]. The Valsalva maneuver, in which the animal exhales against a closed glottis, can also markedly increase IOP (up to 10.2 mmHg in one study) [41] as can holding a panting dog's mouth closed.

Off-center application. In one study in humans IOP was not found to be different if the central cornea was applanated versus the mid-peripheral cornea, even though the mid-peripheral cornea was 40 μm thicker [42]. Of the tonometers most widely used today he TonoVet is probably the most susceptible to off-center application as the tonometer probe must remain parallel to the ground to avoid the effects of gravity on the acceleration and deceleration of the probe tip.

Pharmacologic Pupil Dilation. Pharmacologic pupil dilation with tropicamide or other mydriatics has been reported to have a variable effect on IOP. Some studies suggest pharmacologic pupil dilation does not alter IOP at all whereas others have found increases of up to a few mm Hg in normal dogs [43], cats [44, 45] and humans [46, 47]. Although these differences may sometimes achieve statistical significance, and indicate that IOP should be measured prior to pupil dilation in anti-glaucoma drug efficacy studies, the magnitude of the increase (if any) is clinically unimportant and in the author's experience has not resulted in a toxicologically adverse finding for IOP. Differences between studies showing no effect, and those showing a mild effect, are likely attributable to differences in the statistical power between studies to detect a small change in IOP in many individuals, or the ability of large changes in IOP in few individuals to skew the data set. In anti-glaucoma drug efficacy studies it is also important to recognize that topical mydriatics may alter the pharmacokinetics of the test article by diluting it out, drying the ocular surface (anticholinergics), or vasconstricting the conjunctiva vessels (adrenergic agonists). These drugs may also alter other systemic parameters such as heart rate, blood pressure, and electrocardiographic tracings which may be a component of a toxicity/tolerability component of the study.

Topical Anesthesia. Although generally well tolerated, topical proparacaine may transiently markedly reduce tear production (83 % in beagles in one study) [48], alter corneal thickness [49], corneal epithelial cell adhesion and the corneal penetration of topically applied drugs [50]. Recently, tetracaine was demonstrated to result in a decrease in IOP of 17–29 % for the first 20 min after its application in normotensive rabbits, and 24–31 % in rabbits with ocular hypertension induced by water loading [51]. Repeated use of topical anesthesia over a period of hours to a day, as is typical in many efficacy studies, may result in ocular surface irritation, corneal epithelial cell drying/sloughing, and fluorescein stain uptake. The effect of these disruptions of a major barrier to drug penetration is seldom investigated, but should not be discounted in preclinical safety, efficacy, and especially ADME studies. Topical anesthestics applied soon after the test article may also dilute out the drug, thereby limiting the effective dose administered. The confounding effects of topical anesthesia can be mitigated by the use of smaller volumes (10 μl) or more dilute solutions, using tonometers with smaller tips such as the Tono-Pen, or using the TonoVet which does not require topical anesthesia at all.

Diagnostic Gels and Artificial Tears. Both the Tono-Pen and Tono-Vet are also significantly affected by artificial tears used to lubricate the cornea of anesthetized animals and residual methylcellulose solutions that are used for gonioscopy and certain other diagnostic procedures. In one study residual methylcellulose increased Tono-Pen IOP estimates a mean of 27 %, presumably due to an increase in tear film viscosity [52]. In some animals residual coupling gels will cause both instruments to give either a false measurement or no measurement at all. Because gonioscopy may also alter IOP by compressing the corneal surface and transiently forcing more fluid from the eye, it is important to collect IOP measurements prior to this procedure. Ocular discharge, perhaps attributable to repeated IOP measurements or irritation by the test article, also increases tear film viscosity and may confound results through a similar mechanism.

4.3 Animal-Associated Factors

Diurnal Variations in IOP. Because of diurnal variations in IOP it is important to control the light cycle in the room in which the animals are housed. In general, nocturnal species such as rats, cats, and rabbits tend to exhibit lower IOP during the day and to increase during the night, whereas more diurnal species such as dogs, monkeys, and humans IOP tends to peak in the morning and decrease over the course of the day [53–58]. IOP increases during this circadian rhythm are typically attributable to decreased outflow via the trabecular meshwork. In some species there are also changes in aqueous humor production and uveoscleral outflow. This variation can be statistically significant and, if not properly controlled for, mistaken for a modest drug effect, especially in dogs and nonhuman primates. For example, the IOP difference in dogs between their peak (often around 7 a.m.) at lowest values (in the afternoon) is approximately 20 % (3 mmHg) [57, 58], whereas in rabbits IOP begins to increase with the onset of darkness and may be a change of 6.4–16.6 mmHg [31, 59, 60]. In rabbits it may take 10–14 days for a normal circadian rhythm to be re-established if the animal is stressed, transported substantial distances (i.e. from a supplier to a research facility), or anesthetized [31]. In general an animal can be considered to be acclimated to its environment when a circadian rhythm can be identified.

It is also important to recognize that the peak changes in IOP associated with a diurnal curve can vary greatly between groups of animals for reasons that are not entirely clear and in some groups of animals it may be opposite that which is traditionally expected [31, 59–61]. Therefore it is important to establish the profile of the diurnal curve for each set of animals and not rely entirely on previously published normal values.

Animal Handling Factors. Continuous manometry studies have yielded substantial information about how a variety of factors affect IOP in otherwise unrestrained animals [31, 32, 59]. They have demonstrated why it is critical for conscious animals that are being used in anti-glaucoma drug studies to be acclimated to IOP measurements. It is important to recognize that during blinking IOP transiently increases approximately 15 mmHg during lid closure and that this transient spike is followed by a 1–2 mmHg undershoot for a approximately 1 s [62]. Simply moving a rabbit from one room to another (the room in which the animal is housed to another room for tonometry) can cause a 20 % increase in IOP and it may take some animals 4–5 h to return to baseline [31, 32]. Handling, IOP measurements, exposure to a single stimulus (auditory, visual, tactile, olfactory, or thermal) evokes a transient rise in IOP in rabbits with an amplitude as great as 10 mmHg [31, 32, 63]. Common procedures in the laboratory can also substantially alter IOP. For example the act of performing pneumatonometry or changing a rabbit's cage can increase IOP 3–6 mmHg and this may persist for an hour after the procedure has concluded [32]. Restoring water after 24 h of no water (as may occur if the watering system malfunctions) can increase IOP 6 mmHg for 4–5 h [32].

Additionally, IOP in rabbits is not constant but can vary as much as 3–5 mmHg in a single minute and it can rapidly vary approximately 1 mmHg at intervals that correlate with heart rate [31]. If the animal is resisting tonometry, or is not acclimated to the room and the surrounding environment, these variations in IOP can be further magnified. There is little reason to believe that similar alterations in IOP do not occur in species other than rabbits. In the aggregate these factors indicate that measurements need to be acquired in as consistent and calm an environment as possible.

The Effect of Age on IOP. IOP often decreases with age as an animal reaches maturity. Therefore in long-term studies starting with juvenile animals IOP may decline over time simply because the animal reaches adulthood.

Alterations in Corneal Thickness. Both the Tono-Pen and the TonoVet are affected by alterations in corneal thickness, both in normal eyes and more so in eyes with grossly abnormal corneas. One study of 60 clinically normal dogs found that for every 100 μm in central corneal thickness the estimated IOP was increased 1 and 2 mmHg by the Tono-Pen XL and the TonoVet respectively [64]. Corneal edema and other adverse events associated with toxicity of anti-glaucoma drugs also may significantly alter IOP estimates with all tonometers.

5 Notes

5.1 Efficacy Study Design

IOP efficacy studies should be designed as ocular physiology experiments and not assessments of toxicity or tolerability. It is important to resist the temptation to add a large number of ADME or tolerability/toxicity endpoints such as blood draws (which can ruin acclimation to tonometry), fluorescein staining and dilated pupil examinations (commonly included in many ocular irritation scoring schemes), pupillometry, corneal sensitivity, corneal pachymetry, noncontact specular microscopy, anterior segment optical coherence tomography, electroretinography, and fundus imaging. Although some secondary endpoints do not affect IOP measurements, many do and the addition of any secondary endpoints must be done with the full knowledge of what impact these have on the study achieving its primary objective of determining the ability of the test article to lower IOP. Additional considerations in the design of an anti-glaucoma drug efficacy studies include the following: (1) selecting the most appropriate species, (2) identifying the rate of nonresponders within the study population, (3) determining whether normotensive or glaucomatous animals should be used, and deciding (4) what secondary endpoints (if any) to include, and (5) whether one eye or both should be dosed.

5.2 Species Selection

Selecting the proper test species is one of the most critical aspects in designing an anti-glaucoma drug efficacy study. It is essential to correctly identify the species which possesses the putative target receptors and the physiologic pathways necessary to elicit a response. The considerable differences between species in terms of cost, availability, and housing/handling requirements also are important considerations in getting studies up and running as quickly as possible in as cost-effective manner as possible. For example, some species such as rabbits and dogs are easily housed and cared for, readily available and rapidly acclimated to tonometry, whereas this is less true for cats, pigs, and monkeys. The need for sedation or general anesthesia in some species (such as monkey and sometimes rats/mice) also can introduce confounding variables in a complex and sometimes unpredictable fashion that may ultimately call the validity of the study into question.

If one species is nonresponsive to a promising anti-glaucoma drug it is important to determine if this is a species-specific finding or if a similar lack of response would also translate to humans. There are numerous examples of potent ocular hypotensive drugs in humans that did not meaningfully alter IOP in one or more animal species. This phenomenon is so common that it is very likely that highly effective anti-glaucoma drugs in humans have been prematurely discarded, especially in the early screening stages of new classes of drugs in which the receptor profiles and responsiveness of various species are poorly understood. Examples of the disconnect between humans and animals include the lack of IOP lowering efficacy of latanoprost in rabbits and cats (but its profound reduction of IOP in dogs and monkeys, [65, 66]), and the trivial, if any, reduction in IOP by timolol dogs [67, 68]. The toxicity profile of anti-glaucoma drugs in animals also may not mimic the profile in humans.

If there is not a robust literature base to guide the initial selection of the test species there are three possible approaches: (1) Begin work based on determinations of the target receptor distribution and concentration in several different species and select the one that most closely mimics humans, (2) Conduct pilot studies using two to three animals of several different species to experimentally identify the species that best shows a decrease in IOP, and (3) Begin with nonhuman primates which generally (but not always) best approximate humans. Even with a robust literature base, however, selecting the optimal test species may not be easy. For example, cats were found to be profoundly responsive to the parent compound PGF2α but only marginally, or nonresponsive, to many of its derivatives including those that are currently commercially available [66]. Because of this phenomenon, promising compounds which are well tolerated should not be abandoned until the lack of efficacy in humans is established. This means that often the goal of pre-clinical efficacy studies in animals is to simply demonstrate a reduction in IOP that would enable further studies in humans. It is likely that the variation in species sensitivity to various classes of anti-glaucoma drugs will only increase as drugs are developed to precisely target highly specific cellular pathways.

Another consideration in selecting a test species is the considerable species-associated variations in size of the various compartments of the eye (cornea, anterior chamber, lens, vitreous volume, etc.) which may profoundly affect the pharmacokinetics and ADME of the test article. For example, in mice a topically applied drug needs to pass through only 0.097 mm of cornea and travel 3.3 mm to reach the retina whereas in humans that same drug needs to pass through 0.567 mm of cornea and travel 23.9 mm to reach the retina. Hence achieving a therapeutic level in rodents may not translate to humans simply due to both relative and absolute differences in the various compartments of the eye. Table 1 lists normative data for some compartments of the eye for several species.

Although not comprehensive, some species-specific considerations in designing anti-glaucoma drug efficacy studies are discussed in the following section.

Nonhuman Primates. The Cynomolgus (also known as the crab-eating macaque, *Macaca fascicularis*) and Rhesus macaque (*Macaca mulatta*) are the most widely used and best studied. Their close phylogeny and high homology with humans makes them excellent test species and their responsiveness to

Table 1
Relative comparison of select ocular parameters across species

	Axial length (mm)	Corneal thickness (mm)	Corneal diameter (mm)	Anterior chamber depth (mm)	Anterior chamber volume (ml)	Lens thickness (mm)	Vitreous chamber depth (mm)	Vitreous volume (ml)	References
Human	23.92	0.567	H-11.75 V-10.55	3.03	0.15	4.0	16.32	4.0	[150–153]
Cynomolgus	17.92	0.452	H-9.8	3.24	0.13	2.98	11.30	3.2	[153–156]
Cat	22.3	0.567	H-16.5 V-16.2	4.52	0.82	8.5	8.13	3.5 (est)	[157–161]
Dog	20.8	0.538	H-13–17 V-12–16	4.29	0.79	7.85	10.02	3.2	[156, 162, 163]
Rabbit	18.1	0.366	H-13.4 V-13.0	2.9	0.31	7.9	6.20	1.5	[153, 156, 164–166]
Pig	23.9	0.877	H-14.9 V-12.4	2.7	0.22	7.4	11.9 (est)	2.67	[167, 168]
Rat	5.98	0.170	5.1 (est)	0.87	0.011 (est)	3.87	1.51	0.020	[153, 169–171]
Mouse	3.38	0.097	3.15 (est)	0.40	0.0059	2.0	0.60	0.010 (est)	[171–173]

Values are approximates and derived from published values using a variety of techniques, calculations based on published values for schematic eyes, and data collected by the author. Values in the literature vary by technique, age, strain, and study. The author thanks Dr Christopher J Murphy for assistance in compiling this table

H horizontal corneal diameter, *V* vertical corneal diameter, *Est* estimated values

anti-glaucoma drugs correlates well with that of humans. Like humans, macaques respond to most anti-glaucoma drug classes including adrenergics, cholinergics, beta-blockers, carbonic anhydrase inhibitors, prostaglandins, rho-kinase inhibitors, serotonin-2 receptor agonists, melatonin analogues, vitamin D analogues, cannabinoids, and drugs which alter the actin cytoskeleton [69–78]. Important differences between macaques and humans do exist, however, including a smaller corneal surface area and overall body mass which may affect the pharmacokinetics, ADME, and systemic toxicity of topically applied anti-glaucoma drugs.

Although IOP is traditionally measured in this species under light ketamine anesthesia because of the animal's temperament, this can significantly affect IOP values [79]. In chronic studies repeated anesthesia interferes with normal food and water consumption leading to dehydration, weight loss, and altered IOP [79]. It is possible to train conscious macaques to accept tonometry, but this requires a dedicated staff with substantial experience in handling these species and several weeks to months of acclimation [80]. Females are generally more amenable to training that males, who become much stronger and often more aggressive as they reach sexual maturity. Additional negatives of using macaques for anti-glaucoma efficacy studies is their expense, limited availability, high public profile, temperament, the need to maintain them in special housing facilities, and that they may harbor diseases such as tuberculosis and Herpes B which may be fatal to humans.

Cats (Felis catus). There is an extensive literature base regarding the autonomic innervation of the feline eye and adnexa making it particularly useful for teasing out the mechanism of action of autonomically active drugs. There also is a modest set of data, generally in the veterinary literature, regarding their responsiveness to anti-glaucoma drugs. Although the magnitude of IOP reduction is generally less than monkeys and dogs, cats have been reported to respond to most anti-glaucoma drug classes including adrenergics, cholinergics, beta-blockers (although most cats have little resting adrenergic tone so the response is minimal), carbonic anhydrase inhibitors, and some types of prostaglandins in ways that are not entirely predictable [81–85]. Normal cats, however, do not respond to the commercially available PGF2α derivatives because they lack the FP receptor [65, 66]. Their claws and temperament also can make them difficult to handle and acclimate to tonometry (compared to dogs and rabbits). Additionally, in most studies IOP tends to increase over the course of the day which may mask drug-associated IOP reductions in the afternoon if these values are compared to predose values acquired in the morning. Their large cornea, vertical slit pupil, and relatively small body mass may also cause the pharmacokinetics, ADME, and systemic toxicity profiles of topically applied drugs to not accurately mimic humans. For example, topical application of the alpha-2 agonist apraclonidine usually causes cats to vomit [85], presumably due to systemic interaction with the chemoreceptor trigger zone in the brain, whereas this is not a common finding in dogs or humans.

Dogs (Canis lupus familiaris). This readily available, well studied species is generally easily trained and much less aggressive towards humans than all other laboratory species with the possible exception rabbits. Laboratory beagles of the Marshall strain are particularly passive and amenable to handling. Dogs have a relatively large eye (compared to rodents), allow tonometry without general anesthesia or sedation, and respond to most anti-glaucoma drug classes including adrenergics, cholinergics, beta-blockers, carbonic anhydrase inhibitors, prostaglandins, and cannabinoids [65, 67, 68, 71, 86–90]. However, they have a larger cornea and anterior chamber than humans, greater housing requirements than rabbits, a need for continual acclimation/socialization to maintain acclimation to tonometry, and a diurnal curve in which IOP tends to decline over the course of the day. Without adequate controls the latter may be mistaken for a drug effect. Like cats, the mechanism of action of anti-glaucoma drugs does not always mimic humans, especially in regards to effects of anti-glaucoma drugs on the pupil. For example, apraclonidine dilates the canine pupil and latanoprost constricts it, whereas neither drug consistently alters pupil size in humans [66, 67, 89].

Rabbit (Oryctolagus cuniculus). This relatively docile species has a large eye and an extensive supporting literature base. Tonometry does not require sedation or anesthesia and can often be accomplished by one individual (versus two for the other species discussed here with the possible exception of sedated monkeys). However, they have a number of potentially significant ocular anatomical and physiological differences from humans including relatively low tear production, an increased sensitivity to ocular irritation, a much thinner cornea and sclera which reduces ocular rigidity, a fragile blood:aqueous barrier that is easily broken down, a large lens, a markedly different blood supply to the retina and a naturally deeply cupped optic disc ([91, 92], Table 1). The presence of albinism in some strains may also alter the pharmacokinetics and efficacy of drugs which have significant pigment binding. The thinner cornea tends to cause tonometers to underestimate true IOP and the low ocular rigidity makes the eye very susceptible to artifactual increases in IOP due to compression of the globe by handling, eyelid squeezing, or the animal retracting the globe as it seeks to avoid the probe tip touching the cornea. These factors, plus a somewhat "fearful" demeanor which leads to breath holding and causes rapid changes in systemic blood pressure and heart rate results in IOP that may naturally vary 3–5 mmHg in 1 min [31, 32]. IOP also may be elevated after common handling procedures such as after being handled for tonometry, moving to a different cage or restoring water after a period in which it was not available (Fig. 4). This species can also have a marked diurnal curve with IOP increasing 6.4–16.6 mmHg during the night relative to the daytime [31, 32]. This curve, which is an indicator of how well acclimated the animal is to its surroundings, can take 10–14 days to re-establish if transported, stressed, or anesthetized [32]. The IOP increase at night is mainly due to reduced outflow. Although increased aqueous humor production at night also occurs, this appears to be balanced out by an increase in uveoscleral outflow [60].

Rabbits have been reported to respond to most anti-glaucoma drug classes including adrenergics, cholinergics, beta-blockers, carbonic anhydrase inhibitors, rho-kinase inhibitors, melatonin analogues, some cannabinoid analogues, serotonin-2 receptor agonists, and prostaglandin analogues, although the responsiveness to the latter two classes can be quite variable [62, 66, 70, 71, 75, 93–95].

Rodents. Rats and mice, especially those with transgenic or knockout traits, have been extensively used in glaucoma research, especially in "proof of concept" studies or those investigating fundamental pathophysiologic responses to increased IOP. Additionally their relatively low cost and minimal housing requirements allow for larger sample sizes and greater statistical certainty. Although additional work needs to be done, many instruments and techniques involved in measuring aqueous humor dynamics have recently been optimized for these species [96, 97].

There are substantial differences between rodent and human eyes, not only anatomically in which the relative proportions of the various ocular tissues differ markedly (which affects the pharmacokinetics, ADME, and systemic toxicity profile) but also physiologically (Table 1). There also can be substantial differences in the responsiveness of one strain compared to another. The presence of albinism in both rats and mice, and background retinal degeneration in many mouse strains also can be a significant variable. The small eye and difficulties in restraining them for measurements without introducing technical errors makes accurate IOP measurements challenging. IOP studies involving rats typically requires additional equipment to standardize how the tonometer is applied to ocular surface, the initial use of sedatives to acclimate the animal to the restraint device, and an acclimation period which in the author's experience exceeds that of dogs (Fig. 5). For this, and other reasons previously mentioned, rodent IOP lowering efficacy studies are typically not the primary studies used to support FDA investigational new drug applications.

Gottingen Mini-Pig (Sus scrofa domestica). Mini-pigs have a large eye and have been suggested to mimic humans in many respects, especially dermal, cardiovascular, and gastrointestinal [98] although the eye has not been as well studied. An experimental glaucoma model involving intracameral injection of 4 % methylcellulose [99] or cauterization of episcleral vessels has also been

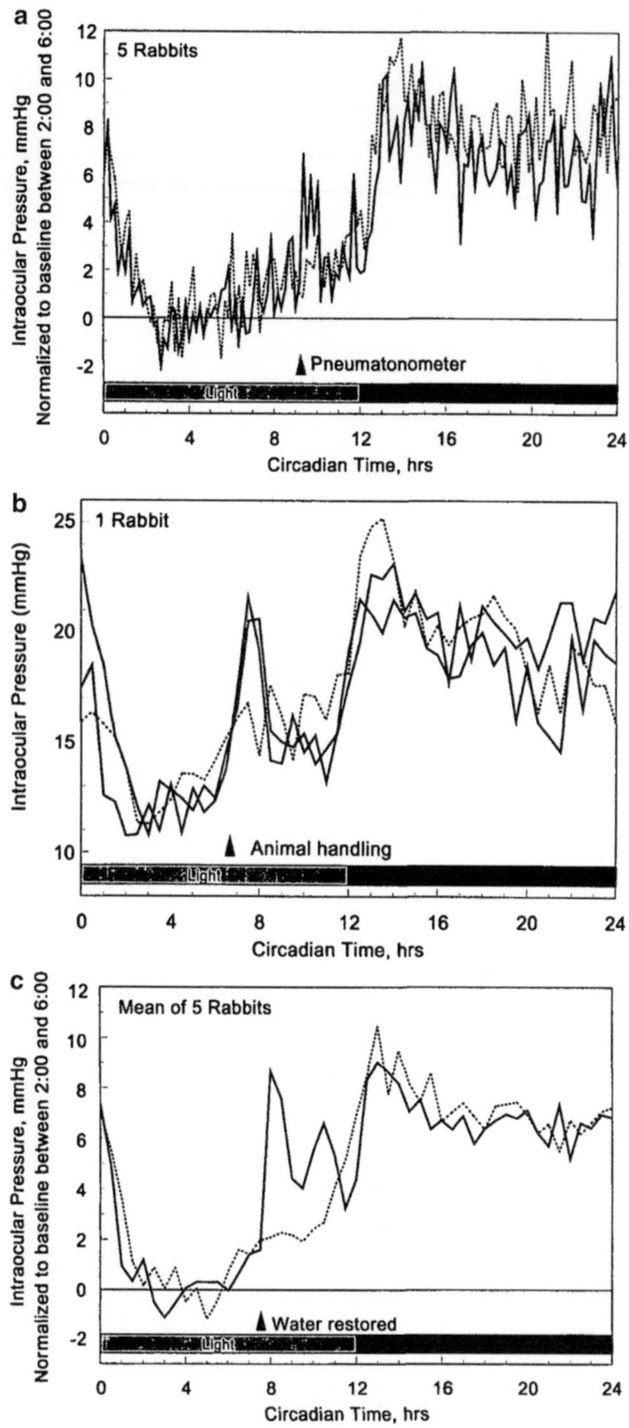

Fig. 4 Effects of environmental disturbance on IOP in rabbits. *Solid line* = day of disturbance at time indicated by *arrow*; *dotted line* = undisturbed day. (**a**) Effect of pneumatonometry. IOP remains elevated for nearly 1 h after tonometry. (**b**) Transferring an animal from one cage to another elevated IOP for 1 h after animal was disturbed on each of 2 days (one animal). (**c**) Effects of drinking water after a 24-h period of water deprivation. Just after animals beginning to drink IOP rose and remained elevated for several hours. From: Dinslage S, McLaren J, Brubaker R (1998) Intraocular pressure in rabbits by telemetry II: effects of animal handling and drugs. Invest Ophthalmol Vis Sci 39 (12):2485–2489

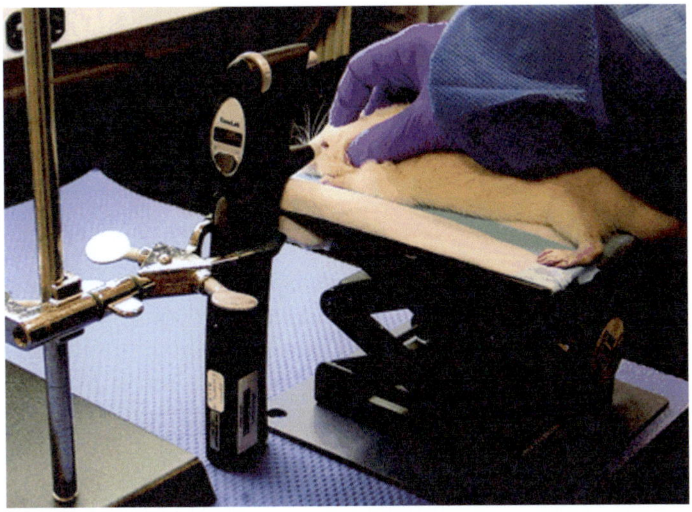

Fig. 5 Experimental setup for measuring IOP in conscious rats with the rebound tonometer. The animal is gently manually restrained on a platform of adjustable height and the instrument is mechanically stabilized for the measurements. From: Wang WH, Millar JC, Pang IH et al (2005) Noninvasive measurement of rodent intraocular pressure with a rebound tonometer. Invest Ophthalmol Vis Sci 46:4617–4621

reported [100]. Substantial impediments to their routine use in anti-glaucoma drug efficacy studies include a paucity of data regarding their responsiveness to anti-glaucoma drugs, their temperament (especially when restrained which can markedly alter systemic blood pressure, heart rate, respiratory effort, and breath holding), physical size (up to 50 kg), physical strength, rapid growth rate, and greater housing requirements compared to other laboratory animal species. Often several handlers and possibly additional equipment such as slings are required to collect IOP measurements from pigs. In the author's experience IOP in pigs can spontaneously vary considerably over a period of seconds to minutes. Their deep set eye, relatively thick cornea, oily tear film, and strong eyelids also pose challenges in accurately measuring IOP.

5.3 Responders

The percentage of the population that exhibits reduced IOP after application of the drug is an another important consideration in designing efficacy studies, determining a dose:response curve, or making comparisons between related drugs to identify the "lead" compound. This is important because the type and distribution of the receptors varies not only by species but by individuals within that species, and this distribution plays a critical role in determining the sample size needed to detect a meaningful difference in IOP [101, 102]. Studies which include large number of "nonresponders," either by chance or because of relative nonresponsiveness of the species as a whole, are typically unable to identify compounds that would be effective in humans. For example, in dogs the response rate (as defined by a 15 % reduction in IOP) latanoprost is approximately 89 % whereas it is 0–20 % for timolol [67, 68, 103]. In humans the response rate is approximately 82 % for latanoprost and 74 % for timolol after 3 months of use [104]. In one study using cynomolgus monkeys, 72 % were found to respond to latanoprost whereas the remaining 28 % exhibited no IOP reduction at all [101].

Often it is valuable to use only "responders" to conduct studies which are designed to make comparisons between various concentrations, formulations, or congeners. If the test article is closely related to a commercially available compound, or is a derivative of a parent compound, it may be possible to assess the potential for responsiveness by using the commercial or parent compound, but this is not a foolproof approach [101]. For example, PGF2α lowers IOP in normal cats but the commercially available PGF2α derivatives does not, and the commercially available PGF2α analogue talfluprost can lower IOP in monkeys that are unresponsive to the closely related PGF2α analogue latanoprost [66, 101]. For truly novel compounds often the nonresponse rate of a given species can only be experimentally derived. In studies involving repeated or prolonged exposure to one or more test articles it may also be important to periodically conduct a single-dose efficacy trial using the parent compound (or class standard) to verify that tachyphylaxis has not occurred.

5.4 Normotensive or Hypertensive?

Another consideration is whether the test animals should be normotensive or if one of the ocular hypertension models should be used. Advantages of normotensive animals is their ready availability, the ability to relatively rapidly initiate a study without the need for additional interventions, decreased animal care requirements, reduced costs, and the high probability that if IOP lowering is seen in normotensive animals that an even greater reduction in IOP is likely in glaucomatous patients. Normotensive animals, however, have fully intact aqueous humor dynamics and compensatory pathways that often blunt IOP decreases. Their numerically lower IOP values also leave less room for IOP to decrease. (To get around this some researchers only use normal animals with IOPs at the higher end of the normal range). These two factors increase the risk that a modest IOP reduction in a specific animal species would be lost in the ±2 mm inherent variability in the tonometer. Additionally, the need to overcome intact aqueous humor dynamics in preclinical studies often leads to an overestimation of the therapeutic dose that will be required in glaucomatous patients. Because of this it is often advisable in definitive preclinical toxicity and safety studies to include dose levels that are lower than those required to achieve peak efficacy in normal animals (or even normal humans).

Ocular hypertensive models have abnormal aqueous humor dynamics which magnify minor changes in aqueous production or outflow, thereby increasing the reduction in IOP and the ability to detect these changes. Additionally, the resting IOP levels are numerically higher in these models making it mathematically easier to detect a reduction in IOP over the ±2 mmHg inherent "noise" in the tonometer itself. They are, however, more difficult to maintain, slower studies to be able to get "up and running" and much more expensive to conduct. Additionally, no single model mimics all aspects of glaucoma in humans and each model has its own unique limitations. For example, increased IOP due to photocoagulation and scarring of the trabecular meshwork may not be a good model for evaluating drugs which increase outflow through this tissue. In most of these models IOP also spontaneously and rapidly makes large swings from day-to-day, making studies lasting longer than a few hours to a day difficult to conduct. All of these factors together usually results in ocular hypertensive models being used when IOP lowering is minimal in normotensive animals, to show "proof of concept," to work out a potential mechanism of action or to screen a series of compounds in a weakly responsive species in an effort identify potentially promising new drugs.

5.5 Spontaneous Versus Experimentally Induced Models of Increased IOP

Spontaneous, genetically based, glaucoma has been reported in a number of species including New Zealand White rabbits [105–108], beagle dogs [109], Siamese cats [110], a group of rhesus monkeys at the Cayo Santiago monkey colony in Puerto Rico [111], transgenic mice [112–115], and rats [116, 117]. Although these are useful models for teasing out various pathophysiologic events in the genesis of glaucoma, they are typically not commercially available and often their populations are limited to a few dozen animals or less. Therefore, most anti-glaucoma efficacy studies utilize nonhuman primates or rabbits with experimentally increased IOP versus one of the spontaneous models. Although there are experimentally induced models of glaucoma in rats and mice, the primary endpoint for studies using these species is typically to identify specific molecular or cellular alterations involved in the pathogenesis of the glaucoma and not to determine the efficacy of anti-glaucoma drugs intended for use in humans. The following is a brief summary of some of the more common ocular hypertension models used in anti-glaucoma efficacy studies.

5.6 Primate Models of Ocular Hypertension

The most widely used and best described nonhuman primate model involves diode or argon laser photocoagulation of the trabecular meshwork [118]. In this model one eye is lasered and the fellow eye serves as the normal control. Several laser treatments over a period of weeks to months are usually required. Although IOP is typically chronically elevated in most animals, IOP may vary considerably from day-to-day and some animals may have marked IOP increases whereas others may have little to none [118]. Therefore, most studies usually only measure IOP for a few hours to a day or two after a single application of a drug. IOP may be measured either in anesthetized animals, or better yet, in animals that have been trained to accept tonometry while conscious [80]. Although poorly described in the literature, persistent breakdown of the blood: aqueous barrier may occur in this model and the effect this has on the pharmacokinetics or distribution of topically applied drugs remains to be elucidated. These features, plus the expense and time required to create the model, makes this model most useful for screening a series of formulations, concentrations, or related compounds. Washout periods between drugs vary with the drug being evaluated, but typically are 2 weeks as treatment periods are usually short. Other less widely used experimental monkey models of chronic IOP elevation involve obstruction of the trabecular meshwork by intracameral injection of latex microspheres [119] or autologous fixed red blood cells [120, 121].

5.7 Rabbit Models of Ocular Hypertension

A number of rabbit models of ocular hypertension exist and the following are some of the more widely used. Rabbit models of ocular hypertension can either be acute, in which IOP is transiently elevated for a few hours by creating osmotic shifts within the eye, or chronic in which more sustained (although potentially unstable) IOP increases occur.

Intravitreous Hypertonic Saline. Intravitreous injection of 0.1 ml of 5 % sodium chloride draws water into the vitreous and causes a short-lived IOP spike [122]. In this model the test article is typically administered prior to the injection and IOP is measured at 0 (predose), 0.5, 1.0, 1.5, 3, and 5 h after dosing. IOP spontaneously normalizes in several hours as the solute is absorbed. Efficacy is based on the ability of the test article to inhibit the IOP increase rather than on the ability to lower IOP from baseline values.

Water Loading. This is a well-established model which also gives a transient IOP spike due to osmotic shifts in the eye [123–125]. Food and water are withheld for 24 h and a 12 french catheter is used as an orogastric tube to deliver 60–70 ml/kg of tap water orally. Some researchers do this with the animal anesthetized (ketamine/xylazine) whereas others do not. Most investigators warm the water to 37 °C to avoid substantial drops in body temperature (which can lead to a number of other potentially confounding physiologic alterations). IOP generally increases from approximately 15 mmHg at baseline to low 30's, peaking at 20–30 min after administration of the water bolus and lasting for 2–3 h. With this model the test article is typically given prior to water loading and IOP is measured at various intervals depending on the pharmacokinetics of the test article. In some studies the water bolus is repeated in 4–5 h. Examples of common time points include −30 min (predose), 0, 5, 10, 15, 20, 25, 30, 35, 40, 55, 70, 85, 100, and 115 min and −30, 0, 30, 60, 90, 120, 180, 240, 300, 360, and 420 min. Efficacy is measured by the ability of the test article to blunt the IOP spike rather than to lower IOP from baseline values [123–125].

5 % Glucose Infusion. Rapid administration of 15 ml/kg of 5 % glucose intravenously via the marginal ear vein (usually over 20 s) also gives a transient IOP spike [126, 127]. Like oral administration of water, this hypotonic solution reduces blood osmolality which leads to transfer of water into the eye. In theory this spike is more predictable than that generated by administering water orally because it is not dependent on the rapid absorption of large amounts of water across the gastrointestinal tract. As with water loading, IOP typically doubles from baseline values with the peak increase occurring approximately 30 min post infusion. IOP values usually return to near baseline values by 50–135 min post-infusion. The test article is typically administered prior to infusion and IOP is measured at 0 (predose), 30, 45, 60, 75, 90, 105, 120, and 135 min after infusion; or until IOP returns to baseline values. Efficacy is measured by the ability of the test article to blunt the IOP spike rather than to lower IOP from baseline values.

Corticosteroid-Induced Hypertension. Corticosteroids increase IOP in some individuals by inducing biochemical alterations in the trabecular meshwork which leads to increased resistance to aqueous humor outflow and increased IOP [128]. The IOP increase in this model is typically more chronic than that seen in the previously described osmotic models [128]. Although the concept behind this model is well established, there are a number of permutations that vary from researcher to researcher and no single method dominates the literature. Common methodologies include: a single intravitreous injection of 0.1 ml of 4 mg/ml preservative free suspension of triamcinolone acetonide (this led to increased IOP within days in one study [129], but is quite variable in the author's experience), weekly subconjunctival injections of 4 mg of a repository betamethasone repeated over 3 weeks (reported to increase IOP in 96 % of rabbits with limited systemic toxicity in one study [130]), and once/week unilateral subconjunctival injection (into the lower conjunctival cul-de-sac) for 4–7 weeks of 0.7 ml of a betamethasone suspension which contains betamethasone sodium phosphate (3 mg/ml) and betamethasone acetate (3 mg/ml) [131, 132]. The latter was reported to lead to a relatively consistent IOP increase starting after two to three injections [132]. Topical application of 0.1 % dexamethasone phosphate three times daily for 5 weeks also has been reported to increase in IOP in some studies [133], but others have found topical dexamethasone was no better than placebo at increasing IOP in rabbits [134]. A portion of the variability described in the literature may stem from the fact that not all rabbits are genetically predisposed to develop increased IOP after corticosteroid administration and that this percentage probably varies from strain to strain and even by cohort within a strain. The usefulness of the animal may also be limited by ocular toxicity (cataracts or corneal ulceration) or systemic toxicity. Usually only animals with an IOP of 25 mmHg or more are used in the dosing phase of the study. Efficacy is determined by the ability of the test article to lower IOP in the corticosteroid-treated eye.

A corticosteroid-induced glaucoma model with a 100 % "responder" rate has been described in sheep and cattle [135–138]. Topical application of 0.5 % prednisolone acetate three times/day in one eye increased IOP from baseline values of 16–17 mmHg to 30–35 mmHg in cattle and from baseline values of 11–23 mmHg in sheep [135–138]. IOP in these animals returned to normal within a few weeks after treatment was discontinued. Although the IOP increase was predictable, the utility of this model is limited because few laboratory facilities are designed to house, handle, and care for these species and their responsiveness to anti-glaucoma drugs is largely unknown.

Intracameral α-Chymotrypsin. A single injection of α-chymotrypsin, typically into the posterior chamber, also results in a chronic elevation in IOP which may last a year or more [62, 126, 131, 140–142]. IOP is usually increased into the 30's, and is seldom greater than 50 mmHg [139]. The exact mechanism by which IOP is increased (important in determining the suitability of the model for a drug with a specific mechanism of action) is unclear, but may be associated with obstruction of the trabecular meshwork by lysed lens zonular proteins, inflammatory debris, or peripheral anterior synechia [139, 140]. Other work, however, suggests that the IOP increase is due to a 1.5× increase in the rate of aqueous humor inflow due to breakdown of the blood aqueous barrier [141].

As for the corticosteroid-induced model, this model has several permutations. Commonly reported doses of α-chymotrypsin include: 45 UAE in 100 μl [62], 50 UAE in 100 μl of saline [131], 50 UAE in 200 μl of saline [142], and 150 units in 0.5 ml of sterile saline [126]. In the latter study stable increased IOP was achieved at 15 days (instead of at 1 month in the other studies). In one paper [140], elevated IOP was produced in 50 % of rabbits given 75 units into the posterior chamber. One approach is to constrict the pupil with one to two drops of pilocarpine 15 min prior to the injection [62], induce anesthesia with intramuscular ketamine HCL (35 mg/kg) and xylazine (5 mg/kg), enter the anterior chamber with a 25–30 g needle and inject α-chymotrypsin into the posterior chamber through the pupil with a 27–30 g needle or a comparably sized blunt cannula. The tip of the needle/cannula should be swept so as to distribute the enzyme evenly throughout the posterior chamber and left in the posterior chamber for at least 1 min before being carefully withdrawn to avoid the enzyme coming into contact with the cornea (especially the corneal stroma which may melt if the enzyme contacts it, [142]). The external surface of the eye should then be rinsed with 10 ml of sterile saline to remove any residual enzyme [142]. Some authors inject 60 units in 0.2 ml of saline into the anterior chamber and leave the needle in the anterior chamber for 2 min to minimize leak back [141], but corneal injury may be increased with this technically simpler approach. Another approach is to pressurize the anterior chamber to approximately 25 mmHg with a 30 g needle attached to an elevated bag of saline and then do the injection with a separate 30 g cannula [126]. Appropriate analgesics and topical anti-inflammatory drugs are typically used for 4–5 days after the procedure. More prolonged used of anti-inflammatories may reduce the number of animals with elevated IOP. Daily examinations may be required for weeks after the injection so as to identify complications and ensure the animal's welfare [62].

Compared to corticosteroid-induced models this model is more difficult to manage as complications may be high, inflammation may be severe, and intraocular damage may be considerable. Because of these alterations this model is best suited for studies in which the only endpoint is IOP (i.e. the model is generally not used to assess drug tolerability, the effect of the test article on intraocular structures or to investigate the pathophysiology of glaucoma). Common complications that may render the animal not useful for the study include lens luxation, severe intraocular inflammation (5–10 % of animals, [62, 142]), severe corneal inflammation (17 % in one study, [126]), and failure to develop a sustained increase in IOP (up to 50 % of animals). Most studies wait 4 weeks after administration of α-chymotrypsin to evaluate the utility of a given animal, and only use rabbits with an IOP which is at least 15 mmHg higher than the fellow control eye or has an IOP of 25 mmHg or more. The IOP levels, however, may vary greatly from animal to animal and from day-to-day. Because of the high complication rate, α-chymotrypsin may need to be administered to at least twice (or more) as many animals as will be needed during the efficacy phase of the study. Because corneal edema is common in this model (which may affect tonometric estimates of IOP) only relative changes in IOP should be used for data analysis purposes, as absolute IOP values may not be directly comparable to those acquired prior to injection or in the un-injected fellow eye. Efficacy of anti-glaucoma drugs is determined by the ability of the test article to lower IOP [62, 126, 131, 140–142].

5.8 Other Considerations in Designing Efficacy Studies

Other Biomarkers. Although ADME studies typically will indicate whether the test article actually gets into the eye in some instances additional endpoints may be used to confirm that pharmacologically active drug is reaching the eye. Secondary biomarkers that may be easily and noninvasively observed include alterations in pupil size and conjunctival hyperemia [143].

One Eye Versus Two. A common dilemma in efficacy studies is whether one or both eyes should be dosed. Arguments can be made for both approaches but it is essential to have a clear understanding of what is to be the control value. When dosing relatively small animals (versus humans) it is possible that systemic absorption may produce a contralateral reduction on IOP and this may mask a drug effect if values in the treated eye are compared to the contralateral untreated eye (which may also decrease). Examples of systemically mediated effects in small animals include bilateral decreases in IOP with unilateral dosing of timolol and apraclonidine in cats and a kappa opioid agonist in monkeys [84, 85, 144]. In general, in early phase efficacy studies there should be a separate control group which receives vehicle control and the test article should be administered to only one eye in the treated group(s). This allows for the detection of a contralateral reduction in IOP and avoids potentially discarding an effective compound because it does not alter IOP in the treated eye relative to the contralateral control (i.e., it lowers IOP in both eyes roughly equally after unilateral administration). In subsequent studies bilateral dosing may be initiated to better mimic the clinical situation or to maximize systemic exposure to the test article. In general, for statistical analysis purposes, the "N" in an IOP efficacy study is the animal and not the eye. In studies with bilateral dosing the data from the two eyes should be averaged (provided the tonometrist has no inherent bias in measurements from one side versus the other) to create a single value for that animal at each time point.

5.9 Phases of an Efficacy Study

There are several distinct phases in an efficacy study

Acclimation Phase. This phase typically lasts several days to several weeks depending on species and the set of animals. It is absolutely essential that conscious dogs, monkeys, and rats be fully acclimated to the entire process of tonometry as IOP typically decreases as the animals become better adjusted to the process. The extent of this decrease may exceed that of a highly effective ocular hypotensive drug and must not be underestimated. Rabbits also must be acclimated to the process, but they tend to adjust more quickly than other species. Studies which show a decrease in IOP in the control groups during the dosing phase typically suffer from a lack of adequate acclimation and the data in the treatment groups should be viewed with suspicion.

The animals should be acclimated to the entire process from start to finish including the room, the table, application of topical anesthesia, the instrument approaching and touching the eye and ideally the reward at the end of the procedure. Acclimation typically begins by allowing the animal to become adjusted to the room, the handlers, and the table or chair (in the case of nonhuman primates) without IOP measurements. Positive reinforcement, usually with a unique and highly desired food treat, is essential. In the author's experience females tend to acclimate faster than males. The room should be quiet with no distractions such as the presence of other animals, music, or unnecessary personnel. This can be a challenge in a busy facility with the need for cage cleaning, rack changes, and other activities in adjacent animal rooms. Once the animal is adjusted to the room they are acclimated to the application of topical anesthetics (which may briefly sting), the process of tonometry, and data recording. In studies with multiple readings/day the acclimation process should mimic the dosing phase of the study in terms of frequency and intervals. Adequate acclimation can usually be verified by observing a diurnal variation in IOP or by noting that over a several day period IOP is stable at a given time of day. Ideally this acclimation would occur prior to the induction of an increase in IOP if one of the ocular hypertensive models is to be used.

Predose Phase. Once the animal is acclimated data from the predose phase is collected for statistical comparison purposes. Baseline values should be collected at the same time of day as during the dosing phase, and are often done over 1–3 days depending on the duration of the dosing phase. It is also important to understand what values constitute the baseline values. For short-term studies this is typically the data collected during the predose phase, but for longer term studies (many weeks to months) IOP may spontaneously vary over time. This may because of changes in the seasons, variation in the estrus cycle, continued physical maturation of the animal or the animal developing anticipatory behaviors to unpleasant events (such as the induction of anesthesia, blood draws, or the development of drug hypersensitivity responses to topical anesthesia or the test article). Although rarely described in the literature, it is also possible that the calibration of the tonometer may drift over a period of months or that different lots of protective tonometer tips may give slightly different readings (a phenomenon described for the Tono-Pen by the manufacturer). Therefore, for long-duration studies comparison to the untreated control group may be more appropriate than comparing to predose values.

Dosing Phase. This phase typically lasts for a few hours to several days, but occasionally can be a year or more. If the dosing phase is to last for several weeks and IOP is being collected from conscious animals it is important to continue with acclimation training to ensure that the animal remains accustomed to the process. Ideally the same tonometrist and restrainer should collect measurements over the course of the study.

If the drug is highly effective a lowering IOP proof of efficacy may be obvious within a few hours after application. Because of this, many screening studies which are simply looking for IOP lowering effects last only a few hours to a day or two. Lack of efficacy in this time frame, however, does not necessarily mean the drug is ineffective, especially in drugs which have complex mechanisms of action involving alterations in the metabolic profile of the cell. Additionally, the full magnitude of the reduction may not become apparent for several days or more until steady state concentrations are achieved. Alternatively, tachyphylaxis may rapidly occur.

To address these possibilities a common design is to conduct a multiday study [145]. With this approach a full IOP "curve" is usually collected at one or more intervals during the predose phase, on Day 1, and on the last day of the dosing phase. IOP is usually measured two to four times per day on the intervening days. Statistically the treated eyes may be compared to the contralateral eye (as a concurrent control), to predose values (to verify adequate acclimation), or to a separate control group if the possibility of a contralateral effect on IOP exists. A variety of study designs have been used to make comparisons between multiple concentrations, formulations, or related compounds. Although some studies sequentially expose the set of animals to various concentrations, formulations, or congeners there is the risk that previous exposure may either heighten or impair subsequent responsiveness [146]. Because of this, the ideal approach would be to randomly assign individuals to various control or treatment groups and evaluate all permutations simultaneously, but the logistics of making numerous simultaneous comparisons are daunting and the risk for a mis-dose is high.

Recovery Phase or "Wash-Out" Period. Because of the expense associated with acquiring and acclimating animals to IOP measurements and determining their responsiveness to the class of test article, it is often desirable to re-use the same animals to compare different concentrations, formulations, or related compounds. The time for the drug to "wash-out" from the animal's system varies considerably, ranging from only a few hours to several weeks or more. The pharmacokinetics of the test article and the duration of therapy play important roles in determining the duration of the washout period. Prostaglandins and rho-kinase inhibitors, which alter complex metabolic pathways such as the extracellular matrix or cytoskeletal elements, often require a washout period of 2–6 weeks, whereas a week or two may be adequate for the beta-blockers [147–149]. Usually, but not always, return to baseline IOP is a good indicator that the drug has "washed-out". During the recovery phase delayed effects of exposure to the drug may also be evaluated.

5.10 A Note on Design of Toxicity Studies for Anti-glaucoma Drugs

Although the design of toxicity studies is covered elsewhere in this text, there are a few unique considerations in the design of anti-glaucoma drug toxicity studies. It is important to resist the temptation to collect IOP lowering efficacy data in toxicity studies because of the large number of confounding variables that are introduced with a toxicity study design and because supra-therapeutic drug concentrations are typically included in toxicity studies. IOP reduction should not be a primary endpoint in a toxicity study but instead IOP should be measured only to demonstrate that a toxicologically adverse alteration in IOP did not occur. Because it is easy to identify these marked alterations in IOP, extensive predose, and dosing phase assessments of IOP are not required. Additionally, the large number of potentially confounding end-points required in a toxicity study can frequently create so much "noise" in IOP values that even a clinically meaningful reduction can be masked, thereby creating confusion as to whether the test article actually lowers IOP or not.

Endpoints meriting consideration in toxicity studies of anti-glaucoma drugs include Hackett-McDonald or McDonald-Shaddock ocular irritation scoring (which involve the application of fluorescein stain and a topical mydriatic), corneal pachymetry, anterior segment optical coherence tomography to evaluate changes in corneal thickness and anterior segment morphology, noncontact specular microscopy to measure corneal thickness and assess changes in the corneal endothelium, gonioscopy, electroretinography to assess retinal effects, electrocardiography, and systemic blood pressure changes, a wide range of toxicokinetic samples and histopathology of the eye and other organs.

References

1. Miller PE (2013) The glaucomas. In: Maggs DJ, Miller PE, Ofri R (eds) Slatter's fundamentals of veterinary ophthalmology, 5th edn. Elsevier, St. Louis, MO
2. Casson RJ, Chidlow G, Wood JP et al (2012) Definition of glaucoma: clinical and experimental concepts. Clin Experiment Ophthalmol 40(4):341–349. doi:10.1111/j.1442-9071.2012.02773.x
3. Nickells RW, Howell GR, Soto I et al (2012) Under pressure: cellular and molecular responses during glaucoma, a common neurodegeneration with axonopathy. Annu Rev Neurosci 35:153–179. doi:10.1146/annurev.neuro.051508.135728
4. Klein BE, Klein R, Sponsel WE et al (1992) Prevalence of glaucoma: the Beaver Dam Eye study. Ophthalmology 99(10):1499–1504
5. Quigley HA, Broman A (2006) The number of persons with glaucoma worldwide in 2010 and 2020. Br J Ophthalmol 90:151–156
6. Rudnicka AR, Mt-Isa S, Owen CG et al (2006) Variations in primary open-angle glaucoma prevalence by age, gender, and race: a Bayesian meta-analysis. Invest Ophthalmol Vis Sci 47(10):4254–4261
7. Resnikoff S, Pascolini D, Etya'ale D et al (2004) Global data on visual impairment in 2002. Bull World Health Organ 82:844–851
8. Collaborative Normal-Tension Glaucoma Study Group (1998) Comparison of glaucomatous progression between untreated patients with normal-tension glaucoma and patients with therapeutically reduced intraocular pressures. Am J Ophthalmol 126:487–497
9. The AGIS Investigators (2000) The advanced glaucoma intervention study (AGIS):7. The relationship between control of intraocular pressure and visual field deterioration. Am J Ophthalmol 130:429–440
10. Goel M, Picciani RG, Lee RK et al (2010) Aqueous humor dynamics: a review. Open Ophthalmol J 4:52–59. doi:10.2174/1874364101004010052
11. Brubaker RF (2004) Goldmann's equation and clinical measures of aqueous dynamics. Exp Eye Res 78(3):633–637
12. Johnson TV, Tomarev SI (2010) Rodent models of glaucoma. Brain Res Bull 81(2–3):349–358. doi:10.1016/j.brainresbull.2009.04.004

13. Knollinger AM, La Croix NC, Barrett P et al (2005) An evaluation of a rebound tonometer for measuring intraocular pressure in dogs and horses. J Am Vet Med Assoc 227:244–248
14. Miller PE, Pickett JP, Majors LJ et al (1991) Clinical comparison of the Mackay-Marg and Tono-Pen applanation tonometers in the dog. Prog Vet Comp Ophthalmol 1:171–176
15. Stuckey GC (2004) Application of physical principles in the development of tonometry. Clin Experiment Ophthalmol 32(6):633–636
16. McCulloh RJ, Holley GP, Miller PE et al (2008) Pachymetery in New Zealand white rabbits, Beagle dogs, and Cynomologus monkeys. In: Abstracts of the 2008 annual meeting of the association for research in vision and ophthalmology, Fort Lauderdale, Florida, May 2008. Electronic abstract
17. Liu J, Roberts CJ (2005) Influence of corneal biomechanical properties on intraocular pressure measurement: quantitative analysis. J Cataract Refract Surg 31(1):146–155
18. Hessemer V, Rössler R, Jacobi KW (1989) Tono-Pen, a new tonometer. Int Ophthalmol 13(1–2):51–56
19. Abrams LS, Vitale S, Jampel HD (1996) Comparison of three tonometers for measuring intraocular pressure in rabbits. Invest Ophthalmol Vis Sci 37(5):940–944
20. Ahn JT, Jeong MB, Park YW et al (2012) Accuracy of intraocular pressure measurements in dogs using two different tonometers and plano therapeutic soft contact lenses. Vet Ophthalmol 15(Suppl 1):83–88. doi:10.1111/j.1463-5224.2011.00979.x
21. Peterson JA, Kiland JA, Croft MA et al (1996) Intraocular pressure measurement in cynomolgus monkeys. Tono-Pen versus manometry. Invest Ophthalmol Vis Sci 37(6):1197–1199
22. Gelatt KN, Peiffer RL Jr, Gum GG et al (1977) Evaluation of applanation tonometers for the dog eye. Invest Ophthalmol Vis Sci 16(10):963–968
23. Bito LZ, Merritt SQ, DeRousseau CJ (1979) Intraocular pressure of rhesus monkey (Macaca mulatta). I. An initial survey of two free-breeding colonies. Invest Ophthalmol Vis Sci 18(8):785–793
24. Andrade SF, Palozzi RJ, Giuffrida R et al (2012) Comparison of intraocular pressure measurements between the Tono-Pen XL® and Perkins® applanation tonometers in dogs and cats. Vet Ophthalmol 15(Suppl 1):14–20. doi:10.1111/j.1463-5224.2011.00926.x
25. Takenaka J, Mochizuki H, Kunihara E et al (2011) Evaluation of rebound tonometer for measuring intraocular pressure at deviated angle and position. Curr Eye Res 36(5):422–428. doi:10.3109/02713683.2010.534574
26. Acosta AC, Espana EM, Nose I, Orozco M et al (2007) Estimation of intraocular pressure in rabbits with commonly used tonometers. Ophthalmic Surg Lasers Imaging 38(1):43–49
27. Wang WH, Millar JC, Pang IH et al (2005) Noninvasive measurement of rodent intraocular pressure with a rebound tonometer. Invest Ophthalmol Vis Sci 46(12):4617–4621
28. McGee HT, Fraunfelder FW (2007) Toxicities of topical ophthalmic anesthetics. Expert Opin Drug Saf 6(6):637–640. doi:10.1517/14740338.6.6.637
29. Elsmo EJ, Kiland JA, Kaufman PL et al (2011) Evaluation of rebound tonometry in non-human primates. Exp Eye Res 92(4):268–273
30. McLellan GJ, Kemmerling JP, Kiland JA (2012) Validation of the TonoVet(®) rebound tonometer in normal and glaucomatous cats. Vet Ophthalmol 16(2):111–118. doi:10.1111/j.1463-5224.2012.01038.x
31. McLaren JW, Brubaker RF, FitzSimon JS (1996) Continuous measurement of intraocular pressure in rabbits by telemetry. Invest Ophthalmol Vis Sci 37:966–975
32. Dinslage S, McLaren J, Brubaker R (1998) Intraocular pressure in rabbits by telemetry II: effects of animal handling and drugs. Invest Ophthalmol Vis Sci 39(12):2485–2489
33. Mansouri K, Weinreb RN (2012) Meeting an unmet need in glaucoma: continuous 24-h monitoring of intraocular pressure. Expert Rev Med Devices 9(3):225–231. doi:10.1586/erd.12.14
34. Antonio Z, Miller PE, Taschwer M et al (2009) Telemetry of intraocular pressure in New Zealand White Rabbits. In: Abstracts of the 2009 annual meeting of the association for research in vision and ophthalmology, Fort Lauderdale, Florida, May 2009. Electronic abstract
35. Downs JC, Burgoyne CF, Seigfreid WP et al (2011) 24-hour IOP telemetry in the nonhuman primate: implant system performance and initial characterization of IOP at multiple timescales. Invest Ophthalmol Vis Sci 52(10):7365–7375
36. Chitnis G, Maleki T, Samuels B et al (2012) A minimally invasive implantable wireless

pressure sensor for continuous IOP monitoring. IEEE Trans Biomed Eng 60 (1):250–256

37. Faschinger C, Mossböck G (2010) Kontinuierliche 24-h-Aufzeichnung von Augendruckschwankungen mittels drahtlosem Kontaktlinsensensor Triggerfish™. Ophthalmologe 107(10):918–922
38. Dziezyc J, Millichamp NJ, Smith WB (1992) Comparison of applanation tonometers in dogs and horses. J Am Vet Med Assoc 201 (3):430–433
39. Moses RA, Marg E, Oechsli R (1962) Evaluation of the basic validity and clinical usefulness of the Mackay-Marg tonometer. Invest Ophthalmol 1:78–85
40. Klein HE, Krohne SG, Moore GE et al (2011) Effect of eyelid manipulation and manual jugular compression on intraocular pressure measurement in dogs. J Am Vet Med Assoc 238 (10):1292–1295
41. Brody S, Erb C, Veit R et al (1999) Intraocular pressure changes: the influence of psychological stress and the Valsalva maneuver. Biol Psychol 51(1):43–57
42. Mok KH, Wong CS, Lee VW (1999) Tono-Pen tonometer and corneal thickness. Eye (Lond) 13(Pt 1):35–37
43. Taylor NR, Zele AJ, Vingrys AJ et al (2007) Variation in intraocular pressure following application of tropicamide in three different dog breeds. Vet Ophthalmol 10(Suppl 1):8–11
44. Stadtbäumer K, Frommlet F, Nell B (2006) Effects of mydriatics on intraocular pressure and pupil size in the normal feline eye. Vet Ophthalmol 9(4):233–237
45. Gomes FE, Bentley E, Lin TL et al (2011) Effects of unilateral topical administration of 0.5% tropicamide on anterior segment morphology and intraocular pressure in normal cats and cats with primary congenital glaucoma. Vet Ophthalmol 14(Suppl 1):75–83. doi:10.1111/j.1463-5224.2011.00927.x
46. Kim JM, Park KH, Han SY et al (2012) Changes in intraocular pressure after pharmacologic pupil dilation. BMC Ophthalmol 12:53. doi:10.1186/1471-2415-12-53
47. Tsai IL, Tsai CY, Kuo LL et al (2012) Transient changes of intraocular pressure and anterior segment configuration after diagnostic mydriasis with 1% tropicamide in children. Clin Exp Optom 95(2):166–172. doi:10.1111/j.1444-0938.2011.00677.x
48. Hamor RE, Roberts SM, Severin GA et al (2000) Evaluation of results for Schirmer tear tests conducted with and without application of a topical anesthetic in clinically normal dogs of 5 breeds. Am J Vet Res 61 (11):1422–1425
49. Herse P, Siu A (1992) Short-term effects of proparacaine on human corneal thickness. Acta Ophthalmol (Copenh) 70(6):740–744
50. McGee HT, Fraunfelder FW (2007) Toxicities of topical ophthalmic anesthetics. Expert Opin Drug Saf 6(6):637–640
51. Sarchahi AA, Bozorgi H (2012) Effect of tetracaine on intraocular pressure in normal and hypertensive rabbit eyes. J Ophthalmic Vis Res 7(1):29–33
52. Holec-Iwasko S, Shin DH, Parrow KA et al (1990) The influence of residual methylcellulose solution on Tono-Pen readings. Am J Ophthalmol 109(5):602–603
53. Liu JHK, Shieh BE, Alston CS (1994) Short-wavelength light reduces circadian elevation of intraocular pressure in rabbits. Neurosci Lett 180:96–100
54. Del Sole MJ, Sande PH, Bernades JM et al (2007) Circadian rhythm of intraocular pressure in cats. Vet Ophthalmol 10:155–161
55. Nickla DL, Wildsoet C, Wallman J (1998) The circadian rhythm in intraocular pressure, axial length, and choroidal thickness in a primate model eye growth, the common marmoset. Invest Ophthalmol Vis Sci 43:2519–2528
56. Anjou CIN (1961) Influence of light on the 24-hour variation in aqueous flare density and intra-ocular pressure in normal rabbits' eyes. Acta Ophthalmol 39:852–873
57. Gelatt KN, Gum GG, Barrie KP et al (1981) Diurnal variations in intraocular pressure in normotensive and glaucomatous Beagles. Glaucoma 3:21–24
58. Giannetto C, Piccione G, Giudice E (2009) Daytime profile of the intraocular pressure and tear production in normal dog. Vet Ophthalmol 12(5):302–305
59. Akaishi T, Ishida N, Shimazaki A et al (2005) Continuous monitoring of circadian variations in intraocular pressure by telemetry system throughout a 12-week treatment with timolol maleate in rabbits. J Ocul Pharmacol Ther 21(6):436–444
60. Zhao M, Hejkal JJ, Camras CB et al (2010) Aqueous humor dynamics during the day and night in juvenile and adult rabbits. Invest Ophthalmol Vis Sci 51(6):3145–3151. doi:10.1167/iovs.09-4415
61. Bar-Ilan A (1984) Diurnal and seasonal variations in intraocular pressure in the rabbit. Exp Eye Res 39(2):175–181
62. Percicot CL, Schnell CR, Debon C et al (1996) Continuous intraocular pressure

measurement by telemetry in alpha-chymotrypsin-induced glaucoma model in the rabbit: effects of timolol, dorzolamide and epinephrine. J Pharmacol Toxicol Methods 36:223–228

63. Collins CC (1962) Evoked pressure response in the rabbit eye. Science 155:106–108
64. Park YW, Jeong MB, Kim TH et al (2011) Effect of central corneal thickness on intraocular pressure with the rebound tonometer and the applanation tonometer in normal dogs. Vet Ophthalmol 14(3):169–173. doi:10.1111/j.1463-5224.2010.00859.x
65. Studer ME, Martin CL, Stiles J (2000) Effects of 0.005% latanoprost solution on intraocular pressure in healthy dogs and cats. Am J Vet Res 61(10):1220–1224
66. Stjernschantz JW (2001) From PGF(2alpha)-isopropyl ester to latanoprost: a review of the development of xalatan: the Proctor Lecture. Invest Ophthalmol Vis Sci 42(6):1134–1145
67. Smith LN, Miller PE, Felchle LM (2010) Effects of topical administration of latanoprost, timolol, or a combination of latanoprost and timolol on intraocular pressure, pupil size, and heart rate in clinically normal dogs. Am J Vet Res 71(9):1055–1061. doi:10.2460/ajvr.71.9.1055
68. Gelatt KN, Larocca RD, Gelatt JK et al (1995) Evaluation of multiple doses of 4 and 6% timolol, and timolol combined with 2% pilocarpine in clinically normal beagles and beagles with glaucoma. Am J Vet Res 56 (10):1325–1331
69. Kaufman PL (2008) Enhancing trabecular outflow by disrupting the actin cytoskeleton, increasing uveoscleral outflow with prostaglandins, and understanding the pathophysiology of presbyopia interrogating Mother Nature: asking why, asking how, recognizing the signs, following the trail. Exp Eye Res 86 (1):3–17
70. Tokushige H, Inatani M, Nemoto S et al (2007) Effects of topical administration of y-39983, a selective rho-associated protein kinase inhibitor, on ocular tissues in rabbits and monkeys. Invest Ophthalmol Vis Sci 48 (7):3216–3222
71. Sugrue MF (1996) The preclinical pharmacology of dorzolamide hydrochloride, a topical carbonic anhydrase inhibitor. J Ocul Pharmacol Ther 12(3):363–376
72. Woodward DF, Phelps RL, Krauss AH et al (2004) Bimatoprost: a novel antiglaucoma agent. Cardiovasc Drug Rev 22(2):103–120
73. Sharif NA, Xu SX, Crider JY et al (2001) Levobetaxolol (Betaxon) and other beta-adrenergic antagonists: preclinical pharmacology, IOP-lowering activity and sites of action in human eyes. J Ocul Pharmacol Ther 17(4):305–317
74. Kutuzova GD, Gabelt BT, Kiland JA et al (2012) 1α,25-Dihydroxyvitamin D(3) and its analog, 2-methylene-19-nor-(20S)-1α,25-dihydroxyvitamin D(3) (2MD), suppress intraocular pressure in non-human primates. Arch Biochem Biophys 518(1):53–60. doi:10.1016/j.abb.2011.10.022
75. Sharif NA (2010) Serotonin-2 receptor agonists as novel ocular hypotensive agents and their cellular and molecular mechanisms of action. Curr Drug Targets 11(8):978–993
76. Wang RF, Serle JB, Gagliuso DJ et al (2000) Comparison of the ocular hypotensive effect of brimonidine, dorzolamide, latanoprost, or artificial tears added to timolol in glaucomatous monkey eyes. J Glaucoma 9(6):458–462
77. Serle JB, Wang RF, Peterson WM et al (2004) Effect of 5-MCA-NAT, a putative melatonin MT3 receptor agonist, on intraocular pressure in glaucomatous monkey eyes. J Glaucoma 13 (5):385–388
78. Bunch TJ, Tian B, Seeman JL et al (2008) Effect of daily prolonged ketamine anesthesia on intraocular pressure in monkeys. Curr Eye Res 33(11):946–953. doi:10.1080/02713680802447121
79. Chien FY, Wang RF, Mittag TW et al (2003) Effect of WIN 55212-2, a cannabinoid receptor agonist, on aqueous humor dynamics in monkeys. Arch Ophthalmol 121(1):87–90
80. Nilsson SF, Drecoll E, Lütjen-Drecoll E et al (2006) The prostanoid EP2 receptor agonist butaprost increases uveoscleral outflow in the cynomolgus monkey. Invest Ophthalmol Vis Sci 47(9):4042–4049
81. Wang YL, Toris CB, Zhan G et al (1999) Effects of topical epinephrine on aqueous humor dynamics in the cat. Exp Eye Res 68 (4):439–445
82. Wilkie DA, Latimer CA (1991) Effects of topical administration of 2.0% pilocarpine on intraocular pressure and pupil size in cats. Am J Vet Res 52(3):441–444
83. Rankin AJ, Crumley WR, Allbaugh RA (2012) Effects of ocular administration of ophthalmic 2% dorzolamide hydrochloride solution on aqueous humor flow rate and intraocular pressure in clinically normal cats. Am J Vet Res 73(7):1074–1078. doi:10.2460/ajvr.73.7.1074
84. Wilkie DA, Latimer CA (1991) Effects of topical administration of timolol maleate on intraocular pressure and pupil size in cats. Am J Vet Res 52(3):436–440
85. Miller PE, Rhaesa SL (1996) Effects of topical administration of 0.5% apraclonidine on

intraocular pressure, pupil size, and heart rate in clinically normal cats. Am J Vet Res 57 (1):83–86

86. Fischer KM, Ward DA, Hendrix DV (2013) Effects of a topically applied 2% delta-9-tetrahydrocannabinol ophthalmic solution on intraocular pressure and aqueous humor flow rate in clinically normal dogs. Am J Vet Res 74 (2):275–280. doi:10.2460/ajvr.74.2.275
87. Gwin RM, Gelatt KN, Gum GG et al (1977) The effect of topical pilocarpine on intraocular pressure and pupil size in the normotensive and glaucomatous beagle. Invest Ophthalmol Vis Sci 16(12):1143–1148
88. Prasanna G, Carreiro S, Anderson S et al (2011) Effect of PF-04217329 a prodrug of a selective prostaglandin EP(2) agonist on intraocular pressure in preclinical models of glaucoma. Exp Eye Res 93(3):256–264. doi:10.1016/j.exer.2011.02.015
89. Miller PE, Nelson MJ, Rhaesa SL (1996) Effects of topical administration of 0.5% apraclonidine on intraocular pressure, pupil size, and heart rate in clinically normal dogs. Am J Vet Res 57(1):79–82
90. Gwin RM, Gelatt KN, Gum GG et al (1978) Effects of topical 1-epinephrine and dipivalyl epinephrine on intraocular pressure and pupil size in the normotensive and glaucomatous Beagle. Am J Vet Res 39:83–86
91. Barabino S, Chen W, Dana MR (2004) Tear film and ocular surface tests in animal models of dry eye: uses and limitations. Exp Eye Res 79(5):613–621
92. Williams DL (2007) Laboratory animal ophthalmology. In: Gelatt KN (ed) Veterinary ophthalmology, 4th edn. Blackwell Publishing, Ames, IA
93. Gupta SK, Agarwal R, Galpalli ND et al (2007) Comparative efficacy of pilocarpine, timolol and latanoprost in experimental models of glaucoma. Methods Find Exp Clin Pharmacol 29(10):665–671. doi:10.1358/mf.2007.29.10.1147765
94. Alarma-Estrany P, Guzman-Aranguez A, Huete F et al (2011) Design of novel melatonin analogs for the reduction of intraocular pressure in normotensive rabbits. J Pharmacol Exp Ther 337(3):703–709. doi:10.1124/jpet.110.178319
95. Naveh N, Weissman C, Muchtar S et al (2000) Submicron emulsion of HU-211, a synthetic cannabinoid, reduces intraocular pressure in rabbits. Graefes Arch Clin Exp Ophthalmol 238(4):334–338
96. Millar JC, Clark AF, Pang IH (2011) Assessment of aqueous humor dynamics in the mouse by a novel method of constant-flow infusion. Invest Ophthalmol Vis Sci 52 (2):685–694. doi:10.1167/iovs.10-6069
97. Pease ME, Cone FE, Gelman S et al (2011) Calibration of the TonoLab tonometer in mice with spontaneous or experimental glaucoma. Invest Ophthalmol Vis Sci 52 (2):858–864. doi:10.1167/iovs.10-5556
98. Swindle MM, Makin A, Herron AJ et al (2012) Swine as models in biomedical research and toxicology testing. Vet Pathol 49(2):344–356. doi:10.1177/0300985811402846
99. Rosolen SG, Rigaudière F, Le Gargasson JF (2003) Un nouveau modèle d'hyperpression oculaire induite chez le miniporc. J Fr Ophtalmol 26(3):259–267
100. Ruiz-Ederra J, García M, Hernández M et al (2005) The pig eye as a novel model of glaucoma. Exp Eye Res 81:561–569
101. Kurashima H, Asai Y, Aihara M et al (2012) Ocular hypotensive effect of tafluprost in latanoprost low-responder cynomolgus monkeys. J Glaucoma 21(2):123–128. doi:10.1097/IJG.0b013e31820bc9ce
102. Mandić Z, Novak-Laus K, Bojić L et al (2010) Safety and efficacy of monotherapy change to fixed combination (travoprost 0.004%/timolol 0.5%) in 6 months follow up period. Acta Clin Croat 49(4):411–419
103. Wilkie DA, Latimer CA (1991) Effects of topical administration of timolol maleate on intraocular pressure and pupil size in dogs. Am J Vet Res 52(3):432–435
104. Camras CB, Hedman K, US Latanoprost Study Group (2003) Rate of response to latanoprost or timolol in patients with ocular hypertension or glaucoma. J Glaucoma 12 (6):466–469
105. Edward DP, Bouhenni R (2011) Anterior segment alterations and comparative aqueous humor proteomics in the buphthalmic rabbit (an American Ophthalmological Society thesis). Trans Am Ophthalmol Soc 109:66–114
106. Kolker AE, Moses RA, Constant MA et al (1963) The development of glaucoma in rabbits. Invest Ophthalmol 2:316–321
107. Hanna BL, Sawin PB, Sheppard LB (1962) Recessive buphthalmos in the rabbit. Genetics 47:519–529
108. Fox RR, Crary DD, Babino EJ Jr et al (1969) Buphthalmia in the rabbit. Pleiotropic effects of the (bu) gene and a possible explanation of mode of gene action. J Hered 60(4):206–212
109. Kuchtey J, Olson LM, Rinkoski T et al (2011) Mapping of the disease locus and identification

of ADAMTS10 as a candidate gene in a canine model of primary open angle Glaucoma. PLoS Genet 7(2):e1001306

110. Sigle KJ, Camaño-Garcia G, Carriquiry AL et al (2011) The effect of dorzolamide 2% on circadian intraocular pressure in cats with primary congenital glaucoma. Vet Ophthalmol 14(Suppl 1):48–53

111. Dawson WW, Brooks DE, Hope GM et al (1993) Primary open angle glaucomas in the rhesus monkey. Br J Ophthalmol 77 (5):302–310

112. Senatorov V, Malyukova I, Fariss R et al (2006) Expression of mutated mouse myocilin induces open-angle glaucoma in transgenic mice. J Neurosci 26(46):11903–11914

113. Zhou Y, Grinchuk O, Tomarev SI (2008) Transgenic mice expressing the Tyr437His mutant of human myocilin protein develop glaucoma. Invest Ophthalmol Vis Sci 49 (5):1932–1939

114. Mabuchi F, Lindsey JD, Aihara M et al (2004) Optic nerve damage in mice with a targeted type I collagen mutation. Invest Ophthalmol Vis Sci 45(6):1841–1845

115. Aihara M, Lindsey JD, Weinreb RN (2003) Ocular hypertension in mice with a targeted type I collagen mutation. Invest Ophthalmol Vis Sci 44(4):1581–1585

116. Heywood R (1975) Glaucoma in the rat. Br Vet J 131(2):213–221

117. Naskar R, Thanos S (2006) Retinal gene profiling in a hereditary rodent model of elevated intraocular pressure. Mol Vis 12:1199–1210

118. Gaasterland G, Kupfer C (1974) Experimental glaucoma in the rhesus monkey. Invest Ophthalmol 13(6):455–457

119. Weber AJ, Zelenak D (2001) Experimental glaucoma in the primate induced by latex microspheres. J Neurosci Methods 111 (1):39–48

120. Quigley HA, Addicks EM (1980) Chronic experimental glaucoma in primates. I. Production of elevated intraocular pressure by anterior chamber injection of autologous ghost red blood cells. Invest Ophthalmol Vis Sci 19(2):126–136

121. Quigley HA, Addicks EM (1980) Chronic experimental glaucoma in primates. II. Effect of extended intraocular pressure elevation on optic nerve head and axonal transport. Invest Ophthalmol Vis Sci 19(2):137–152

122. Krauss AH, Impagnatiello F, Toris CB et al (2011) Ocular hypotensive activity of BOL-303259-X, a nitric oxide donating prostaglandin F2α agonist, in preclinical models. Exp Eye Res 93(3):250–255. doi:10.1016/j.exer.2011.03.001

123. Vareilles P, Silverstone D, Plazonnet B et al (1977) Comparison of the effects of timolol and other adrenergic agents on intraocular pressure in the rabbit. Invest Ophthalmol Vis Sci 16(11):987–996

124. Nishio M, Fukunaga T, Sugimoto M et al (2009) The effect of the H-1152P, a potent Rho-associated coiled coil-formed protein kinase inhibitor, in rabbit normal and ocular hypertensive eyes. Curr Eye Res 34 (4):282–286. doi:10.1080/02713680902783763

125. Gual A, Mintenig GM, Belmonte C (1989) Intraocular pressure effects of water loading and venous compression tests in normal and denervated pigmented rabbits. Exp Eye Res 48(3):365–374

126. Shah GB, Sharma S, Mehta AA et al (2000) Oculohypotensive effect of angiotensin-converting enzyme inhibitors in acute and chronic models of glaucoma. J Cardiovasc Pharmacol 36(2):169–175

127. Ito Y, Nagai N, Shimomura Y (2010) Reduction in intraocular pressure by the instillation of eye drops containing disulfiram included with 2-hydroxypropyl-β-cyclodextrin in rabbit. Biol Pharm Bull 33(9):1574–1578

128. François J, Benozzi G, Victoria-Troncoso V et al (1984) Ultrastructural and morphometric study of corticosteroid glaucoma in rabbits. Ophthalmic Res 16(3):168–178

129. Song Z, Gong Y, Liu H et al (2011) Glycyrrhizin could reduce ocular hypertension induced by triamcinolone acetonide in rabbits. Mol Vis 17:2056–2064, Published online 2011 August 4. PMCID: PMC3156820

130. Bonomi L, Perfetti S, Noya E et al (1978) Experimental corticosteroid ocular hypertension in the rabbit. Albrecht Von Graefes Arch Klin Exp Ophthalmol 209(2):73–82

131. Stagni E, Privitera MG, Bucolo C et al (2008) A water-soluble carbon monoxide-releasing molecule (CORM-3) lowers intraocular pressure in rabbits. Br J Ophthalmol 93 (2):254–257

132. Melena J, Santafé J, Segarra J (1998) The effect of topical diltiazem on the intraocular pressure in betamethasone-induced ocular hypertensive rabbits. J Pharmacol Exp Ther 284(1):278–282

133. Galassi F, Masini E, Giambene B et al (2006) A topical nitric oxide-releasing dexamethasone derivative: effects on intraocular pressure and ocular haemodynamics in a rabbit

glaucoma model. Br J Ophthalmol 90 (11):1414–1419

134. Hester DE, Trites PN, Peiffer RL et al (1987) Steroid-induced ocular hypertension in the rabbit: a model using subconjunctival injections. J Ocul Pharmacol 3(3):185–189
135. Gerometta R, Spiga MG, Borrás T et al (2010) Treatment of sheep steroid-induced ocular hypertension with a glucocorticoid-inducible MMP1 gene therapy virus. Invest Ophthalmol Vis Sci 51(6):3042–3048
136. Gerometta R, Podos SM, Danias J et al (2009) Steroid-induced ocular hypertension in normal sheep. Invest Ophthalmol Vis Sci 50(2):669–673
137. Tektas OY, Hammer CM, Danias J et al (2010) Morphologic changes in the outflow pathways of bovine eyes treated with corticosteroids. Invest Ophthalmol Vis Sci 51 (8):4060–4066
138. Gerometta R, Podos SM, Candia OA et al (2004) Steroid-induced ocular hypertension in normal cattle. Arch Ophthalmol 122 (10):1492–1497
139. Sears D, Sears M (1974) Blood aqueous barrier and alpha chymotrypsin glaucoma in rabbits. Am J Ophthalmol 77(3):378–383
140. Best M, Rabinovitz AZ, Masket S (1975) Experimental alphachymotrypsin glaucoma. Ann Ophthalmol 7(6):803–810
141. Melena J, Santafé J, Segarra-Doménech J et al (1999) Aqueous humor dynamics in alpha-chymotrypsin-induced ocular hypertensive rabbits. J Ocul Pharmacol Ther 15(1):19–27
142. Campana G, Bucolo C, Murari G et al (2002) Ocular hypotensive action of topical flunarizine in the rabbit: role of sigma 1 recognition sites. J Pharmacol Exp Ther 303 (3):1086–1094
143. Chen J, Dinh T, Woodward DF et al (2005) Bimatoprost: mechanism of ocular surface hyperemia associated with topical therapy. Cardiovasc Drug Rev 23(3):231–246
144. Rasmussen CA, Gabelt BT, Kaufman PL (2007) Aqueous humor dynamics in monkeys in response to the kappa opioid agonist bremazocine. Trans Am Ophthalmol Soc 105:225–238, discussion 238–9
145. Lee PY, Podos SM, Serle JB et al (1987) Intraocular pressure effects of multiple doses of drugs applied to glaucomatous monkey eyes. Arch Ophthalmol 105(2):249–252
146. Millar JC, Kaufman PL (1995) PGF2 alpha/pilocarpine interactions on IOP and accommodation in monkeys. Exp Eye Res 61 (6):677–683
147. Rouland JF, Traverso CE, Stalmans I, T2345 Study Group et al (2013) Efficacy and safety of preservative-free latanoprost eyedrops, compared with BAK-preserved latanoprost in patients with ocular hypertension or glaucoma. Br J Ophthalmol 97(2):196–200. doi:10.1136/bjophthalmol-2012-302121
148. Sonty S, Mundorf TK, Stewart JA et al (2009) Short-term tolerability of once-daily timolol hemihydrate 0.5%, timolol maleate in sorbate 0.5%, and generic timolol maleate gel-forming solution 0.5% in glaucoma and/or ocular hypertension: a prospective, randomized, double-masked, active-controlled, three-period crossover pilot study. Clin Ther 31(10):2063–2071. doi:10.1016/j.clinthera.2009.10.003
149. Dinslage S, Hueber A, Diestelhorst M et al (2004) The influence of latanoprost 0.005% on aqueous humor flow and outflow facility in glaucoma patients: a double-masked placebo-controlled clinical study. Graefes Arch Clin Exp Ophthalmol 242(8):654–660
150. Wang D, Qi M, He M et al (2012) Ethnic difference of the anterior chamber area and volume and its association with angle width. Invest Ophthalmol Vis Sci 53(6):3139–3144
151. O'Donnell C, Hartwig A, Radhakrishnan H (2012) Comparison of central corneal thickness and anterior chamber depth measured using LenStar LS900, Pentacam, and Visante AS-OCT. Cornea 31(9):983–988
152. Deering MF (2005) A photon accurate model of the human eye. ACM Trans Graph 24 (3):649–658
153. Short BG (2008) Safety evaluation of ocular drug delivery formulations: techniques and practical considerations. Toxicol Pathol 36 (1):49–62. doi:10.1177/0192623307310955
154. Lapuerta P, Schein SJ (1995) A four-surface schematic eye of macaque monkey obtained by an optical method. Vision Res 35 (16):2245–2254
155. Kaufman PL, Calkins BT, Erickson KA (1981) Ocular biometry of the cynomolgus monkey. Curr Eye Res 1(5):307–309
156. McCulloh RJ, Holley GP, Miller PE et al (2008) Pachymetry in New Zealand White Rabbits, Beagle dogs, and Cynomologus Monkeys. In: Abstracts of the 2008 annual meeting of the association for research in vision and ophthalmology, Fort Lauderdale, Florida, May 2008. Electronic abstract
157. Moodie KL, Hashizume N, Houston DL et al (2001) Postnatal development of corneal curvature and thickness in the cat. Vet Ophthalmol 4(4):267–272
158. Carrington SD, Woodward EG (1986) Corneal thickness and diameter in the domestic cat. Ophthalmic Physiol Opt 6(4):385–389

159. Rankin AJ, Crumley WR, Allbaugh RA (2012) Effects of ocular administration of ophthalmic 2% dorzolamide hydrochloride solution on aqueous humor flow rate and intraocular pressure in clinically normal cats. Am J Vet Res 73(7):1074–1078
160. Vakkur GJ, Bishop PO (1963) The schematic eye in the cat. Vision Res 61:357–381
161. Konrade KA, Hoffman AR, Ramey KL et al (2012) Refractive states of eyes and associations between ametropia and age, breed, and axial globe length in domestic cats. Am J Vet Res 73 (2):279–284. doi:10.2460/ajvr.73.2.279
162. Mutti DO, Zadnik K, Murphy CJ (1999) Naturally occurring vitreous chamber-based myopia in the Labrador retriever. Invest Ophthalmol Vis Sci 40(7):1577–1584
163. Ward DA, Cawrse MA, Hendrix DV (2001) Fluorophotometric determination of aqueous humor flow rate in clinically normal dogs. Am J Vet Res 62(6):853–858
164. Bozkir G, Bozkir M, Dogan H et al (1997) Measurements of axial length and radius of corneal curvature in the rabbit eye. Acta Med Okayama 51(1):9–11
165. Hughes A (1972) A schematic eye for the rabbit. Vision Res 12(1):123–138
166. Gwon A (2008) The rabbit in cataract/IOL surgery. In: Tsonis PA (ed) Animal models in eye. Research Elsevier Ltd, San Diego, CA, pp 184–205
167. Sanchez I, Martin R, Ussa F et al (2011) The parameters of the porcine eyeball. Graefes Arch Clin Exp Ophthalmol 249:475–482
168. Faber C, Scherfig E, Prause JU et al (2008) Corneal thickness in pigs measured by ultrasound pachymetry in vivo. Scand J Lab Anim Sci 35(1):35–43
169. Yin J, Huang J, Chen C et al (2011) Corneal complications in streptozocin-induced type I diabetic rats. Invest Ophthalmol Vis Sci 52 (9):6589–6596. doi:10.1167/iovs.11-7709
170. Massaf RW, Chang FW (1972) A revision of the rat schematic eye. Vision Res 12 (5):793–796
171. Remtulla S, Hallett PE (1985) A schematic eye for the mouse, and comparisons with the rat. Vision Res 25(1):21–31
172. Aihara M, Lindsey JD, Weinreb RN (2003) Aqueous humor dynamics in mice. Invest Ophthalmol Vis Sci 44(12):5168–5173
173. Mansoor H, Zeng H, Chiao M (2011) Real-time thickness measurement of biological tissues using a microfabricated magnetically-driven lens actuator. Biomed Microdevices 13(4):641–649. doi:10.1007/s10544-011-9534-6

Methods in Pharmacology and Toxicology (2014): 243–265
DOI 10.1007/7653_2013_4

Published online: 29 August 2013

Study Design and Methodologies for Study of Ocular Medical Devices

Joseph W. Carraway and Elaine M. Daniel

Abstract

This chapter focuses on the test methods necessary to demonstrate the safety and "biocompatibility" of ocular medical devices. Biocompatibility has a variety of definitions, but in general it is the quality of the medical device or biomaterial to not have toxic, adverse, or injurious effects on biological systems. The test methods described in this chapter are the commonly used routine test methods for establishing biocompatibility.

Key words Medical devices, Biocompatibility, ISO 10993, Standards, Testing requirements, Safety, Biological effect

1 Introduction

1.1 Regulatory Guidance

The ISO 10993: *Biological evaluation of medical devices* series is an internationally recognized set of standards that define the evaluation process, testing requirements, and test methods for establishing biocompatibility of medical devices regardless of the device type [1–10]. The ISO 10993 series is composed of 20 parts currently. ISO 10993-1: *Evaluation and testing within a risk management process* [1] defines the principles of a safety evaluation, how devices are categorized based on the nature and duration of their contact with the body, biological effects that must be evaluated, and the overall assessment of data to assure safety. The remaining parts of the series primarily relate to the actual test methods. The ISO 10993 series of standards are considered "horizontal" standards as they apply to all devices regardless of type. For ocular devices, additional standards exist that are unique to a specific type of ocular device, such as those for contact lenses (ISO 9394) [11], intraocular lenses (IOLs) (ISO 11797-5) [12], and viscosurgical devices (ISO 15798) [13]. These "vertical" standards define additional testing requirements beyond and in addition to those defined in ISO 10993.

1.2 General Testing Requirements Based on Contact and Duration

ISO 10993–1 [1] defines three broad types of body contact: (1) surface contacting, (2) externally communicating, or (3) implant. Within each of these major categories there are subcategories. Surface contacting includes the skin, mucous membranes, and skin or mucous membranes where the surface is breached or damaged. Contact lenses and lens solutions would be considered examples of devices in the surface contacting, mucous membranes category. Externally communicating includes devices with indirect blood path, tissue/bone/dentin, and circulating blood exposure. Ocular devices in this category could include ophthalmic instruments and fluid sets used during cataract surgery, i.e., an item with contact inside the eye but a portion that remains outside the eye. The final category is implant devices and this is subdivided into those with tissue/bone contact and those with blood contact. An IOL or aqueous shunt would fall into this category.

Devices are categorized based on their duration of tissue/body contact. The three durations are (1) limited exposure (≤24 h), (2) prolonged exposure (>24 h to ≤30 days), and (3) permanent contact (>30 days). These contact durations are based on single, multiple, or repeated exposure. So for a device such as a contact lens, it may be worn for 12–16 h a day (limited exposure), but because of multiple exposures, it is considered to be in a prolonged exposure category.

The combination of type of body contact and contact duration determines the types of biological effects that must be considered for a device. In general, surface contacting, limited exposure devices require assessment of the fewest biological effects. As the body contact becomes more invasive and/or the duration of contact increases, the potential for adverse biological effects increases, prompting the need to evaluate more biological effects.

1.3 Biological Effects to Consider

ISO 10993–1 defines the biological effects that must be considered for a device. These effects include cytotoxicity, irritation/intracutaneous reactivity, sensitization, acute systemic toxicity, subacute/subchronic toxicity, genotoxicity, implantation, and hemocompatibility. These biological effects for consideration are common to all medical devices. Depending on the nature of the device, additional biological effects may require evaluation such as chronic toxicity, biodegradation, toxicokinetics, immunotoxicity, and organ-specific toxicities. ISO 10993–1 requires that you consider what is known about the biomaterials composing the device, the history of use of the material, and the nature and quantity of leachable chemicals/substances that could have biological exposure during use. Based on the information, a determination is made as to whether sufficient data are available to address the biological effects appropriate for the tissue contact and duration of exposure for the device. If sufficient data are not available, testing must be conducted to assure the material does not cause an adverse effect. The following sections describe some of the common test methods used to address those biological effects.

2 Standard Biocompatibility Testing

2.1 Sample Preparation

Many of the in vivo test methods used for evaluation of medical devices are adaptations of established test methods that have been historically used for testing chemicals and pharmaceuticals. The adaptations relate to how the medical device is prepared to deliver a dose. In general, medical devices are mixtures of materials, such as polymers, metals, and ceramics. While most medical devices are essentially insoluble and solid, some can be soluble solids or liquids. For *insoluble solid devices*, these are typically prepared for dosing by creating an extract of the medical device in various solvents. These solvents are used to pull out or extract the chemicals that could be anticipated to leach from the device during clinical use. Since a device can be exposed to polar (aqueous) and nonpolar (lipids) fluid environments during clinical use and the device may have polar and nonpolar chemicals present, extractions are accomplished with polar and nonpolar solvents. The solvents used and extraction conditions (time and temperature for extraction) are spelled out in ISO 10993–12: *Sample preparation and reference materials* [9]. Saline is frequently used as a polar solvent and refined vegetable oil is commonly used as a nonpolar solvent. Following incubation or "extraction" of the device in the solvent, the resultant "device extract" from this process become the test solution used for evaluation. It is important to note that the temperatures used during extraction are not intended to mimic clinical exposure conditions. They are exaggerated to optimize the amount of leachable chemicals extracted for the purposes of hazard identification.

Recently, exhaustive extraction methods based on the Japanese Ministry of Health, Labor, and Welfare (MHLW) testing guidelines for medical devices have been advocated for polymeric materials as an option to typical extraction methods in ISO 10993–12. These extraction methods utilize organic solvents to more aggressively extract leachables from the medical device. The extract is reduced to a residue, which can then be dissolved in a solvent appropriate for the test system. Since the mass of residue is known, the test solution (extract) can be prepared with a defined concentration. In the conventional extraction method, the quantity of leachables in the extract is unknown. It can be argued that the extraction with organic solvents is extreme, does not represent exposure conditions under clinical use, and may result in chemical alterations of possible leachables. However, this more rigorous extraction procedure can improve assay sensitivity with respect to detecting undesirable biological effects.

For *soluble devices*, the device is mixed with an appropriate solvent, if necessary, to create a solution at a concentration that is physiologically compatible. With extracts of devices or solutions created from devices, the mixture is typically used immediately since the stability of the solution or extract is unknown. Soluble devices can be tested as a single dose of the 100 % extract, which could be considered equivalent to the "maximum tolerated dose" (MTD). This single MTD is used for risk assessment purposes since adverse responses associated with extracts of medical devices are rare.

For some of the test methods, the medical device can be tested directly without the need for extraction. For example, an examination glove would be tested directly in a skin irritation test; similarly a contact lens solution would be tested in an eye irritation test. For the assessment of local effects following implantation (ISO 10993–6) [6], the medical device or parts thereof (or the composing materials) are implanted directly in tissues. Tests to evaluate systemic toxicity may utilize extracts of the device for the acute duration studies and implant portions of the device for subacute and subchronic toxicity studies.

2.2 Cytotoxicity

In general, in vitro assays are useful tools for identifying potential hazards associated with chemical compounds or materials. ISO 10993–5: *Tests for in vitro cytotoxicity* [5] describes the various in vitro cytotoxicity assays used to evaluate medical devices. Since cytotoxicity assays are quite sensitive, they are recommended as one of the first screening tests to be done on new biomaterials and medical devices. While the presence of cytotoxicity does not necessarily imply a biomaterial or device lacks biocompatibility, one should understand the possible mechanisms for cytotoxicity and how cytotoxicity may correlate to a tissue response during expected clinical use.

There are various cytotoxicity assays that are commonly used. These assays are categorized by type of cell exposure, method of detection, and the evaluation criteria. The cells in the assays are exposed by three possible approaches: an extract test, a direct contact test, and an indirect contact test. The choice of exposure route depends on the nature of the device exposure and the type of device being tested. Cytotoxicity is determined by evaluation of cell morphology, cell damage, and cell growth or by measurement of cellular activity. Various cell lines are available for cytotoxicity testing, although some cell lines are specified for a given assay in the ISO 10993–5 standard. The L-929 mouse fibroblast cell lines is commonly used. Assay measurement systems for cell detection can include the neutral red assay, the tetrazolium salt assay (e.g. MTT, XTT, WST-1), the colony-forming assay, or the LDH assay detecting primarily membrane damage in cells. The criteria for assessment can be either qualitative or quantitative. In each cytotoxicity assay, positive, negative, and blank controls should be included to allow assessment of normal cell growth, effects of the extraction media, and sensitivity of the test system via response to a known positive control.

Test samples should be prepared as described in ISO 10993–12: *Sample preparation and reference material* [9]. A variety of extraction solvents and extraction conditions can be used, but extraction in serum supplemented culture medium tends to be the most common. The serum added to the tissue culture medium supports cell growth and allows for the extraction of both polar and nonpolar compounds. During the extraction procedure, sterile conditions should be maintained or if the source material is not sterile, sterilization of the extract and/or test sample should be considered. For ocular medical devices (e.g., contact lenses, IOLs, aqueous shunts), in addition to extracts, the devices themselves can also be used in a direct contact or indirect contact cytotoxicity assays.

2.3 Sensitization

Evaluation of a medical device's potential to cause sensitization is required for all devices regardless of tissue contact and contact duration. The tests used are classical models that have a long history of use. Currently, there are three basic models: (1) the guinea pig maximization test (GPMT), (2) the guinea pig closed patch or Buehler method, and (3) the local lymph node assay (LLNA). The GPMT is used most frequently and can be used regardless of the device's tissue contact. This method is covered in detail as it is the most likely method to be used for ocular medical device testing. The Buehler method is typically reserved for devices that only have contact with intact skin. The two guinea pig test methods are qualitative assays, while the LLNA is a quantitative method. The LLNA has a long history of use for chemicals, but has a relatively short history of use in medical device testing. Due to less historical data with medical devices and questions regarding its adaptation and use with medical devices, some regulatory agencies do not fully recognize this method at this time. However, the methodology for the LLNA is discussed as it can provide a good screening tool and may be more widely used in future regulatory testing paradigms.

2.3.1 Guinea Pig Maximization Test

The basic methodology is described in ISO 10993–10: *Tests for irritation and skin sensitization* [7] and is similar to other standard methods such as OECD 406, *Skin Sensitization* [14]. The test is conducted in young guinea pigs weighing 300–500 g at the beginning of the test. Either sex can be used, but all should be the same sex; females should be nonpregnant or nulliparous. The test utilizes ten animals per test extract with five animals for the respective control extract. A study with both saline (polar) and nonpolar (vegetable oil) extracts, a total of 30 animals are used. ISO 10993–10 [7] requires that positive control materials be tested at least once every 6 months utilizing a weak sensitizer to demonstrate sensitivity of the animal model and test methods. The study has three phases: intradermal induction, topical induction, and challenge. For the intradermal induction, animals receive three pairs of intradermal injections over the scapular region. The pairs are as follows:

Site A—A 50:50 mixture of the chosen solvent/extract vehicle and Freund's complete adjuvant. The mixture is well mixed to form a stable emulsion.

Site B—The test sample (undiluted extract); inject the control animals with the solvent alone.

Site C—A 50:50 mixture of the test extract/solution and Freund's complete adjuvant. The mixture is well mixed to form a stable emulsion. Control animals are injected with a 50:50 mixture of the respective solvent/extract vehicle and Freund's complete adjuvant.

Topical induction occurs approximately 1 week after the intradermal injections. One day prior to topical induction, the previous injection site area is clipped to remove excess hair and approximately 0.5 ml of 10 % sodium lauryl sulfate (SLS) in petroleum is applied to the area to cause mild irritation that will improve topical absorption. Twenty-four hours after application of the SLS, it is removed. The test extract/solution is applied to an approximate 8 cm^2 filter paper or absorbant gauze, then applied over the previous injection site area and covered with an occlusive dressing. The patches are removed after 48 h. Two weeks after this topical induction, hair is closely clipped over the back and flank region. In the test animals, the test extract/solution is applied to the right flank and the vehicle control is applied to the left flank. In the control animals, the control vehicle/solution is applied to the right flank and the test applied to the left. Test and control materials are left in place for 24 h, then removed and sites are scored for erythema and edema using a standardized scale (Table 1) at 24 and 48 h following patch removal.

In general, scores of 1 or greater are considered evidence of sensitization. However, scores of 1 or greater may also be seen in the control animals. Response greater than the control are considered a positive indication of sensitization. The overall response in the test animals is compared to the response in the control animals. In the situation of an equivocal response, animals should receive a rechallenge of the topical application. This is accomplished 1–2 weeks following the initial challenge and the materials are applied to fresh skin sites.

2.3.2 Local Lymph Node Assay

The LLNA was validated as an alternative test method to determine the sensitization potential of individual chemicals in 1999. In 2002, it was accepted by OECD as OECD 429—*Skin Sensitisation: Local*

Table 1
Magnusson and Kligman scale

Patch test reaction	Grading scale
No visible change	0
Discrete or patchy erythema	1
Moderate and confluent erythema	2
Intense erythema and/or swelling	3

Lymph Node Assay [15]. After several years, this method was adopted for use with medical device extracts. The current version of ISO 10993–10 [7] contains detailed methods for the conduct of this assay. The assay offers several advantages over the guinea pig sensitization assays. It is a quantitative assay, can be conducted in less than a week, needs relatively small amounts of material for testing, and has animal welfare benefits. The disadvantage is that in recent years there have been questions about: (1) the validity of using this assay with extracts that are by their nature mixtures vs. single chemical, and (2) whether the method is appropriate with aqueous solvents. Due to these questions, some regulatory agencies have not recommended this assay. However, new data have been presented recently supporting that the LLNA is valid with mixtures and an aqueous solvent.

Nonpolar or hydrophobic solvents have been historically used with the LLNA for chemicals. These solvents are readily absorbed through the skin. Aqueous solvents tend to bead up and roll off the skin. To utilize aqueous medical device extracts, it is necessary to improve skin adherence and absorption. This has been accomplished in one of two methods. The first is through either the addition of a thickener such as carboxy methyl cellulose or hydroxyethyl cellulose (0.5 % w/v) or the use of a surfactant such as 1 % pluronic [16]. The addition of either the thickener or surfactant allows for better coating and absorption when using aqueous solvents. Aside from these adaptations for device extracts, the test methods are the same as those for chemicals.

The basic methodology is as follows. Young (8–12-week old), nulliparous, nonpregnant female mice of CBA/Ca or CBA/J strain mice are used. A minimum of four mice per group are used for chemicals. However, for medical device testing, since only one dose level is typically used, five mice per group are recommended. A 25 μl portion of test extract or control solution is painted onto the dorsal surface of both ears of the mouse. This application is repeated daily for three consecutive days. At 72 h following the last application, animals are injected intravenously with the radioisotope, ^{3}H-methyl thymidine. The isotope will be incorporated into rapidly dividing cells. If the test substance is a sensitizer, lymphocyte proliferation will be increased in the lymph nodes that drain the ears and thus radioactivity levels will be higher. At 5 h following the isotope injection, animals are euthanized, lymph nodes are collected, and radioactivity is measured. The radioactivity level in the test animals is divided by the background level of radioactivity in the negative control animals to determine a "stimulation index" (SI). If the SI is $\geq$3.0, the substance is considered a potential sensitizer. It is recommended to use a weak sensitizer (hexyl cinnamic aldehyde, mercaptobenzothiazole, benzocaine) as a concurrent positive control. If a laboratory has a long history of consistent positive responses with their positive controls, they may elect to do periodic positive controls. The positive controls should be run at minimum of every 6 months or less.

2.4 Ocular or Intracutaneous Irritation

Irritation is a biological effect that must be addressed for essentially all medical devices. Irritation tests provide an assessment of the local inflammatory tissue response following direct contact with a medical device or extract of a device. As with other test described, these tests are classic test models that have been historically used for chemicals and have been adapted for medical devices. Detailed methods have been included in this chapter for ocular irritation and intracutaneous irritation testing.

The albino New Zealand White (NZW) rabbit has historically been used to assess ocular irritation, because it is easy to assess ocular reactions due to the lack of ocular pigmentation. The test methods are based on OECD 405 and US Consumer Product Safety Commission test guidelines [17]. Three young rabbits weighing at least 2 kg are typically used for this assay. Test methods involve placing 0.1 ml of the test extract or solution in the lower conjunctival sac of one eye in each rabbit. The eyelid is held closed for 1 s. The opposite eye is similarly treated with the control vehicle or solution. The standard test method involves a single application and observations for 3 days. However, based on the nature of the clinical exposure, repeat applications and longer durations may be appropriate. Eyes are observed and scored for ocular reactions based on a standardized Draize scoring system at 1, 24, 48, and 72 h after treatment. Animals showing severe reactions are humanely euthanized.

Results in the test treated eyes are compared to the control eyes. If more than one test treated eye has a positive response in any of the categories, the material is considered an eye irritant. If only one test treated eye demonstrates a positive response, the results are considered equivocal and the test is repeated in additional animals. A severe reaction in one animal is considered sufficient to consider the material an irritant.

Additional irritation methods can involve the injection of solutions or extracts into the eye. These methods are not specifically defined in the ISO 10993 series. These methods are adapted from the ISO 15798 standard [13] which contains a test method for evaluation of irritation following injection of viscosurgical materials into the anterior chamber. In these test methods, 3–6 rabbits are used and solutions or extracts are injected into either the anterior chamber (intracameral) or into the vitreous body (intravitreous). Evaluation procedures may include ocular examinations (slit-lamp and indirect ophthalmic exams for intravitreal), intraocular pressure measurements, leukocyte counts, and histopathology. The specific test methods are customized based on the nature of the device and exposure duration.

The intracutaneous reactivity test is a standard screening assay for medical devices regardless of their tissue contact during clinical use. This test has a long history of use as part of USP method for evaluating leachables associated with pharmaceutical containers and can be utilized for evaluating irritation from leachables for externally communicating and implantable ocular devices. In the USP version of the test, four extracts are used: saline, 5% alcohol saline, propylene glycol, and vegetable oil. Today for most medical devices, only saline and vegetable oil extracts are evaluated. Materials with a pH ≤ 2.0 or ≥ 11.5 are assumed to be irritants and not tested. In this model, NZW rabbits are used. The current ISO version requires three rabbits weighing at least 2.0 kg. Following closely clipping the fur over the back, 0.2 ml of test and control extracts are injected intradermally with a small gauge needle at five sites. Extracts are injected in rows. In each rabbit, a row of five test saline blebs and five saline control blebs will be placed on one side with the vegetable oil injections placed on the opposite side. The appearance of the blebs is evaluated for erythema and edema immediately after injection, and at 24, 48, and 72 h following injection using a standardized scoring scheme (Table 2).

Scores for erythema and edema for all sites and animals are added and divided by the total observations to arrive at an average irritation score for the test and control extracts. The value of the respective control is subtracted from the test extract score. The extract meets the criteria of the test if the value is ≤ 1.0. An important technical consideration regarding this assay is the use of high quality vegetable oil. If the vegetable used is not refined or has become rancid, it will cause excessive reactivity obscuring a reaction associated with leachables. With refined vegetable oil, scores of 1 for erythema and possibly edema are common at 24 and 48 h, but are reduced or absent by 72 h. Scores of ≥ 2, particularly for erythema with the vehicle control may suggest an issue with the oil.

2.5 Acute Systemic Toxicity

Acute systemic toxicity is defined as adverse effects occurring at any time after single, multiple, or continuous exposures of a test sample within a 24-h period. Typically the observation period is several days to a week. The purpose of this initial toxicity screen is to

Table 2
Skin reaction scoring scheme

Reaction	Irritation score
Erythema and eschar formation	
No erythema	0
Very slight erythema (barely perceptible)	1
Well-defined erythema	2
Moderate erythema	3
Severe erythema (beet-redness) to eschar formation preventing grading of erythema	4
Edema formation	
No edema	0
Very slight edema (barely perceptible)	1
Well-defined edema (edges of area well defined by definite raising)	2
Moderate edema (raised approximately 1 mm)	3
Severe edema (raised more than 1 mm and extending beyond exposure area)	4

determine if leachables or soluble chemicals are present that would cause some degree of toxicity.

The design for the acute toxicity tests used for medical devices can vary, but they are most often based on the United States Pharmacopeia (USP) systemic toxicity test [18]. In this method, device extracts are dosed by the intravenous and intraperitoneal routes. The USP method was originally designed for pharmaceutical containers, i.e., drug vials. Since the vehicle or drug product vehicle for pharmaceuticals can vary, a set of four vehicles is used in this method: (1) saline, (2) 5% alcohol in saline, (3) vegetable oil, and (4) polyethylene glycol (PEG). For ISO 10993–11 testing [8], saline and vegetable oil extracts are considered sufficient for this screening assay. In this test method, mice are used and dosed intravenously (saline-based materials) or intraperitoneally (non-saline solution). Mice are observed for clinical symptoms of toxicity such as lethargy, hyperactivity, convulsions, weight loss, and death. Animals are observed for a minimum of 3 days. For extracts a relatively large dose volume, 50 ml/kg of body weight, is used. While this dose volume is large, it is tolerated by mice. Since the quantity of leachables is generally expected to be low, this high dose volume improves the sensitivity of the assay. However, this high dose volume can present issues when extracting devices that are soluble. When testing a soluble medical device, a physiologically compatible solution should be prepared. The arbitrary 50 ml/kg dose should not apply, but rather the dose should reflect a multiple of the clinical dose on an mg/kg basis. This exaggeration factor is frequently 10–20 times the clinical dose for acute studies.

2.6 Genotoxicity

Genotoxicity is indicated if a review of the medical device composition reveals the possible presence of compounds that might interact with genetic material, or when the chemical composition of the medical device is unknown. The genotoxicity testing of a medical device should start with a series of in vitro tests. The requirement to assess genotoxicity primarily applies to external communicating devices or implant medical devices with a prolonged or permanent contact.

The in vitro tests commonly used evaluate two major classes of genetic damage: gene mutations and chromosomal damage. The specific test methods to detect genetic damage are described in detail for medical devices in the latest edition of the ISO 10993-3 [3] technical specification. These methods have been adapted for medical devices from various OECD test methods [19–21]. A common assay for detection of gene mutations is the bacterial reverse mutation test (Ames test). This assay uses strains of *Salmonella typhimurium* and *Escherichia coli* to detect point mutations, which involve substitution, addition, or deletion of one or a few DNA base pairs. The bacteria in this assay have been modified or mutated such that their ability to synthesize an essential amino acid has been lost resulting in limited growth on amino acid restricted media. When exposed to a mutagene, they can regain their ability to synthesize amino acids resulting in increased growth/numbers of colonies as compared to the control bacteria.

For the in vitro gene mutation test, several mammalian cell lines can be used but the thymidine kinase (TK) deficient mouse lymphoma cell line is the most common and the assay is generally referred to as the Mouse Lymphoma Assay (MLA). The TK deficient mutant cells are able to proliferate in the presence of the pyrimidine analogue trifluorothymidine (TFT), whereas normal cells, which contain thymidine kinase, cannot. The mutation frequency is determined by seeding known cell numbers in medium containing device extracts or solutions. After a suitable incubation time, colonies are counted, and cloning efficiency (viability) is determined. The mutation frequency is compared between cells exposed to the device extract/solution and those exposed to the control vehicle.

For detection of chromosomal damage with an in vitro mammalian cell test, colony sizing as an endpoint in the MLA can be used or the chromosomal aberration (CA) assay is used. In the CA assay, either human lymphocytes or Chinese hamster ovary cells are grown in culture media dosed with device extracts or solutions. After appropriate incubation periods, cells are arrested in metaphase and prepared on slides for evaluation of numeric or structural chromosomal changes. The chromosomal changes in the test exposed cells are compared to the vehicle exposed cells to determine the presence of chromosomal damage.

Under the testing recommendations of ISO 10993–3 [3], in vivo genotoxicity testing is not required unless a genotoxic response is noted in one of the in vitro assays for the device. As a note, some countries do not recognize ISO 10993–3 as a consensus standard and require in vivo genotoxicity assays as part of the overall genotoxicity assessment regardless of the response in the in vitro assays. When in vivo genotoxicity assays are required, in vivo tests for chromosomal damage in rodent hematopoietic cells are typically used. The two most common assays in this category are (1) the in vivo mouse micronucleus assays and (2) the in vivo chromosomal aberration assay.

The in vivo mouse micronucleus assay currently is the more popular of the two in vivo assays. The methodology is based on OECD 474, *Mammalian Erythrocyte Micronucleus Test* [22]. The assay is conducted in young rodents, either mice or rats, but mice are used most commonly. Assays are conducted with concurrent negative (vehicle) and positive controls. A minimum of five males and five females per group are used. Both sexes are used unless a single sex is justified. Animals are dosed with the device extract or solution by an appropriate route. The intravenous route is typically used for saline extracts (insoluble devices) and the intraperitoneal route for other extracts and solutions. The oral route of administration may be applicable for devices that have exposure through the gastrointestinal system. If bone marrow is used, the animals are sacrificed at appropriate times after treatment, the bone marrow extracted, and preparations made and stained. When peripheral blood is used, the blood is collected at appropriate times after treatment and smear preparations are made and stained. For studies with peripheral blood, smears can be prepared as with bone marrow specimens or samples can be analyzed by flow cytometry. With both methods, preparations are analyzed for the presence of micronuclei. Numbers of micronuclei in test animals are compared to the negative control to determine whether the treatment caused an increase in micronuclei.

The basic methodology for the in vivo chromosomal aberration assay is based on OECD 475, *Mammalian Bone Marrow Chromosome Aberration Test* [23]. As with the mouse micronucleus assay, the test is conducted in young rodents with similar numbers and groups. Animals are dosed once daily for two consecutive days (multiple or split dosing may be justified) and the dose is based on a maximum volume per kg body weight or mg/kg with extract residues. Animals are sacrificed at 1.5 cell cycle hour times after the last treatment, which is approximately 12–18 h for mice. Prior to sacrifice (3–5 h for mice), animals are treated with a metaphase-arresting agent (Colchicine). Bone marrow cells are harvested, slides are prepared, and metaphase cells are scored for different types of chromosomal aberrations. The percentage of metaphase cells with aberrations in the test group is compared to the negative control to determine whether the treatment caused an increase in aberrations.

2.7 Implantation

For devices placed within tissues, the ISO 10993-1 standard [1] requires that the local pathological effects on living tissue be evaluated. This evaluation is accomplished through gross and microscopic examination of tissues [6]. The preferred site for evaluating the local tissue response for ocular devices is the actual site of intended clinical use. This could involve implanting an actual ocular device or simply a biomaterial used within the device. Rabbits tend to be a commonly used animal model for implants, although the smaller size of the rabbit eye can present limitation, prompting the use of larger animals.

Following implantation in an ocular site, the eye offers the advantage of being able to monitor local tissue responses over the course of the study. At the end of the study, ocular tissues are examined grossly and microscopically. Besides ocular implantation, devices can also be implanted in muscle tissue for screening studies or shorter duration implantation studies (e.g., 2 weeks) to assess local tolerance in this surrogate, highly vascular tissue. The rabbit paravertebral muscle implantation model is a commonly used implant model for evaluation of the local tissue response to materials.

Since a tissue response changes over time and even more so with degradable materials, evaluations of the local responses at multiple implant durations are typically required. For permanent implants, implant intervals should encompass short-term and long-term intervals. Ideally, the long-term interval should be sufficient that the local tissue response has reached homeostasis or steady state. With non-degradable materials steady state is typically reached by approximately 12 weeks in soft tissues. For degradable materials, the intervals should be carried out to the point of complete material degradation, resorption, and tissue restoration. Short-term intervals are typically considered 1–4 weeks in duration, although 2 weeks as an early interval is preferred to avoid changes associated with surgical trauma. Long-term intervals typically range from 12 to 56 weeks. In implantation studies, control materials are implanted for comparison. Since any implanted material will elicit some response, it is necessary to compare test materials to negative control materials with well-known accepted local reactions, e.g., (certified) high density polyethylene or commercially available predicate ocular devices. The macroscopic assessment is based on the zone of tissue response and/or encapsulation surrounding the implanted specimen. For the microscopic evaluation, implant sites are scored based on the inflammatory cells that have migrated to the site (number per high powered field and width of zone surrounding the implant), presence of necrosis, fibrosis, vascularization, and other tissue alterations. In some scoring schemes, the reaction for the control material is subtracted from the reaction of the test material. The resultant score is correlated to a scale and defined as slight to severe irritant.

When addressing local effects following implantation, these data may be obtained from other studies where the primary endpoint is not a local effect. For example, during ocular device functional, efficacy or toxicity studies, these implant sites are also evaluated, providing, local effects data at these intervals. In these cases where the local effects can be evaluated, specific studies to examine only local effects are then not needed. Therefore, it is prudent to consider practical design of ocular implantation studies so irritation and other endpoints are possible in the same study.

2.8 Subchronic Toxicity

The testing guideline in ISO 10993 has both subacute and subchronic toxicity in the same general biological effect category [1, 8]. Subacute and subchronic differ in duration of exposure. Subacute systemic toxicity is defined as adverse effects occurring after multiple or continuous exposure between 24 h and 28 days. Subchronic systemic toxicity is defined as adverse effects occurring after the repeated or continuous administration of a test sample for up to 90 days or not exceeding 10 % of the animals lifespan. The rationale for selection of either a subacute or subchronic test should be based on the biomaterial comprising the device, clinical duration of use for the medical device, the nature of exposure, and the overall testing strategy. The method of exposure is usually by implantation subcutaneously to provide the exposure dose. For ocular medical devices, this type of study is usually only needed if a risk assessment shows that the biomaterial of the device has not been adequately characterized for leachables systemically.

For subacute/subchronic studies where the device is implanted, rats are most often used for these studies and parts of the device are implanted subcutaneously. The subcutaneous tissue along each side of the back is used most often as it can more readily accommodate larger pieces of a device. Selection of a "dose" should be based on the clinical dose of the device. This is best determined on a weight basis. Using the device weight and patient weight (70 kg as a standard weight for adults), a clinical dose is calculated (mg or g of device/kg body weight). To improve the sensitivity of the assay, a safety factor is assigned to the animal dose, 100× if possible. The size of the device will dictate the safety factor that is possible. As a general guideline, samples for subcutaneous implantation should be no more than approximately 1.5–2 cm across and 2–3 mm thick with rounded edges. To achieve a given dose, multiple specimens, up to three per side, can be placed in each animal. The duration of these studies range from 4 weeks to 3 months. The parameters evaluated throughout the course of the study include clinical observations, body weight measurements, implant site observations, necropsy observations, and clinical and anatomic pathology. An advantage of the implant design is the implanted specimens provide tissues for the evaluation of local effects following implant. Therefore, this design can address both subchronic toxicity and implantation (ISO 10993–6) [6] requirements.

3 Specialized Testing Requirements

3.1 Contact Lenses and Lens Care Products

In addition to standard biocompatibility testing, a specific guidance was drafted by ISO for the evaluation of both novel contact lens material and contact lens care products (ISO 9394) [11]. The purpose of this in vivo test method is to evaluate the degree of ocular irritation produced by a device applied to rabbit eyes daily over 22 days.

The NZW rabbit is the prescribed animal model. Rabbits of either sex or both sexes weighing at least 2.5 kg and having eyes free from ocular irritation and corneal retention of fluorescein stain are used. Six rabbits are recommended for use; one eye receives the test article and contra-lateral eye receives the control article. The control article should be a device with defined safety and performance characteristics such as a currently marked product. In the case of contact lens testing, the rabbits receive test and control lenses; whereas, for contact lens products, the rabbits receive the same type of lens but test and control lens solutions are used. Contact lenses should be of sufficient thickness to represent human use extremes or the manufacturing conditions. In addition, the contact lenses should fit a rabbit's eye well enough to be retained over the daily treatment period.

If contact lens care products are to be used in the evaluation, the lenses should be prepared, cleaned and disinfected, stored, and rinsed according to the lens manufacturer's instructions for use. Any lenses that fall out during the daily treatment period should be rinsed with a rinsing solution and reinserted into the appropriate eye. Damaged or lost lenses should be replaced. Hydrogel lenses that have dried out can be cleaned, rehydrated, and reused for testing.

Within 24 h prior to study start, each rabbit eye should be examined by fluorescein stain and slit lamp and scored according to the McDonald-Shadduck system. The contact lenses are placed in the appropriate rabbit eyes for 7–8 h periods daily for 21 consecutive days. On day 22, the lenses are worn for 4 h prior to the study end. During the daily treatment period, the eyes are examined hourly to monitor the lens placement. After removal each day, the lenses are stored and subsequently treated as per the instructions for use. Cases for storage and the lenses themselves need to be used for the same rabbit over the course of the study if possible. Rewetting solutions may be incorporated into this study design when they are considered the test article on the study.

Examinations of the rabbit eyes are done using a Draize scoring system on days 1–7, 9–14, and 16–21 just prior to lens removal. Additional examinations of the eyes can be performed based on any findings noted during the study. On days 8, 15, and 22 after lens removal, eyes are fluorescein stained and slit-lamp examinations using the McDonald-Shadduck scoring system are conducted. The animals are euthanized after the eye examinations on day 22, and the eyes are fixed in an appropriate fixative (e.g. Davidson's solution, 10% neutral-buffered formalin). Microscopic examination of the cornea, conjunctivae, iris, and lens is conducted.

Evaluation of corneal metabolism may be important safety data based on the nature of the test article (e.g., extended wear contact lenses). It is suggested that a minimum of three additional rabbits (test and control eyes) are used if the effects on corneal metabolism are tested in this 22-day study.

3.2 Intraocular implants

A specific ISO standard 11979–5 [12] was written to address the biocompatibility evaluation of IOLs. The requirements in this standard include evaluation of physicochemical properties that are relevant to biocompatibility and guidance on conducting an ocular implantation study.

Prior to biocompatibility testing for any device, an initial risk assessment (ISO 14971) [24] should be conducted also taking into account the history of material in clinical use and animal models to test the long-term stability of the materials. To address any gaps in the risk assessment, the following physicochemical tests, which are described in the ISO standard for IOLs, should be considered.

1. Exhaustive extraction test
   The IOL material should be tested for extractables under exhaustive conditions, and the extraction media should be analyzed.
2. Test for leachables
   The purpose of this testing is to detect and quantify extractable additives and other leachables from IOL material under physiologic conditions.
3. Test for hydrolytic stability
   This test should determine the stability of an IOL material in an aqueous environment through detection and quantification of possible degradation products from hydrolysis and changes in physical appearance, optical properties, and chromatographic characteristics.
4. Photostability test
   The purpose of this test is to determine the photostability of IOL materials when irradiated over a wavelength of 300–400 nm.

5. Nd-YAG laser exposure test
   Laser therapy may be given to patients with IOLs, and this test is designed to evaluate any physical or chemical effects or leakage from IOLs after Nd-YAG laser exposure.
6. Evaluation of insoluble inorganics
   The IOL material should be evaluated for the presence of residual insoluble inorganics on and in the lens from manufacturing and process aids. If any are identified, then the residuals should be identified.

Based on risk assessment of the materials, the following biocompatibility endpoints should be considered for IOLs: cytotoxicity, genotoxicity, local effects after implantation, and sensitization potential. Since IOLs are extremely small (approximately 20 mg), no testing is required to evaluate systemic or chronic toxicity. Details on the conduct of the cytotoxicity, genotoxicity, and sensitization studies were discussed earlier in this chapter.

Because of the target tissue for IOLs, an ocular implantation study is the likely choice for evaluation of local effects. This specific guidance on IOLs describes an ocular implantation study in rabbits. As is ideal for biocompatibility studies, the test article should be a finished IOL, and the control article should be an IOL of a similar design with at least 5 years of successful marketed use. A minimum of six test IOL eyes and six control IOL eyes should be evaluated for the study; the control IOL should be implanted in contra-lateral eye from the test IOL.

If the rabbit is chosen as the model, then the implantation study duration should be 6 months; the rabbit is prone to fibrin formation and rapid lens regrowth which complicates a longer-term assessment. Any other animal model used for this study should have a duration of 1 year. The implantation procedure should be as close to the clinical use as possible; however, due to the rabbit model and ocular geometry, the IOL material can alternatively be located at another ocular site with adequate justification.

After implantation, slit-lamp biomicroscopy is used to monitor the eyes after 7 days, 4 weeks, 3 months, 6 months, and at the end of the follow-up period (if longer than 6 months). The observations should include fibrin, flare, cells, adhesions, neovascularization, corneal edema, material clarity, location of the haptic, and centration of the IOL. At the conclusion of the study, the eyes are enucleated, dissected, examined, and fixed for histopathologic examination. During dissection, the IOLs are removed and examined by light microscopy for cells, debris, and fibrinous deposits. Half of the lenses are cleaned and examined for optical properties as described in ISO standard 11979–2 [12]. The remaining lens samples are evaluated by scanning electron microscopy for signs of calcification.

3.3 Ophthalmic Viscosurgical Devices

A specific ISO standard (ISO 15798) [13] was developed for testing ocular surgical implants with viscous and/or viscoelastic properties intended for use during surgery in the anterior chamber. As with all device materials, a risk assessment should be conducted to determine if there are any potential ocular hazards in the finished device from raw materials (e.g., biological origin) or contaminants (e.g., manufacturing processes). Based on the results of the risk assessment, biocompatibility studies as described in ISO 10993–1 [1] should be conducted to fill in the testing gaps.

An intraocular implantation test for ophthalmic viscosurgical devices (OVD) is described in Annex A of the ISO 15798 guidance [13] which is focused on intraocular pressure and inflammatory response evaluations. The control OVD should be one that has at least 5 years of successful clinical use without related adverse events. The study design uses six NZW rabbits which are young adults. Pre-operatively, the animals are examined using applanation tonometry, slit-lamp biomicroscopy, and pachmetry. Only animals with healthy eyes should be used for this surgical study. The surgery is done by removing approximately 25 % of the liquid volume of the anterior chamber and exchanging it with the test OVD in one eye and the control OVD in the contra-lateral eye. After the surgery, intraocular pressure is measured by applanation tonometry at 2, 4, 6, 8, 12, and 24 h and at 7 days. Inflammatory response is measured by slit-lamp biomicroscopy at 6, 24, 48, and 72 h and at 7 days postsurgery. The study is not described as having a histopathology phase, but this could be a valuable option if unexpected findings are observed.

3.4 Aqueous Shunt Devices

The US FDA has a specific guidance regarding 510(K) submissions for Aqueous Shunts [25], intended to reduce intraocular pressure in neovascular glaucoma or glaucoma that was not treatable by conventional medicine or surgery. As is usually recommended for all devices, aqueous shunts should be tested in the final form, sterilized as intended for ocular implantation. The resistance and pressure/flow characteristics of the test device should be substantially equivalent to the predicate device serving as the control.

Biocompatibility testing for the aqueous shunt should include cytotoxicity, genotoxicity, and sensitization studies as well as intramuscular implantation and intracutaneous irritation studies. Another recommended test is a 6-month ocular implantation study which is described in detail in the following paragraphs.

Several animal species have been used for aqueous shunt implantation studies including rabbits, cats, and primates. The rationale for species selection should be based on being able to adequately evaluate: inflammatory response of the eye to the material, adhesion of cells to the implant surface, and biodegradation of the material. However, rabbits are the most frequently chosen species for this test. For the test to be considered valid, a minimum of six test eyes is needed for evaluation at the end of a 6-month implantation period. Therefore, one extra animal each for the test and control groups (total of seven) should be considered to account for any inadvertent animal loss during the study.

The study animals should be anesthetized, prepared, and draped under aseptic techniques. After insertion of a lid speculum, a fornix-based conjunctival flap is dissected between the insertions of two adjacent rectus muscles. The shunt is sutured to the sclera an appropriate distance posterior to the limbus and is inserted into the anterior chamber through an appropriately sized needle tract. A patch graft may be placed over the anterior portion of the tube. The conjunctival wound is closed, and the eye is treated with an antibacterial or steroid ointment.

Gross examination of the eyes should be done at 1 and 3 days postsurgery; both slit-lamp biomicroscopic and indirect ophthalmoscopic examinations should be at done 1 and 4 weeks, and at 3 and 6 months postsurgery. The observations should include at a minimum flare, cell adhesions, neovascularization, corneal edema, and location of the tube and implant. After the 6-month interval, the animals should be euthanized; at least three enucleated eyes should be immediately fixed in neutral-buffered formalin for storage. The retrieved eyes should be sectioned equatorially and examined noting the location/placement of the shunt. Histopathological evaluations should be done at the anterior and posterior segments of the eyes. The explanted shunts should be examined for cellular and fibrinous deposits, especially inside and at the tube/implant junctions. At least two shunts should have pressure/flow testing, and the structural integrity of the shunts should be evaluated. The aqueous shunt material will be judged biocompatible if implantation in the eye does not produce a significant local response, and does not have any detectable changes in flow properties.

3.5 Ophthalmic Instruments

The US FDA uses a classification system (Class 1, 2, and 3) for ophthalmic medical devices [26] which is based on how much regulatory control or risk is applicable for clinical use. For example, Class 1 devices require the least regulatory control such as distometers, visual acuity charts, ophthalmic trial lens sets, and a corneal radius measuring device. Class 2 devices require a 510(k) premarket application and have functions that either contact the eye directly (e.g., corneal electrode or thermal cautery unit) or have impact on eye care if there are malfunctions (e.g., ophthalmoscope, AC-powered slit-lamp biomicroscope, or visual field laser). Class 3 ophthalmic devices have the most stringent testing requirements, and a Premarket application is needed that assures that the device is safe and effective for its clinical use. Examples of Class 3 ophthalmic devices include excimer lasers, intraocular pressure measuring device, and intraocular gas.

3.6 Combination Products (Drug and Device)

According to the 21 CFR 3.2(e), there are four types of combination devices [27].

1. One type of combination product is comprised of two or more regulated components (i.e., drug/device, biologic/device, drug/biologic, or drug/device/biologic) that are physically, chemically, or otherwise combined or mixed and produced as a single product. Examples of this combination device include drug-eluting stents, catheters with microbial coating, skin substitutes with cellular components, prefilled syringes, or metered inhalers.
2. Combination products by definition can also consist of two or more separate products (i.e., drugs, biologics, and/or devices) packed together in a single package or as a unit. Examples of this type of combination product include a drug or biological product packaged with a delivery device or a surgical tray with surgical instruments, drapes, and lidocaine.
3. A combination device can be a drug, device, or biological product packaged separately that are intended of use only with an approved individually specified drug, device, or biological product. Both entities are required to achieve the intended use, indication, or effect and where, upon approval of the proposed product, the labeling of the approved product needs to be changed. A photosensitizing drug and activating laser/light source combination is an example as well as an iontophoretic drug delivery patch and controller.
4. A combination product may also be any investigational drug, device, or biological product packaged separately that is for use only with another individually specified investigational drug, device, or biological product. Both entities are required to achieve the intended use, indication, or effect.

The Office of Combination Products at the US FDA makes the determination of whether a product candidate is a combination product, and also determines which agency center (CDER, CBER, or CDRH) at the FDA will have the lead responsibility for the product approval process. The determination is based on the primary mode of action of the combination product, and other associated agencies can serve as a consulting center based on the combination product constituents.

3.6.1 Study Design Considerations

Testing requirements for a combination product are based on the testing required for each component. If a drug is in the combination product, then its testing will be based on the CDER requirements. Likewise, if a biological component is in the combination product, its testing will need to be according to the CBER requirements. Any device components will need to be evaluated based on

CDRH requirements. Some specific combinations may have unique guidance documents such as drug-eluting stents.

When using existing drugs in a combination device, the combination product drug should be compared with existing toxicity data and previous therapeutic uses of the drug. If the device provides targeted delivery of the drug, then local exposure is usually more of a consideration than systemic exposure. For well-characterized drugs, the safety profile for systemic exposure may be sufficient to assess risk, and no additional systemic toxicity evaluations may be needed. However, if the drug has not been previously evaluated for safety in the target location (e.g., eye), then tissue-specific toxicity testing may be required to assess any local effects.

Using an existing device in a combination product could require limited testing if indications for use are unchanged from the original device. Additional testing could be required if there are any interactions between the drug and the device which could create a new chemical entity; if the manufacturing process has the potential to introduce unknown chemicals in the finished product; or if the drug alters a local or systemic biological response to the device.

There are additional considerations for biocompatibility testing of a combination product device. The combination product is likely to be extracted for testing, and potential adverse effects of extraction on any product components need to be taken into account. If a drug is a component, multiple dose levels may need to be tested in some assays with the device to characterize the drug toxicity. Depending on the assay, the drug component may need to be excluded from testing because of its method of action. For example, drugs that affect cell division or have antimicrobial properties are inappropriate for cytotoxicity or bacterial mutagenicity assays. Lastly, the use of appropriate controls is important to provide a comparator of the anticipated response in the assays.

Testing requirements for a new device and an existing drug combination product may be similar to testing just the device. Safety evaluation may be required for the device alone so there is no possibly of toxicity being masked by the drug in the combination product. Functional studies will be needed to support the claims made by the combination product.

Combination ocular products which have drugs as a component may require an evaluation of drug exposure or a toxicokinetic profile over the conditions of clinical use [10]. Considerations for measuring drug exposure include the drug dose in the final product, how well the drug has been previously characterized, and the route and duration of drug exposure. If the drug component is used commercially via a variety of routes and has been well characterized (e.g., triamcinolone), a risk assessment is likely to demonstrate that low doses do not pose a safety concern and as such no toxicokinetic evaluation is necessary. Based on the drug dose or if the delivery route is novel, limited drug exposure data might be needed. For example, if an intraocular implant is used as a drug delivery device, the analysis of eluting drug concentration may be required in the eye (aqueous and vitreous humor), tears as well as limited time points in the systemic circulation.

Toxicokinetic studies should be considered if substantial quantities of potentially toxic or reactive degradation products and leachables are likely or known to be released from a medical device during clinical use. However, toxicokinetic data would not be needed if a risk assessment shows that the rates of release of degradation products and leachables have been judged to have safe limits by clinical exposure or historical references.

References

1. ISO 10993-1:2009. Biological evaluation of medical devices—Part 1: evaluation and testing within a risk management process, ISO, Geneva, Switzerland, 2009
2. ISO 10993-2:2006. Biological evaluation of medical devices— Part 2: animal welfare requirements, ISO, Geneva, Switzerland, 2006
3. ISO 10993-3:2003. Biological evaluation of medical devices—Part 3: tests for genotoxicity, carcinogenicity and reproductive toxicity, ISO, Geneva, Switzerland, 2003
4. ISO 10993-4:2002/Amd 1:2006. Biological evaluation of medical devices—Part 4: selection of tests for interactions with blood. ISO, Geneva, Switzerland, 2002, 2006
5. ISO 10993-5:2009. Biological evaluation of medical devices—Part 5: tests for *in vitro* cytotoxicity, ISO, Geneva, Switzerland, 2009
6. ISO 10993-6:2007. Biological evaluation of medical devices—Part 6: tests for local effects after implantation, ISO, Geneva, Switzerland, 2007
7. ISO 10993-10:2010. Biological evaluation of medical devices—Part 10: tests for irritation and skin sensitization, ISO, Geneva, Switzerland, 2010
8. ISO 10993-11:2006. Biological evaluation of medical devices—Part 11: tests for systemic toxicity, ISO, Geneva, Switzerland, 2006
9. ISO 10993-12:2012. Biological evaluation of medical devices—Part 12: sample preparation and reference materials, ISO, Geneva, Switzerland, 2012
10. ISO 10993-16:2010. Biological evaluation of medical devices—Part 16: toxicokinetic study design for degradation products and leachables, ISO, Geneva, Switzerland, 2010
11. ISO 9394:1998, Ophthalmic optics – Contact lenses and contact lens care products—determination of biocompatibility by ocular study with rabbit eyes, ISO, Geneva, Switzerland, 2011
12. ISO 11979-5:2006(E). Ophthalmic implants—intraocular lenses—Part 5: biocompatibility, ISO, Geneva, Switzerland, 2006
13. ISO 15798: 2009(E). Ophthalmic implants—ophthalmic viscosurgical devices, ISO Geneva, Switzerland, 2009
14. OECD Guidelines for the Testing of Chemicals. Test No. 406: Skin sensitization. OECD, Paris, France, 1992
15. OECD Guidelines for the Testing of Chemicals. Test No. 429: Skin sensitization: local Lymph Node Assay. OECD, Paris, France, 2010
16. Ryan CA, Cruse LW, Skinner RA, Dearman RJ, Kimber I, Gerberick GF (2002) Examination of a vehicle for use with water soluble materials in the murine local lymph node assay. Food Chem Toxicol 40:1719–1725
17. OECD Guidelines for the Testing of Chemicals. Test No. 405: Acute eye irritation/corrosion. OECD, Paris, France, 2012
18. United States Pharmacopeia. General chapter <88> biological reactivity tests, in vivo. Rockville, MD, USA, 2013
19. OECD Guidelines for the Testing of Chemicals. Test No. 471: Bacterial reverse mutation test. OECD, Paris, France, 1997
20. OECD Guidelines for the Testing of Chemicals. Test No. 476: In vitro mammalian cell gene mutation test. OECD, Paris, France, 1997
21. OECD Guidelines for the Testing of Chemicals. Test No. 473: In vitro mammalian cell

Chromosomal Aberration Test. OECD, Paris, France, 1997

22. OECD Guidelines for the Testing of Chemicals. Test No. 474: Mammalian erythrocyte micronucleus test. OECD, Paris, France, 1997
23. OECD Guidelines for the Testing of Chemicals. Test No. 475: Mammalian bone marrow chromosome aberration test. OECD, Paris, France, 1997
24. ISO 14971:2007. Medical devices—application of risk management to medical devices, ISO, Geneva, Switzerland, 2007
25. Guidance for Industry and for the US FDA Reviewers and Staff. Aqueous Shunts—501(k) Submissions, U.S. Department of Health and Human Services, Food and Drug Administration, Center for Devices and Radiologic Health. November 16, 1998
26. Code of Federal Regulations, Title 21, Volume 8, Chapter I, Subchapter H, Part 886 Ophthalmic Devices, April, 2012
27. Code of Federal Regulations, Title 21, Volume 1, Subchapter 1, Part 3.2 Definitions, April 2012

Methods in Pharmacology and Toxicology (2014): 267–289
DOI 10.1007/7653_2013_5

Published online: 29 August 2013

Methodologies for Microscopic Characterization of Ocular Toxicity

Leandro B.C. Teixeira and James A. Render

Abstract

The eye is unique in being composed of different types of structures with various functions. One needs to be aware of these unique aspects and changes due to spontaneous, iatrogenic, or environmental conditions in order to detect toxicologic ocular changes. Since most ocular structures can be examined clinically, with or without specialized instruments, it is important to obtain microscopic correlates for clinical findings. This requires special attention to the techniques involved in obtaining good histologic sections for evaluation. Findings in standard histologic sections may be further characterized by use of immunohistochemistry or electron microscopy and appropriate terminology is important when identifying findings. This chapter will review all of these aspects of the microscopic examination for ocular toxicity.

Key words Ocular, Histopathology, Fixation, Immunohistochemistry, Plastic embedding, Electron microscopy

1 Introduction

1.1 Goals of Toxicity Study

Since the eye is an organ with multiple unique structures that may vary depending on the location within the eye, one needs to clearly understand the goal of the toxicity study as it pertains to the eye. Is the study a general toxicity study and just a sample of the eye will be examined for toxicity, or is the toxicity study focused on a particular aspect of the eye (e.g., intravitreal implant). A clear understanding of the purpose of the toxicity study begins with the study protocol.

1.2 Protocol Design

The choice of methodologies for microscopic characterization of ocular toxicity depends on the purpose of the study and choices should be clearly indicated in the study protocol.

The purposes of the microscopic examination of ocular tissue are to further describe ocular findings noted clinically and to detect additional findings not observed clinically. To have microscopic correlates to clinical findings, one must be aware of the types of clinical examination techniques used and the results of those examinations at the time of an experimental animal's death and enucleation, at the time of trimming the globe and ocular tissue, and at the time of microscopic section evaluation. To discover microscopic findings, one must choose methods, which will prepare the ocular tissue for the various types of microscopic examinations.

There are various ways of obtaining pristine ocular sections for evaluation. What works for one laboratory may not work for another laboratory. Therefore, if a histotechnology laboratory is performing a technique for the first time, it is best if a method development study is performed first. This study will help to determine if the laboratory personnel will have some difficulties with obtaining acceptable ocular sections. Results often are better when there are fewer technical staff handling the ocular tissue, but regardless, good results depend on good communication among the study director, study pathologist, study ophthalmologist, and pathology laboratory personnel.

Ocular studies may involve ocular medical devices, including those that are used for drug delivery [1–4]. An ocular medical device is a device that comes in contact with the exterior of the eye (e.g., contact lens and nasal canalicular plug) and those devices that are implanted within the structures of the globe (e.g., subconjunctiva, sclera, suprachoroid, vitreous, and lens). These devices are tested for evidence of biocompatibility (i.e., an absence of localized tissue irritation or toxicity) by following established international standards [5–8]. The in-life phase of these studies involves the use of standard methods such as the Draize scale for scoring ocular findings. This includes biomicroscope slit-lamp examination in accordance with criteria established by McDonald et al. [9]. These findings are used in an attempt to determine microscopic correlates.

For standard systemic toxicity studies, there is generally a fairly standard approach used to examine the globe, which is designed to detect ocular findings associated with systemic toxicity [10]. This approach is generally used for studies which involve ophthalmic examinations consisting of direct ophthalmoscopy, slit-lamp biomicroscopy, and fundoscopy, and studies which have no clinical ophthalmic findings. The test article would be a systemically administered small molecule or biologic entity and the approach involves examination of paraffin-embedded, midsagittal sections of globes that are a few microns in thickness and stained with hematoxylin and eosin (H&E) [10–14]. If the test article is applied topically, injected or implanted, then the standard approach needs to be modified to look for localized effects, as well as, systemic effects.

2 Microscopic Examination of the Eye

Light microscopic examination of the eye requires several factors including (1) knowledge of the clinical ophthalmic findings, (2) an understanding of comparative ocular anatomy and histology, (3) an awareness of iatrogenic ocular findings and artifacts, (4) an awareness of toxicologic changes that may occur in ocular tissues, (5) accurate terminology, (6) good histologic sections of globes, and (7) evaluation of extraocular tissues [4, 10, 15–21].

2.1 Awareness of Clinical Ophthalmic Findings and Type of Test Article Administration

Basic and advanced techniques are used in the clinical examination of the eye and are covered in previous chapters, as well in other references [10, 18, 20, 22–24]. The pathologist needs to be aware of the test method (e.g., topical, oral gavage, etc.) and clinical ophthalmic findings in order to provide an accurate microscopic evaluation of the ocular structures, including microscopic correlates [10]. This may be accomplished by reviewing ophthalmic examination narrative reports or by the use of diagrams or images [25]. To accomplish this goal, protocol and clinical information needs to be available to the study pathologist at the time of enucleation, trimming, and ocular section evaluation.

2.2 Awareness of Comparative Ocular Anatomy

The differences in ocular anatomy among laboratory animals have been well documented in the scientific literature and reviewed in Chapter 2 [19, 24, 26]. Extraocular tissue associated with the eye includes the ocular adnexa, eyelids, and other contents within the orbit. Ocular adnexa include extraocular muscles, ocular glands, and the structures of the lacrimal drainage apparatus. The extraocular muscles are generally not examined, but may be retained with the globe. Examples of when they may be examined include sites of injection into the subTenon's space or muscular issues. Ocular glands vary among laboratory animal species. Many large laboratory animals have a main lacrimal gland located in the superior, temporal, and anterior aspect of the orbit, but some species (e.g., the rabbit) have a large accessory lacrimal gland. Animals with third eyelids have a lacrimal gland associated with that structure and other modified lacrimal glands are present in some laboratory animals. Rabbits have a Harder's gland with two distinct lobes, the white lobe and the pink lobe [27]. Rodents have a harderian gland that fills much of the posterior aspect of the orbit. Secretion of the lacrimal gland contributes to the precorneal tear film and drains away through the puncta that open up to canaliculli which eventually form the nasolacrimal duct.

2.3 Iatrogenic Findings

Iatrogenic findings are those that are caused by the human involvement or environmental exposure that are independent of the effect of the test article. Examples of iatrogenic findings include needle tracts in the cornea, sclera or uvea, orbital lesions following orbital venipuncture, and light-induced photoreceptor degeneration [13, 28–37]. Albino rodents housed on the top shelf of racks may be exposed to an excessive amount of light, even though the illumination in the room may be within acceptable limits [38] and consequently develop light-induced outer retinal (photoreceptor) degeneration.

2.4 Spontaneous Background Findings

Spontaneous background findings involving the globe are findings that occur as a result of a congenital defect, trauma, inherited condition, or aging change and are well described in the literature [13, 35, 39–52]. Some spontaneous ocular findings are reversible, such as cold cataracts in anesthetized mice [53, 54], and others may be a background finding or may be a toxicologic finding, such as corneal calcification in rodents [55–59]. Spontaneous changes may also involve the optic nerve, such as idiopathic bilateral optic neuropathy in monkeys [60].

2.5 Toxicologic Findings

Preclinical toxicologic findings are findings that occur as a result of the administration of a test article and are well described in the literature [13, 14, 22, 35, 40, 47, 61–68]. Any of the ocular structures may be affected, including some findings that occur in ocular structures not present in the human eye, such as tapetum lucidum in dogs and the harderian gland in rodents [69, 70].

2.6 Ocular Terminology

With the different types of ocular tissues and the various methods of identifying specific findings in the structures of the eye, the use of descriptive terms is necessary. Findings need to be identified as to their location. The following terms may be used: superior, inferior, nasal, temporal, inner (internal), outer (external), anterior, posterior, central, or peripheral. The anterior central aspect of the globe (or lens) is the anterior pole and the posterior central aspect of the globe (or lens) is the posterior pole. A vertical plane through these poles is the median or midsagittal plane and planes parallel with the midsagittal plane are sagittal planes. A plane that divides a globe into an anterior and posterior portion is a coronal (frontal) plane, such as a plane through the equator of the globe (or lens). Some terms indicate that a finding is adjacent to another structure (e.g., peripapillary, meaning close to the optic nerve).

If specific cells or areas of the eye are involved, then those terms should be used. For example, minimal diffuse retinal degeneration is nonspecific and implies a change in some part of the retina. Since any change in the retina is important, even minimal ones, the portion of the retina or retinal cells involved should be indicated. Another example is displaced photoreceptor cell nuclei (PDN). These PDN may be observed in retinas with photoreceptor degeneration or they may be observed in retinas with no evidence of photoreceptor degeneration [71, 72]. Since the presence of PDN does not always signify degeneration, PDN should be a separate diagnosis.

Clinical observations should also be specific. Opacification of the lens may be an indication of lenticular irreversible degeneration (i.e., cataract) or it may be a reversible change [73]. Additionally, microscopically, swelling of a few lenticular fibers with no other lenticular changes may be a reversible finding. An accurate assessment and management of the ocular finding can be obtained by use of the correct term for the location and the diagnosis of a microscopic finding.

2.7 Good Histologic Sections of Globes

2.7.1 Enucleation

Getting pristine ocular sections for microscopic examination is essential for detecting microscopic ocular findings. This begins with enucleation [10–13, 25, 74]. Enucleation should be performed on all experimental animals, including rodents, as soon as possible after death of the animal [74]. A small portion (5 mm, if possible) of retrobulbar optic nerve should remain with the globe. These sections of optic nerve will be trimmed to obtain cross sections for evaluation (especially of axons of retinal ganglion cells). All extraocular tissue should be removed, unless there is a need to keep the tissue attached (e.g., deposit in Tenon's capsule). For rodents, the harderian gland should be removed. Removal of extraocular tissue not only enhances fixation, but it also exposes landmarks (e.g., long posterior ciliary body) that are used for trimming. Any tissue removed should be saved in fixative and labeled with the study number, animal number, and left (OS) or right (OD) eye.

To perform an enucleation the medial and lateral commissures of the eyelids may be cut to provide more exposure to the globe. The eyelids and adjacent skin may be removed and the orbital bone removed with rongeurs, if more exposure to the globe is needed. Gentle tension may be applied to connective tissue attached to the globe to aid in the removal of the globe from the orbit. Rough handling of the globe may result in artifact (e.g., sensory retinal separation). Excessive tugging on the globe results in artifactual spaces or hyalinized deposits within the optic nerve [75, 76]. Cutting the optic nerve too close to the globe may result in another artifact, myelin within the subretinal space [77, 78]. Once the globe has been removed from the orbit and cleaned of extraocular tissue, it should be put in a container for fixation. The identification of the globe, including study number, animal number, and right or left globe, should be maintained. If the orientation (i.e., superior, inferior, nasal, and temporal) of the globe may be lost during fixation (e.g., opaque albino rodent globe fixed in Davidson's fixative), then the globe may be marked with tissue dye, tattoo ink, or a fine suture (see Trimming for Light Microscopy below).

2.7.2 Fixation for Light Microscopy

Although 10 % neutral-buffered formalin (NBF) is used in the fixation of extraocular tissues of animals for toxicity studies, it is not ideal for immersion fixation of globes and may result in artifacts (e.g., sensory retinal separation) [25]. Since there is no ideal fixative for ocular fixation, several different fixatives are used on a routine basis (Table 1) [10–13, 79, 80]. Ocular fixatives are the ones in which the globes are entirely immersed after enucleation (e.g., Zenker's, Bouin's, Davidson's, or Modified Davidson's fixatives) or a fixative, like glutaraldehyde (e.g., 4 % glutaraldehyde mixed 1:1 with 10 % NBF), that involves an intravitreal injection of the fixative or initially submerged in the fixative for a brief (5–30 min) period of time then having a small (5 mm) window created. With this type of fixation, the globe is resubmerged for the set period of time. Regardless of the fixative used, the volume of globe to fixative should be at least 1:10 and wide mouth jars with the name of the study, number of the animal, and what globe (right or left) should be used. Gauze may be used to cover the globes to ensure that they stay submerged in the fixative.

Zenker's and Bouin's fixatives have been used in the past for fixation of globes, but require more involvement in processing of the ocular tissue and have issues with disposal. Zenker's fixative contains mercury and Bouin's fixative contains picric acid that is corrosive, potentially explosive, and is difficult to completely remove from the tissue [25]. These fixatives have generally been replaced with Davidson's fixative or Modified Davidson's fixative [11, 21, 78, 79, 81]. These fixatives are used only for fixation for light microscopy and none are used for electron microscopy.

Davidson's fixative or Modified Davidson's fixative is often used for the fixation of rodent globes generally with good results. Fixation time is dependent upon the size of the globe [82, 83]. For globes of rodents, the time is 6–24 h, but for globes of larger animals (i.e., rabbit, dog, monkey) the time is 24–48 h. Globes may be then transferred to 10 % NBF (or 70 % alcohol, but excess exposure to alcohol will harden the lens) until the time of trimming. During this period, the cornea and sclera become firm which helps during trimming. Excess exposure to these fixatives may result in artifacts which may include (1) diffuse opaque gross appearance of globes of albino rats and mice, (2) vacuolation of the corneal epithelium, (3) oblong spaces in the corneal stroma, (4) vacuolation of the corneal endothelium, (5) shattering of the lens, (6) swelling of the lens with rupture of the lens capsule, (7) swelling of lens fibers, (8) fragmentation and globule formation in the lens of monkeys, and (9) indistinct appearance of photoreceptor inner and outer segments. An advantage of Davidson's fixative and Modified Davidson's fixative is the enhancement of lenticular cell outlines.

Table 1
Common ocular fixatives

Fixative solution	Composition		Purpose/characteristics
10 % Formalin, neutral buffered (NBF)	Formaldehyde (37–40 %) Distilled water Disodium diphosphate Monosodium phosphate	10 % 90 % 6.5 g 4.0 g	LM, IHC Readily available, gold standard for IHC
Davidson's fixative	Ethanol (95 %) Formaldehyde (37–40 %) Glacial acetic acid Distilled water	35 % 2 % 10 % 53 %	LM Good histological preservation of the retina
Modified Davidson's fixatives	Ethanol (95 %) Formaldehyde (37–40 %) Glacial acetic acid Distilled water	15 % 30 % 5 % 50 %	LM Good histological preservation of the retina
Bouin's fixative	Picric acid (saturated aqueous) Formaldehyde (37 % w/w) Glacial acetic acid	75 % 25 % 5 %	LM Good histological preservation of the retina, decalcifies tissues
Glutaraldehyde and 10 % NBF	Glutaraldehyde (4 %) 10 % NBF	50 % 50 %	LM, EM Good histological preservation Slow penetration, requires intravitreal injection or a window
Karnovsky's fixative	16 % paraformaldehyde 10 % glutaraldehyde 0.2 M phosphate buffer (pH 7.4) Distilled water	17 % 31 % 50 % 2 %	EM Good tissue penetration and fixation
Zenker's	Distilled water Potassium dichromate Mercuric chloride Glacial acetic acid	1l 25 g 50 g 50 g	LM Excellent fixation of nuclear chromatin, connective tissue fibers and some cytoplasmic features

LM light microscopy, *IHC* immunohistochemistry, *EM* electron microscopy

Another commonly used fixative is 1–6 % glutaraldehyde buffer with monobasic or dibasic sodium phosphate, which is often mixed with another fixative [84, 85]. For example, a 1:1 mixture of 4 % glutaraldehyde and 10 % NBF is used for light microscopy and a mixture of glutaraldehyde and paraformaldehyde has been used for transmission electron microscopy. Advantages of using glutaraldehyde include (1) minimizes vacuolation of the corneal epithelium and endothelium, (2) fewer oblong spaces in the corneal stroma, (3) visualize lenticular cell outlines, and (4) visible outlines of photoreceptor inner and outer segments. Potential artifacts associated with glutaraldehyde fixation include (1) a few oblong shaped spaces in the corneal stroma, (2) lenticular cracks, (3) distorted shape of the cornea and lens in the globes of rodents due to osmolarity [77, 86], (4) vacuolation of the inner layers of the retina, and (5) vacuolation in the layer of photoreceptor inner and outer segments. There appears to be fewer artifacts associated with prolonged fixation in glutaraldehyde, but in general rodent globes are fixed for 12–24 h and larger globes (i.e., rabbit, dog, monkey) for 24–48 h. After the initial fixation, globes should be transferred to 10 % NBF for a minimum of 24 h to help firm the outer tunics (i.e., cornea and sclera) for trimming (especially for the globes of rabbits and monkeys).

As mentioned earlier, emersion fixation of the larger, non-rodent globes may need to be enhanced for a fixative, such as glutaraldehyde, but is not needed for Davidson's fixative or Modified Davidson's fixative. Importantly, no holes should be created in a globe that has not been in fixative. Instead the globe should be placed in fixative for 5–30 minutes and then a small window may be created near the equator to allow better penetration of fixative into intraocular structures.

Another method is the intravitreal injection of fixative. This may be accomplished by use of a small (25–27 ga) needle gently introduced into the vitreous cavity through the sclera just posterior to the equator. The needle should be angled toward the posterior pole to avoid hitting the lens and should be performed in an area that is 90° away from the plane of section to avoid seeing the injection area. For larger, nonprimate globes, this is at a nasal or temporal location. For primate globes this is at a superior or inferior location. With one hand holding the globe, the fixative should be slowly injected until the globe feels firm. This usually involves a volume of 0.15–0.3 ml of fixative. The injected globe should then be immersed in the fixative. When done gently, artifacts, such as retinal detachment, are not observed.

2.7.3 Trimming for Paraffin Embedding

There are many references for trimming globes and the method used will depend on the purpose of the toxicity study [10–13, 78, 79]. For standard systemic toxicity studies using globes from dogs, minipigs, and rabbits, generally one section of the globe through the optic disc and pupil that is parallel to a vertical median (midsagittal) plane is usual. If the test animal is a primate, the desired plane of section is one that is slightly superior to a horizontal plane in order to have the temporal macula and the optic disc in the same section. Although it would be ideal to have the fovea included with the macula, it is generally not required unless it is a specific point of interest. If the globes are fixed well, the lens and vitreous should remain intact. These sections of globes should be accompanied with a cross section of the retrobulbar optic nerve.

An alternative method for trimming primate globes often used in human ocular pathology is to trim the globe along horizontal planes that are parallel with the long posterior ciliary body, but a few millimeters superior and inferior to this horizontal median plane [25, 84]. Two potential disadvantages of this trimming method are the additional facing of the block in order to have the macula in the section and the danger of trimming the globe too thin, thus causing artifacts (e.g., retinal detachment).

If the test article is administered into the vitreous body of a primate, then the trimming method may be a vertical midsagittal section accompanied by a nasal sagittal section and a temporal sagittal section. The temporal section would contain the macula. For standard systemic toxicity studies, the globes of mice are usually not trimmed and the globes of rats often have just one small (~5 mm) window made along a nasal or temporal sagittal plane near the equator of the globe. If intraocular devices or masses are present, globes may be transilluminated (candled) to determine the location of the object of interest [79, 84].

When trimming a larger globe the cornea is faced down and the blade is positioned next to or 1–3 mm away from the optic disc (Fig. 1a–c). The blade should be long and very sharp (e.g., tissue slicer blades or disposable microtome blades). Razors may be used for trimming globes of rats and creating small windows with no sawing motion. Razors are short resulting in a sawing motion that may cause artifacts (e.g., retinal detachment). The edge of the blade near one end should be put in position and then gently push down and slightly forward allowing the sharp blade to cut into the globe. When the blade gets to the lens, there will be some resistance. At this point the long blade is approximately half way through the globe. With one hand holding the blade on each side of the globe, the blade should be pushed down with even force. When the blade cuts through the globe it should be pulled backward out of the globe along the cutting board. For well-fixed globes, all ocular structures should be in place with no detachments. The larger globes should have a small window placed in the center of the domed half of the globe. The window should be just large enough to fit into a mega-cassette. Artifacts occur when globes of larger animals (e.g., rabbit, dog, monkey) are trimmed too thin in order to fit them in standard cassettes or are too thick for the cassette resulting in crushing artifacts. Only one globe should be put in a cassette and cross sections of optic nerve should be put in standard

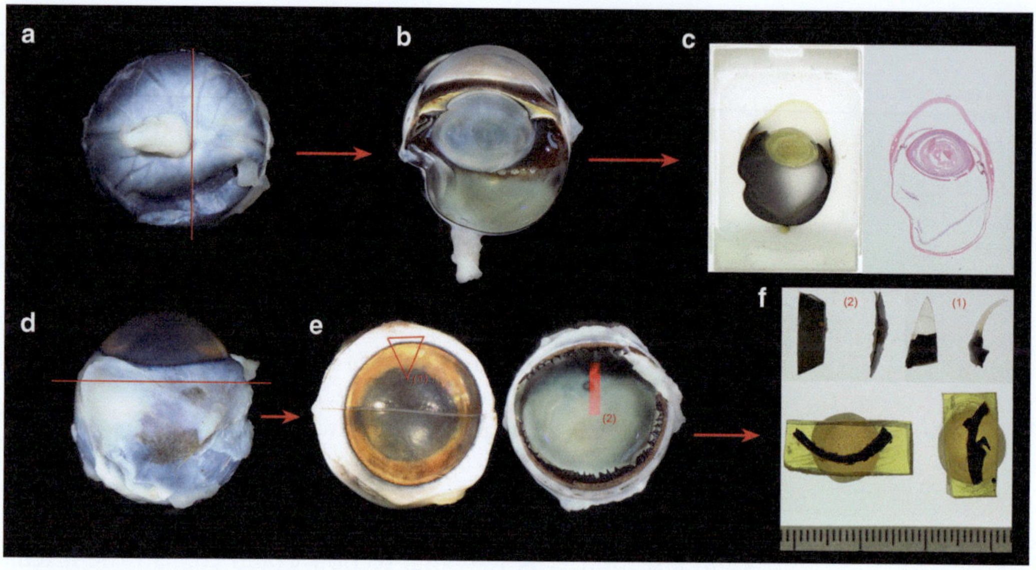

Fig. 1 (**a–c**) Schematic diagram for trimming a feline globe as an example of trimming large animal (nonprimate) globes. The plane of section is generally perpendicular to the long posterior ciliary artery, except for primate globes which are generally trimmed parallel to the long posterior ciliary artery. (**a**) The globe is balanced on the corneal surface while held at the equator. Using a tissue slicer blade an incision is made on the caudal (posterior) surface of the sclera adjacent to the optic nerve or 1–3 mm away from the optic nerve (*red line*), depending on the size of the globe. Using the whole length of the blade cut the sclera until you hit the lens, using a gentle linear motion. With one hand holding the blade on each side of the globe, the blade should be pushed down with even force to cut through the lens. (**b**) A second incision is made parallel to the first, but on the opposite side of the optic nerve and just big enough to allow the trimmed globe to fit into a mega-cassette. (**c**) The globe is embedded in paraffin with the cut surface facing down the block and sectioned with a microtome. (**d**, **e**) Trimming diagram for sectioning the anterior segment and retinal samples for transmission electron microscopy. (**d**) A cut is made along a coronal (frontal) plane at the equator of the globe (posterior to the limbus) dividing the globe into anterior and posterior segments (**e**). At this point the lens is removed. Sections of the anterior segments can be then obtained by placing the cornea facing down on the cutting surface and dividing the tissue into quarters (*1*) using a clean and fresh razorblade. Sections of the posterior segment can be obtained through a similar process with the optic nerve being used as an orientation landmark (*2*). (**f**) Sections from the anterior and posterior segment can be further sectioned in smaller, triangle-shaped wedges not larger than 0.5 × 1.5 mm. Tissues are processed and embedded in plastic molds, which are trimmed and mounted to be cut in an ultramicrotome

cassettes with dividers. Globe or any ocular tissue should be identified as right or left and that identification should persist from gross tissue to histologic section.

Landmarks (e.g., long posterior ciliary body) to aid in trimming albino rat globes may be difficult to see with the naked eye, especially when the globes are fixed in Davidson's fixative or Modified Davidson's fixative. It may be helpful at the time of fixation to mark the globe with tissue dye, tattoo paste, or a fine suture. The dye and tattoo should be very pasty and allowed to dry for best results.

By placing a mark on the superior aspect of the albino rat globe and a mark on the optic nerve, it is possible to get uniform vertical midsagittal sections. With these uniform sections, layers of the sensory retina (e.g., outer nuclear layer) may be measured at set intervals and spider graphs can be created [36, 78, 87].

2.7.4 Paraffin Embedding and Processing of Ocular Tissues

After the globe or extraocular tissue is trimmed, the tissue is processed which involves the removal of water from the tissue and infiltration with paraffin wax [11, 77, 84, 88, 89]. After processing is complete the tissues are embedded in molds filled with paraffin wax. The globes are oriented in the same direction as the mold. The histotechnologist must ensure that the lens (especially of larger globes) comes in complete contact with the bottom of the mold; otherwise the posterior portion of the lens will be absent (Fig. 1c).

2.7.5 Sectioning and Staining Paraffin-Embedded Ocular Tissue

After the paraffin in the molds hardens, ribbons of tissue sections in paraffin are cut from the face of the block by using a microtome (Fig. 1c) [11, 13, 89]. The most common difficulty in sectioning the globe is getting good sections of the lens. There are various techniques used by histotechnologists, such as cooling the block face with ice or applying a substance, that will soften the lens and allow for better ocular sections. After a ribbon has been obtained, it is floated on a water bath. The temperature of the water bath is important. It should not be too warm because the globe will expand quickly and not too cool because the ocular section will not expand enough and artifacts will be present. The ocular section is picked up from the water bath with a glass slide. Adherence to the slide is assisted by applying an adhesive (e.g., poly-L-lysine) to the water bath. After the section is on the slide, there is a drying period before staining. Temperature during drying is important to ensure good adhesion of the section to the slide. In addition to the standard stain combination of hematoxylin and eosin, a silver stain may be used for examining axons; luxol fast blue may be used for examining myelin and periodic acid Schiff helps in the examination of Descemet's membrane, the corneal endothelium, and lenticular capsule.

2.8 Extraocular Tissue Evaluation

Microscopic evaluation of the extraocular tissues involves the same techniques used for the microscopic examination of routine tissues evaluated in toxicity studies. It is important to clearly label the tissue, being as specific as possible, and to indicate if the tissue is from the right or left eye.

3 Ocular Immunohistochemistry (IHC)

Immunohistochemistry has been long used to identify cell types, structures, cell-secreted materials and organisms, such as *Encephalitozoon cuniculi* in the lens of rabbits [90]. Immunohistochemistry is an important tool in eye research and toxicology. Common applications for IHC in the eye are the localization of specific proteins (e.g., outer segments of the retinal photoreceptors), identification of cells types (e.g., characterization of inflammatory cells), and altered pattern of protein expression (e.g., increase expression of Glial fibrillary acidic protein [GFAP] on activated retinal Müller cells). Antibodies useful for labeling ocular tissues are the same ones applied in other organs with exception of antibodies against cell molecules unique to the eye as photoreceptor opsins (Anti-Opsin red, green, and blue and anti-rhodopsin) and against RPE cell proteins (anti-RPE65).

While choosing an antibody for ocular IHC the embryological origin of the ocular tissues should be kept in mind. Developmentally, the tissues of the eye are derived from multiple progenitor sources like neural crest, mesoderm, neuroectoderm (neural tube epithelium), and surface ectoderm creating unexpected patterns of IHC expression when compared to other organs [14]. As an example the pigmented and non-pigmented epithelial layers of ciliary body derived from the neural ectoderm and contrary to epithelial cells in other organs are immunohistochemically positive for neural markers like neuron-specific enolase (NSE) and mesenchymal cell markers like vimentin and are negative for epithelial cells markers like cytokeratins [91, 92].

Another important pitfall while analyzing any IHC reactions is the presence of adequate positive and negative controls [78, 93, 94]. Controls allow you to access the real significance of an IHC signal and to interpret if the signal is a specific or nonspecific reaction. Positive controls are usually sections of tissue known to express the antigen in question in high levels. There are multiple types of negative controls which are used to access the specificity of multiple components of the IHC reaction. The use of tissues or cells expected to be negative for the antibody is a great way to test the antibody specificity [95]. The presence of nonspecific staining can be accessed by using (1) a section of the same tissue incubated only with the secondary antibody, (2) another section incubated with the serum of the animal where the antibody was produced, and (3) another incubated with antibody pre-adsorbed with antigen [78, 95]. It is important to process and stain all control sections together with the tissues been analyzed in order to correctly interpret possible problems.

3.1 Fixation for Immunohistochemistry

Fixation of ocular tissues for immunohistochemistry may require attention to the type of fixative and the length of the fixation time. The main goals of fixation for IHC are to prevent autolysis and displacement of cellular antigens and enzymes facilitating the immunologic and chemical reactions while maintaining tissue morphology [78, 96].

Although 2–4 % paraformaldehyde has been used for fixation, formaldehyde (10 % buffered formalin) is the gold standard of fixatives for IHC, conferring good morphological and antigenic preservation with low cost [14, 95, 96]. Formalin fixation is progressive and time and temperature dependent. There is no standard fixation time for every antigen but most protocols suggest fixation times between 24 and 48 h depending on the size of the globe. As mentioned before, formalin produces cross-linking of cellular peptides that can mask epitopes and results in decreased immunoreactivity [96–98]. Postfixation with 70 % ethanol helps in controlling the deleterious effects of formalin fixation cross-linking. Also, soaking the tissues in concentrated ammonia and 20 % chloral hydrate can partially correct prolonged fixation and antigen retrieval techniques (see later) help re-expose cross-linked antigens [78, 95, 96]. Although the effects of prolonged formalin fixation are well known, one study demonstrated that the immunoreactivity of the majority of the antibodies used in routine veterinary diagnostic pathology was preserved in canine tissues fixed with formalin for up to 7 weeks [97].

Protocols for IHC in Davidson's-fixed rat retinas are reported in the literature and described to present good staining quality compared to formalin-fixed tissues [99]. But in reality IHC protocols for ocular tissues using Davidson's fixative are not common, and technicians typically are reluctant to develop new techniques to optimize IHC for this solution [14].

3.2 Processing the Globe and Ocular Tissues for Immunohistochemistry

Tissue processing for IHC follows the same initial steps previously described for paraffin embedding. Detailed protocols for IHC are extensively described elsewhere [95, 96] and antibody-specific procedures can be found on the technical documents that accompany the specific antibodies. The most delicate steps on the process such as antigen retrieval, choice of primary antibody, and detection system are described below. The main steps of IHC for paraffin-embedded tissues are summarized in Table 2.

3.2.1 Antigen Retrieval

Antigen retrieval is a necessary step on protocols using formalin-fixed tissue and its main goal is to reverse the effects of molecule cross-linking during fixation, releasing antigens for antibody binding [100, 101]. The two most common antigen retrieval procedures are enzymatic and heat-based retrieval [95, 100]. The enzymatic methods use proteases like trypsin, proteinase K, pronase, and pepsin to dissolve peptides and expose hidden epitopes. Its main disadvantages

Table 2
Main steps on standard IHC protocol

Step	Material	Purpose
Antigen retrieval	Enzymatic (proteases) or heat-based (microwave or laboratory steamer)	Re-expose antigens after formalin fixation
Endogen peroxidase blocking	Incubation with hydrogen peroxide	Avoid nonspecific staining due to endogenous peroxidase
Primary antibody incubation	Antibody directed against specific antigen	Recognize antigens and initiate the IHC reaction
Secondary antibody (detection system)	Avidin–biotin or peroxidase-antiperoxidase-based reactions	Label the immune reaction with an enzymatic reporter molecules
Chromogens	Peroxidase and alkaline phosphatase	Reveal the reaction for light microscopy
Counterstain	Toluidine blue or H&E	Lightly stain background tissue

are the low numbers of antigens that are optimized for this retrieval method, the possibility of morphological alterations on the tissues and epitope destruction [95]. The heat-induced epitope retrieval methods are the most commonly used and rely on high temperatures, created by a microwave oven or a laboratory steamer, to partially reverse the chemical reactions between protein and formalin [95, 101].

3.2.2 Primary Antibodies

Along with tissue fixation, the choice of the primary antibodies is the most important factor for success of an IHC protocol. Antibodies are made by immunizing animals (usually mouse, rabbit, goat, or horse) with purified antigens. Those who are produced in multiple species are called polyclonal and those produced in only one species (usually mouse) are called monoclonal [96]. Polyclonal antibodies present the advantage of identifying multiple epitopes of the desired antigen, thus increasing the chance of reaction, but present the disadvantage of an increased likelihood of nonspecific cross-reactivity with similar antigens, causing false-positive reactions [95, 96]. Polyclonal antibodies (which in fact are an antiserum) also contain multiple macromolecules that cause more intense nonspecific background staining when compared to monoclonal antibodies. Monoclonal antibodies are highly specific for a single epitope of an antigen thus the possibility of cross-reactivity is markedly reduced. On the other hand monoclonal antibodies might pose problems in reacting to "hard to detect" antigen in fixed tissues [95].

The availability of effective antibodies for specific antigens should be thoroughly researched either on the literature or with commercial sources. Manufacturer's data is usually a good point for starting. Many aspects need to be accounted while choosing an antibody. Among them are the species in which it was developed and species it is intended for (e.g., Rabbit-anti human), possible species cross-reactivity (antibodies specific for humans usually cross react and can be used in other species like non-human primates or dogs), application intended (IHC, Western blotting, Flow cytometry), methods of tissue preparation tested (frozen or fixed tissue), clone of the antibody, etc. Once a commercial relationship is established manufacturers can be helpful in troubleshooting technical issues.

3.2.3 Detection Systems

In order for the antigen–antibody reaction to be visualized by light microscopy it needs to be labeled with a visible molecule. Detection systems allow the labeling of the immune reaction by attaching fluorescent or color-expressing enzymatic reporter molecules to the primary and secondary antibodies [95, 96]. Detection methods can be classified as direct or indirect. Direct methods are composed of a one-step process with the antibody conjugated with a reporter molecule [95, 102]. Indirect methods are more sensitive and are characterized by the presence of a secondary labeled antibody that presents high affinity with the primary antibody. This renders the primary antibody unlabeled, retaining its original conformation and activity and results in a stronger signal with larger number of antigen–antibody bindings [96, 102]. Common indirect methods are the avidin–biotin methods (avidin–biotin complex [ABC], labeled streptavidin–biotin [LSAB]), and the peroxidase-antiperoxidase (PAP) method) [102]. Another indirect method called polymeric labeling two-step method (EnVision™, PowerVision™) presents a simpler, although more expensive, alternative to ABC or LSAB methods with similar if not higher sensitivity and lack of background staining. It consists of a polymer that harbors multiple molecules of enzymes and the secondary antibody that binds directly to the primary antibody [103, 104].

After the secondary antibody is incubated the reaction needs to be revealed by an enzyme–chromogen reaction. The most commonly used enzymes are peroxidase and alkaline phosphatase and the most commonly used chromogens are 3,3′ diaminobenzidine tetrachloride (DAB) that imparts a brown color to the reaction, 3-Amino-9-ethylcarbazole (AEC) that gives a red color, and 4-Chloro-1-naphthol that causes a blue reaction [102]. DAB is the most popular chromogen but if the IHC protocol targets highly pigmented (particularly with melanin) tissues like the uvea this chromogen should be avoided (due to its brown color) and replaced by a chromogen that results in a more contrasting color, like AEC (red) or 4-Chloro-1-naphthol (blue) [78, 95, 96, 105].

4 Plastic Embedding of Ocular Sections

Soft plastics as methyl methacrylate (MMA) and the preferred glycol methacrylate (GMA) may be used for embedding ocular tissues. Soft ocular tissues containing hard implants or bone require the use of a hard plastic, such as polymethylmethacrylate (PMMA) [1, 106]. In addition, methacrylate-based material such as intraocular lenses may dissolve or become deformed in MMA resin, thus the monomer of PMMA or GMA-based resins may be used as substitutes in these cases [1].

For GMA, the ocular tissue is fixed by systemic perfusion with glutaraldehyde, and then globes are trimmed along a medial plane as for paraffin embedding, and then processed following a schedule with monomer infiltration. This involves agitation to facilitate infiltration and eventual embedding in a mold for polymerization with an oven. The blocks are removed from the molds and the GMA is trimmed from the edges (Fig. 1f). Trimmed blocks are mounted on a chuck of a microtome and sections are collected, placed on a water bath, and adhered to glass slides for staining. Embedding in GMA results in a reduction in shrinkage artifacts and provides better preservation of the cellular detail. Limitations of using GMA include a limit on the size of the tissue embedded requiring trimming of intact globes in smaller tissues and the generation of heat by the GMA blocks during processing that may result in tissue artifacts such as vacuolation of the retinal nerve fiber layer. Also, special equipment is needed and staining of GMA sections may be more challenging.

Processing ocular tissues that contain hard medical devices requires initial fixation followed by dehydration to prepare for plastic infiltration and embedding in a hard plastic, such as PMMA [1]. The ocular tissue is initially trimmed to decrease the size of the tissue and to have the implanted hard medical device near the sectioning surface. This is followed by infiltration, placement in embedding molds, and polymerization. The polymerized block is removed from the embedding mold and the side of the block that is not of interest is mounted on a glass slide using a mounting media. The block mounted on a glass slide undergoes a grinding process to obtain the desired location within the block using coarse to fine grit of sandpaper through a microgrinding system. Following grinding, a parallel glass slide is affixed onto the block and the block is cut with a specialized saw. The sections obtained from the block by the saw are about 200 μm thick. These are then ground to about 45–60 μm thick using the microgrinding system. Tissue sections are stained with stains used for paraffin-embedded sections, generally after etching the slide face.

5 Ocular Electron Microscopy

Electron microscopy is a powerful tool for imaging the ultrastructure of tissues, allowing for characterization of fine details of cellular and extracellular components. Even after losing popularity to molecular methods and newer imaging technologies, electron microscopy still remains an essential resource that provides direct and unequivocal data to explain and address safety concerns in preclinical toxicity studies [64, 107, 108]. Transmission electron microscopy (TEM) and scanning electron microscopy (SEM) are generally applied in order to respond specific questions that usually involve subcellular alteration that can be linked to cellular and tissue changes [1, 107]. For example, TEM can be used to confirm an intracellular structure identified on light microscopy (e.g., lipofuscin in retinal pigment epithelium), to evaluate a normal process (e.g., engulfment of shed membranes from photoreceptor outer segments), to evaluate cellular and extracellular changes in ocular tissues exposed to test articles (e.g., corneal endothelium after intracameral injections) or in the characterization of animal models (e.g., optic nerve and trabecular meshwork of animal models of glaucoma). SEM may be used to determine the degradation of an implanted medical device or to analyze the ultrastructural surface topography of multiple ocular tissues.

5.1 Fixation for Electron Microscopy

In order to obtain high quality images of the ultrastructure of the ocular tissues optimal fixation is of paramount importance. The main goals of fixation for electron microscopy are to preserve the structure of the cells with minimal alteration from the normal state regarding volume, morphology, and spatial relationship between organelles and macromolecules while protecting the tissue from subsequent treatments [105].

The most commonly used fixative for both TEM and SEM is glutaraldehyde [11, 78, 105, 109]. Formalin is adequate but not ideal for both TEM and SEM. Formalin-fixed tissues can be post-fixed in glutaraldehyde, although it should never be the fixative of choice for protocols in which electron microscopy is a primary morphological endpoint [14]. Since glutaraldehyde slowly penetrates tissues it is usually used in conjunction with 10 % buffered formalin in a mixture known as "Karnovsky's fixative." A common mixture for ocular tissues is 16 % paraformaldehyde, 10 % glutaraldehyde, and 0.2 mol/l phosphate buffer (pH 7.4) in a 1:2:4 proportion [14, 78, 109] (Table 1). As mentioned before fixation with glutaraldehyde is obtained by immersion fixation with intravitreal injection of fixative or creation of a window on the sclera after fixation to increase fixative penetration. Vascular perfusion fixation helps to ensure that the structure of interest will be optimally preserved. It is largely used for fixation of the brain and other large parenchymal organs; however, studies comparing the tissue morphology of immersion and perfusion fixed eyes suggest that these methods are equivalent [78]. Perfusion fixation of the eye has been recommended for optimal analyses of the Schlemm's canal and trabecular meshwork [109]. Vascular perfusion can be accomplished by the intracardiac route; by first removing the blood from the circulatory system using a clearing solution like phosphate-buffered saline (PBS) and then injecting freshly prepared fixative. The amount of clearing solution used is usually 15 % of body weight for whole body perfusion and 5 % of body weight for perfusion of the head only and should be performed for at least 10–30 s. The amount of fixative varies between species and can range from 4 to 8 ml in mice to 1,000–1,200 ml in non-human primates [105, 109]. Care is needed to provide a steady pressure, since pressures too high may result in artifacts, such as dilated subretinal space.

Following initial fixation, specimens are postfixed in 1–2 % osmium tetroxide in a phosphate buffer [11]. Specimens are then rinsed, stained with uranyl acetate, washed with acetate buffer, and dehydrated using graded ethanol. Samples are then incubated with propylene oxide and infiltrated with a hard plastic resin. Sadun et al. [110] developed a method using paraphenylenediamine (PPD) along with osmium tetroxide for staining neural processes, especially axons in the optic nerve.

5.2 Trimming for Electron Microscopy

Regardless of the type of animal or type of ocular tissue, ocular tissues fixed for examination by TEM should be small (<2 mm) to allow optimum fixation and penetration [11, 78, 105]. The trimming protocol can vary widely depending on the tissue of interest. Generally a coronal (frontal) cut is made at the level of the posterior chamber (posterior to the limbus) dividing the globe into anterior and posterior segments. At this point the lens is removed. Sections of the anterior segments can be then obtained by placing the cornea facing down on the cutting surface and dividing the tissue into quarters using a clean and fresh razorblade [78]. Sections of the posterior segment can be obtained through a similar process with the optic nerve being used as an orientation landmark. Sections from the anterior and posterior segment can be further sectioned in smaller, triangle-shaped wedges not larger than 0.5 × 1.5 mm (Fig. 1d–e). When the localization of specific, not grossly appreciable, lesions, tissues, or cells is necessary, larger tissue fragments (e.g., half of the anterior or posterior segment of a rodent) can be processed (see next) and prior to the final sectioning, a semithin section can be obtained and analyzed with light microscopy allowing the area of interest to be selected [111, 112].

Since scanning electron microscopy is used to analyze the surfaces of tissues (natural or cut surfaces) and thus do not require embedding and ultrathin sectioning, the tissue selected for analysis can be much larger than for TEM. As an example, for small rodent globes, the whole endothelial (inner) surface of the cornea can be analyzed by cutting the anterior segment into two pieces [113].

5.3 Processing the Globe and Ocular Tissues for Electron Microscopy

After aldehyde fixation, tissues for TEM are postfixed in osmium tetroxide, which cross-links lipids and thereby stabilizes cellular membranes. Subsequent processing steps are analogous to those used for light microscopy, that is, dehydration, embedment (in epoxy resin), sectioning, and staining. Blocks are sectioned on an ultramicrotome to produce 80-nm-thick sections that are picked up on a copper grid and stained using heavy metals such as lead and uranium [11, 105]. As mentioned before, orientation (semithin) sections are made for light microscopy first (generally stained with toluidine blue) to ensure that the area of interest is present and to further select areas for thin sectioning. Many excellent publications of standard TEM methods exist [109, 111, 112, 114, 115].

For SEM, aldehyde fixed-tissues are postfixed in osmium tetroxide and dehydrated through an ethanol series. The tissue is then dried through critical point drying (using a CPD machine), mounted in aluminum specimen mounts with the surface of interest facing up and Sputter-coated with a thin layer of conducting material, typically a metal, such as a gold/palladium (Au/Pd) alloy [113, 116].

References

1. Alves A, Metz A, Render J (2012) Microscopic and ultrastructural pathology of medical devices. In: Boutrand JP (ed) Biocompatability and performance of medical devices. Woodhead Pub, Cambridge
2. Short BG (2008) Safety evaluation of ocular drug delivery formulations: techniques and practical considerations. Toxicol Pathol 36:49–62
3. Weiner AL, Gilger BC (2010) Advancements in ocular drug delivery. Vet Ophthalmol 13:395–406
4. Wilkie DA, Wyman M (1991) Comparative anatomy and physiology of the mammalian eye. In: Hobson DW (ed) Dermal and ocular toxicology: fundamentals and methods. CRC, Boca Raton, FL
5. FDA (1998) Guidance for Industry and for the US FDA Reviewers and Staff. Aqueous Shunts—501(k) Submissions, U.S. Department of Health and Human Services, Food and Drug Administration, Center for Devices and Radiologic Health. November 16
6. ISO 9394 (1998) Ophthalmic optics—contact lenses and contact lens care products—determination of biocompatibility by ocular study with rabbit eyes
7. ISO-11979–5 (2006) E Ophthalmic implants—intraocular lenses—part 5: biocompatability, ISO, Geneva, Switzerland
8. ISO-15798 (2010) Ophthalmic implants—ophthalmic viscosurgical devices—biocom patability, ISO, Geneva, Switzerland
9. McDonald TO, Seabaugh V, Shadduck JA et al (1987) Eye irritation. In: Marzulli FN, Maibach HI (eds) Dermatology. Hemisphere, Cambridge
10. Somps CJ, Greene N, Render JA (2009) A current practice for predicting ocular toxicity of systemically delivered drugs. Cutaneous Ocular Toxicol 28:1–18
11. Ramos M, Reilly CM, Bolon B (2011) Toxicological pathology of the retina and optic nerve. In: Bolon B, Butt MT (eds) Fundamental neuropathology for pathologists and toxicologists: principles and techniques. Wiley, Hoboken, NJ
12. Render JA, Dubielzig RR, Dunn DG, Hardisty JF, Moore RR (2009) Ocular collection protocol of the laboratory rabbit, dog and monkey. Exp Toxicol Pathol 61:403–404
13. Schafer KA, Render JA (2013) Toxicologic pathology of the eye: Histologic preparation and alterations of the anterior segment. In:

Weir AB, Collins M (eds) Assessing ocular toxicology in laboratory animals, molecular and integrative toxicology. Springer Science + Business Media, New York

14. Teixeira LBC, Dubielzig RR (2013) Eye. In: Haschek WM, Rousseaux CG, Wallig MA (eds) Haschek and Rousseaux's handbook of toxicologic pathology, 3rd edn. Elsevier, Missouri
15. Millichamp NJ (1992) Toxicity in specific ocular tissues. In: Chiou GCY (ed) Ophthalmic toxicology. Raven, New York
16. Millichamp NJ (1992) Factors affecting the interpretation of species differences in toxic responses of ocular tissues. In: Chiou GCY (ed) Ophthalmic toxicology. Raven, New York
17. Riley MV, Green K (1992) Comparative physiology and biochemistry of the eye. In: Hockwin O, Green K, Rubin LF (eds) Manual of oculotoxicity testing of drugs. Gustav Fischer, Stuttgart
18. Rubin LF (1992) Comparative anatomy of the eye. In: Hockwin O, Green K, Rubin LF (eds) Manual of oculotoxicity testing of drugs. Gustav Fischer, Stuttgart
19. Rubin LF, Weisse I (1992) Species differences relevant for ocular toxicity studies. In: Hockwin O, Green K, Rubin LF (eds) Manual of oculotoxicity testing of drugs. Gustav Fischer, Stuttgart
20. Schiavo DM (1992) Special topics about the use of laboratory animals in toxicology—an ophthalmoscopic assessment. In: Hockwin O, Green K, Rubin LF (eds) Manual of oculotoxicity testing of drugs. Gustav Fischer, Stuttgart
21. Weisse I (1992) Microscopic examination of the eye. In: Hockwin O, Green K, Rubin LF (eds) Manual of oculotoxicity testing of drugs. Gustav Fischer, Stuttgart
22. Harroff HH (1991) Pathological process of the eye related to chemical exposure. In: Hobson DW (ed) Dermal and ocular toxicology. Fundamentals and methods. CRC, Boca Raton, FL
23. Kuiper B, Boeve MH, Jansen T et al (1997) Ophthalmologic examination in systemic toxicity studies: an overview. Lab Anim 31:177–183
24. Rubin LF (1974) Atlas of veterinary ophthalmoscopy. Lea & Febiger, Philadelphia, PA
25. Saunders LZ, Rubin LF (1975) Ophthalmic pathology of animals. S. Karger, New York
26. Vézina M (2012) Comparative ocular anatomy in commonly used laboratory animals. In: Weir AB, Collins M (eds) Assessing ocular toxicology in laboratory animals, molecular and integrative toxicology. Springer Science + Business Media, New York
27. Eglitis I (1964) The Glands. In: Prince JH (ed) The rabbit in eye research. Charles C. Thomas Pub, Springfield
28. Bellhorn RW (1980) Lighting in the animal environment. Lab Anim Sci 30:440–450
29. Dureau P, Jeanny JC, Clerc B et al (1996) Long term light-induced retinal degeneration in the miniature pig. Mol Vis 2:7
30. Herck HV, Baumans V, van der Craats NR et al (1992) Historical changes in the orbital region of rats after orbital puncture. Lab Anim 26:53–58
31. McGee MA, Maronpot RR (1979) Harderian gland dacryoadenitis in rats resulting from orbital bleeding. Lab Anim Sci 29:639–641
32. Noell WK, Albrecht R (1971) Irreversible effects on visible light on the retina: role of vitamin A. Science 172:76–79
33. Organisaciak DT, Winkler BS (1994) Retinal light damage: practical and theoretical considerations. In: Chader G, Osborne N (eds) Progress Retinal Res. Pergammon, New York
34. Peiffer RL, Porter DP (1991) Light-induced retinal degeneration, rat. In: Jones TC, Mohr U, Hunt RD (eds) Monographs on pathology of laboratory animals: eye and ear. Springer, Berlin
35. Render J, Schafer K, Altschuler R (2013) Special senses. In: Sahota PS, Popp JA, Hardisty JF, Gopinath C (eds) Toxicologic pathology in nonclinical safety assessment. CRC, Boca Raton, FL
36. Tanito M, Li F, Elliott MH et al (2007) Protective effect of TEMPOL derivatives against light-induced retinal damage in rats. Invest Ophthalmol Vis Sci 48:1900–1905
37. Weisse I, Stotzer H, Seitz R (1974) Age- and light-dependent changes in the rat eye. Virchows Arch A Pathol Anat Histol 362:145–156
38. Greenman DL, Bryant P, Kodell RL et al (1982) Influence of cage shelf level on retinal atrophy in mice. Lab Anim Sci 32:353–356
39. Geiss V, Yoshitomo K (1999) Eyes. In: Maronpot RR, Boorman GA, Gaul BW (eds) Pathology of the mouse. Cache River, St. Louis, MO
40. Greaves P (2000) Histopathology of preclinical toxicity studies: interpretation and relevance in drug safety evaluation. Elsevier Science B.V., New York
41. Hubert MF, Gillet JP, Durand-Cavagna G (1994) Spontaneous retinal changes in Sprague Dawley rats. Lab Anim Sci 44:561–567

42. Katsuta O, Shinomiya K, Mochizuki T (2008) Pseudopterygium: Unique conjunctival stricture observed in Japanese White rabbit. J Toxicol Pathol 21:239–241
43. Kuno H, Usui T, Eydelloth RS et al (1991) Spontaneous ophthalmic lesions in young Sprague–Dawley rats. J Vet Med Sci 53:607–614
44. Lai YL, Jacoby RO, Jonas AM (1978) Age-related and light-associated retinal changes in Fischer rats. Invest Ophthalmol Vis Sci 17:634–638
45. Moore CP, Dubielzig R, Glaza SM (1987) Anterior corneal dystrophy of American Dutch Belted rabbits: biomicroscopic and histopathologic findings. Vet Pathol 24:28–33
46. O'Steen WK, Anderson KV, Shear CR (1974) Photoreceptor degeneration in albino rats: dependency on age. Invest Ophthalmol 13:334–339
47. Schafer KA, Render JA (2013) Toxicologic pathology of the eye: alterations of the lens and posterior segment. In: Weir AB, Collins M (eds) Assessing ocular toxicology in laboratory animals, molecular and integrative toxicology. Springer Science + Business Media, New York
48. Shibuya K, Satou K, Sugimoto K et al (1999) Background data on spontaneous ophthalmic lesions in Crj:CD(SD)IGS rats. In: Matsuzawa T, Inoue H (eds) Biological reference data on CD(SD) IGS rats. Best Printing Co. Ltd., Yokohama
49. Sinha DP, Cartwright ME, Johnson RC (2006) Incidental mononuclear cell infiltrate in the uvea of cynomolgus monkeys. Toxicol Pathol 34:148–151
50. Taradach C, Greaves P (1984) Spontaneous eye lesions in laboratory animals: incidence in relation to age. Crit Rev Toxicol 12:121–147
51. Taradach C, Regnier B, Perraud J (1981) Eye lesions in Sprague–Dawley rats: type and incidence in relation to age. Lab Anim 15:285–287
52. Tucker MJ (1997) Special sense organs and associated tissues. In: Tucker MJ (ed) Diseases of the Wistar rat. Taylor and Francis, London
53. Bermudez MA, Vicente AF, Romero MC et al (2011) Time course of cold cataract development in anesthetized mice. Curr Eye Res 36:278–284
54. Delaye M, Clark JI, Benedek GB (1982) Identification of the scattering elements responsible for lens opacification in cold cataracts. Biophys J 37:647–656
55. Carlton WW, Render JA (1991) Calcification of the cornea. In: Jones TC, Mohr U, Hunt RD (eds) Monographs on pathology of laboratory animals: eye and ear. Springer, Berlin
56. Fabian RJ, Bond JM, Drobeck HP (1967) Induced corneal opacities in the rat. Br J Ophthalmol 51:124–129
57. Losco PE, Troup CM (1988) Corneal dystrophy in Fischer 344 rats. Lab Anim Sci 38:702–710
58. Mittl R, Galin MA, Opperman W (1970) Corneal calcification in spontaneously diabetic mice. Invest Ophthalmol 9:137–145
59. Van Winkle TJ, Balk MW (1986) Spontaneous corneal opacities in laboratory mice. Lab Anim Sci 36:248–255
60. Fortune B, Wang L, Bui BV et al (2005) Idiopathic bilateral optic nerve atrophy in rhesus macaque. Invest Ophthalmol Vis Sci 46:3943–3956
61. Chiou GCY (1992) Ophthalmic toxicology. Raven, New York
62. Davidson SI, Rennie IG (1986) Ocular toxicity from systemic drug therapy. An overview of clinically important adverse reactions. Med Toxicol 1:217–224
63. Grant WM (1986) Toxicology of the eye, 3rd edn. Charles C. Thomas, Springfield
64. Heywood R (1982) Histopathological and laboratory assessment of visual dysfunction. Environ Health Perspect 44:35–45
65. Hockwin O, Green K, Rubin LF (1992) Manual of oculotoxicity testing of drugs. Gustav Fischer, Stuttgart
66. Lüllmann H, Lüllmann-Rauch R (1981) Tamoxifen-induced generalized lipidosis in rats subchronically treated with high doses. Toxicol Appl Pharmacol 61:138–146
67. Massa T, Davis GJ, Schiavo D et al (1984) Tapetal changes in beagle dogs: II. Ocular changes after intravenous administration of a macrolide antibiotic—rosaramicin. Toxicol Appl Pharmacol 72:195–200
68. Santaella RM, Fraunfelder FW (2007) Ocular adverse effects associated with systemic medications: recognition and management. Drugs 67:75–93
69. Dillberger JE, Peiffer RL, Dykstra MJ et al (1996) The experimental antipsychotic agent 1192U90 targets tapetum lucidum in canine eyes. Toxicol Pathol 24:595–601
70. Schiavo DM, Green JD, Traina VM, Spaet R, Zaidi I (1988) Tapetal changes in beagle dogs following oral administration of CGS 14796C, a potential aromatase inhibitor. Fund Appl Toxicol 10:329–334

71. Lai YL (1980) Outward movement of photoreceptor cells in normal rat retina. Invest Ophthalmol Vis Sci 19:849–856
72. Lai YL, Masuda K, Mangum MD et al (1982) Subretinal displacement of photoreceptor nuclei in human retina. Exp Eye Res 34:219–228
73. Fraunfelder FW (2003) Ocular adverse drug reactions. Exp Opin Drug Safety 2:411–420
74. Smith RS, Hawes NL, Miller J et al (2002) Photography and necropsy. In: Smith RS (ed) Systematic evaluation of the mouse eye: anatomy, pathology, and biomethods. CRC, Boca Raton, FL
75. Fix AS, Garman RH (2000) Practical aspects of neuropathology: a technical guide for working with the nervous system. Toxicol Pathol 28:122–131
76. Thompson SW, Luna LG (1978) An atlas of artifacts encountered in the preparation of microscopic tissue sections. Charles C. Thomas Pub, Springfield
77. Lee WR (2002) Ophthalmic histopathology. Springer, London
78. Smith RS, Zabeleta A, John et al (2002) General and special histopathology. In: Smith RS (ed) Systematic evaluation of the mouse eye: anatomy, pathology, and biomethods. CRC, Boca Raton, FL
79. Dubielzig RR, Ketring KL, McLellan GJ et al (2010) The principles and practice of ocular pathology. Saunders, New York
80. Saby JA, Sigler RE, Klaus S (1991) Comparison of fixatives for histologic evaluation of the canine eye. J Histotechnol 14:251–255
81. Luna LG (1968) Manual of histology staining methods of the armed forces institute of pathology. McGraw-Hill Book Co, New York
82. Latendresse JR, Warbrittion AR, Jonassen H et al (2002) Fixation of testes and eyes using a modified Davidson's fluid: comparison with Bouin's fluid and conventional Davidson's fluid. Toxicol Pathol 30:524–533
83. Humason GL (1979) Histochemistry and special procedures. Animal tissue techniques. Freeman, San Francisco
84. Menocal NG, Ventura DB, Yanoff M (1980) Eye techniques. In: Sheehan DC, Hrapchak BB (eds) Routine processing of ophthalmic tissue for light microscopy. The CV Mosby Company, St. Louis, MO
85. Yanoff M, Fine BS (1967) Glutaraldehyde fixation of routine surgical eye tissue. Am J Ophthalmol 63:137–140
86. Margo CE, Lee A (1995) Fixation of whole eyes: the role of fixative osmolarity in the production of tissue artifact. Graefe's Arch Clin Exp Ophthalmol 233:366–370
87. Michon JJ, Li Z, Shioura N et al (1991) A comparative study of methods of photoreceptor morphometry. Invest Ophthalmol Vis Sci 32:280–284
88. Mecklenburg L, Schraermeyer U (2007) An overview on the toxic morphological changes in the retinal pigment epithelium after systemic compound administration. Toxicol Pathol 35:252–267
89. Prophet EB (1992) AFIP laboratory methods in histotechnology. American Registry of Pathology, Washington, DC
90. Giordano C, Weigt A, Vercelli A et al (2005) Immunohistochemical identification of Encephalitozoon cuniculi in phacoclastic uveitis in four rabbits. Vet Ophthalmol 8:271–275
91. Labelle P, Reilly CM, Naydan DK, Labelle LA (2012) Immunohistochemical characteristics of normal canine eyes. Vet Pathol 49:860–869
92. Dubielzig RR, Steinberg H, Garvin H et al (1998) Iridociliary epithelial tumors in 100 dogs and 17 cats: a morphological study. Vet Ophthalmol 1:223–231
93. Walker RA (2006) Quantification of immunohistochemistry—issues concerning methods, utility and semiquantitative assessment I. Histopathology 49:406–410
94. Eagle RC (2008) Immunohistochemistry in diagnostic ophthalmic pathology: a review. Clin Experiment Ophthalmol 36:675–688
95. Dabbs DJ (2002) Diagnostic immunohistochemistry. Churchill Livingstone, London
96. Ramos-Vara JA (2005) Technical aspects of immunohistochemistry. Vet Pathol 42:405–426
97. Webster JD, Miller MA, DuSold D, Ramos-Vara J (2009) Effects of prolonged formalin fixation on diagnostic immunohistochemistry in domestic animals. J Histochem Cytochem 57:753–761
98. Berod A, Hartman BK, Pujol JF (1981) Importance of fixation in immunohistochemistry: use of formaldehyde solutions at variable pH for the localization of tyrosine hydroxylase. J Histochem Cytochem 29:844–850
99. McKay JS, Steele SJ, Ahmed G et al (2009) An antibody panel for immunohistochemical analysis of the retina in Davidson's-fixed, paraffin-embedded eyes of rats. Exp Toxicol Pathol 61:91–100
100. Ramos-Vara JA, Beissenherz M (2000) Optimization of immunohistochemical methods using two different AR methods on formalin-fixed, paraffin-embedded tissues: experience with 63 markers. J Vet Diagn Invest 12:307–311

101. Shi SR, Key ME, Kalra KL (1991) Antigen retrieval in formalin-fixed, paraffin-embedded tissue: an enhancement method for immunohistochemical staining based on microwave oven heating of tissue sections. J Histochem Cytochem 39:741–748
102. Polak JM, Van Noorden S (2003) Introduction to immunocytochemistry. Bios Scientific Publishers Ltd, Oxford
103. Petrosyan K, Tamayo R, Joseph D (2002) Sensitivity of a novel biotin-free detection reagent (Powervision™) for immunohistochemistry. J Histotechnol 25:247–250
104. Sabattini E, Bisgaard K, Ascani S et al (1998) The EnVision™ system: a new immunohistochemical method for diagnostics and research: critical comparison with the APAAP, ChemMateTM CSA, LABC, and SABC techniques. J Clin Pathol 51:506–511
105. Bancroft JD, Gamble M (2002) Theory and practice of histological techniques. Churchill Livingstone, London
106. Nalbandian RM, Nagy DW, Vassallo JM (1990) Artifact-free ocular sections: a controlled comparison study between paraffin and glycol methacrylate techniques. J Histotechnol 13:35–41
107. Fagerland JA, Wall HG, Pandher K et al (2012) Ultrastructural analysis in preclinical safety evaluation. Toxicol Pathol 40:391–402
108. Zaki FG, Keysser CH (1973) Application of electron microscopy to drug safety evaluation. Toxicol Pathol 1(4):4–5
109. Hayat MA (2000) Principles and techniques of electron microscopy: biological applications. Cambridge University Press, Cambridge
110. Sadun AA, Smith LE, Kenyon KR (1983) Paraphenylenediamine: a new method for tracing human visual pathways. J Neuropathol Exp Neurol 42:200–206
111. Dykstra MJ, Reuss LE (2003) Biological electron microscopy: theory, techniques and troubleshooting. Kluwer, New York
112. Dykstra MJ, Mann PJ, Elwell MR et al (2002) Suggested standard operating procedures (SOPs) for the preparation of electron microscopy samples of toxicology/pathology samples for toxicology/pathology studies in a GLP environment. Toxicol Pathol 30: 735–743
113. Braet F, De Zanger R, Wisse E (1997) Drying cells for SEM, AFM and TEM by hexamethyldisilazane: a study on hepatic endothelial cells. J Microsc 186:84–87
114. Bozzola JJ, Russell LD (1999) Electron microscopy: principles and techniques for biologists, 2nd edn. Jones and Bartlett, Sudbury
115. Glauert AM, Lewis PR (1998) Biological specimen preparation for transmission electron microscopy. Princeton University Press, Princeton, NJ
116. Wolf T (2011) Preparation of drosophila eye specimens for scanning electron microscopy. Cold Spring Harbor Protoc 2011 (11):1383–1385. doi:10.1101/pdb.prot066506

Methods in Pharmacology and Toxicology (2014): 291–316
DOI 10.1007/7653_2013_11

Published online: 19 September 2013

Nanoparticles for Drug and Gene Delivery in Treating Diseases of the Eye

Shreya S. Kulkarni and Uday B. Kompella

Abstract

Using biodegradable polymeric nanoparticles as model systems for drug and gene delivery, this chapter describes commonly used methods for preparing and characterizing nanoparticles. This chapter focuses on emulsion solvent evaporation-based methods for encapsulating hydrophilic as well as lipophilic drugs in polymeric nanoparticles. In order to describe methods for preparing nanoparticles, we have chosen poly (lactide) (PLA)/poly(lactide-co-glycolide) (PLGA) as the carrier materials for nanoparticles intended for drug and gene delivery. Nanoparticles intended for drug and gene delivery can be characterized for various parameters including particle size, size distribution, morphology, zeta potential, drug loading, syringeability and injectability, in vitro drug release, and stability. Methods for the measurement of these parameters, which influence the performance characteristics of nanoparticles in vivo, are also discussed in this chapter.

Key words Nanoparticles, Manufacturing, Drug delivery, Gene delivery, Emulsion solvent evaporation, Particle size, Zeta potential, Drug loading, Drug release, Stability

1 Introduction

Currently, the incidence of diseases of the anterior as well as posterior segments of the eye is on the rise [1]. Some of the common anterior eye diseases are cataract, glaucoma, and uveitis while some of the posterior eye diseases are diabetic retinopathy, retinal degenerations including age-related macular degeneration (AMD) and retinitis pigmentosa. Although not life threatening, these conditions negatively affect the quality of life by causing ocular discomfort, blurring of vision and ultimately complete blindness [2]. To treat these diseases, several therapeutic agents including conventional small molecule drugs as well as macromolecules including proteins and nucleic acid therapies are under development. While treating ocular pathologies, efficient delivery of therapeutic agent to the target tissues is a critical parameter in developing safe and effective drug candidates. Both anterior and posterior segment diseases are lifelong diseases and therefore, sustained drug levels at the target site are desirable. Indeed, sustained drug delivery systems are known to maintain therapeutic drug concentrations within the therapeutic window at the target site for a prolonged period of time, thereby reducing the dosing frequency and potential systemic side effects. Delivery systems such as implants, scleral plugs, microparticles, and nanoparticles have been developed for treating chronic ocular diseases that require frequent drug dosing [3–5].

Nanoparticle-based delivery systems, particularly those based on polymers, have shown great potential in ocular drug and gene delivery over the past 10 years [5]. Depending on the polymer type employed to design the nanoparticles, these systems can be classified based on polymer origin (natural, synthetic, semi-synthetic), stability (biodegradable, non-biodegradable), charge (cationic, anionic), lipophilicity (hydrophilic, hydrophobic, amphiphilic), and release profile (sustained, controlled). Poly(lactide) (PLA) and poly(lactide-co-glycolide) (PLGA) polymers that are synthetic, biodegradable, and anionic are available in a range of molecular weights and hydrophobicities. These polymers are biocompatible with a long history of human use. They are present in the commercially available microparticle products such as Lupron Depot®, Decapeptyl® SR, and Nutropin® [6]. Hence, these polymers have been widely used for synthesizing nanoparticles. PLA/PLGA nanoparticles can perform the dual function of releasing the drug in a controlled manner while simultaneously protecting the remaining drug still present inside the particle from enzymatic degradation and physiological clearance, thereby providing sustained action. Moreover, PLA/PLGA nanoparticles are amenable to surface functionalization, allowing their use for targeted delivery [7, 8]. Although PLA/PLGA nanoparticles have yet to be tested in clinical trials for ocular diseases, there is growing evidence supporting their use in targeted and sustained drug delivery in treating chronic eye diseases. Hence, this chapter will primarily focus on the methods for preparing PLA/PLGA nanoparticles for ocular drug and gene delivery. Although several methods including those based on emulsions, nanoprecipitation, salting out, and supercritical fluid technology can be used for preparing PLA/PLGA nanoparticles, emulsion solvent evaporation techniques are most commonly used. Further, emulsion-based approaches are used for the commercially available microspheres, suggesting scalability of this method. Therefore, this chapter focuses on the preparation of PLA/PLGA nanoparticles by the emulsion solvent evaporation method. Emulsion solvent evaporation method can be employed for entrapping both hydrophilic and hydrophobic drugs. It involves two major steps, first being the emulsification of the drug in the polymer solution followed by solvent evaporation to precipitate the drug and polymer as nanoparticles [9]. Based on the nature of the drug, this method has two primary variants, namely the single

Table 1
Characterization parameters for nanoparticles and the relevant methods

Parameters	Method
Particle size	Dynamic light scattering
Morphology	Scanning electron microscopy and transmission electron microscopy
Zeta potential	Laser doppler micro-electrophoresis
Drug loading	Drug extraction and quantification
In vitro drug release	Dialysis-based method
Syringeability and injectability	In-house method
Physical Stability	Assessment of long-term physical stability by determining particle size, zeta potential, and amount of drug retained in the particles

emulsion and double emulsion methods, which are detailed in this chapter. Since nanoparticle properties including particle size, particle charge, drug loading and drug release (Table 1) influence the targeting ability and efficacy of nanoparticles, methods for characterizing these parameters are also described in this chapter.

2 Materials

2.1 Materials for Preparing Nanoparticles

L-Poly(lactide) (L-PLA) (Lactel®) having intrinsic viscosity 0.90–1.2 dl/g and molecular weight of about 140,000 Da in chloroform and poly(D, L-lactide-co-glycolide) (DL-PLGA 50:50) (Resomer® RG 503H) that is acid terminated, having a molecular weight of 24,000–38,000 Da and intrinsic viscosity of 0.32–0.44 dl/g in chloroform can be used for preparing nanoparticles (*see* **Note 1**). Poly(vinyl alcohol) (PVA), 87–89 % hydrolyzed and with average molecular weight of 31,000–50,000 Da can be used as the surfactant for emulsification. Dichloromethane (DCM) of HPLC grade can be used as the organic solvent to solubilize the polymer. 50 ml Nalgene oak ridge high speed centrifuge tubes or 250 ml Nalgene centrifuge bottles can be used for settling the particles using a centrifuge.

2.2 Materials for Characterizing Nanoparticles

2.2.1 Materials for Particle Size

0.2 μm Millipore filter is useful for filtering distilled and de-ionized water. Zetasizer Nano ZS (Malvern® Instruments, Westborough, MA, USA) can be used for determining the particle size.

2.2.2 Materials for Morphology

Aluminum stubs are required for sample loading in scanning electron microscope (SEM) and carbon-coated grids are required for transmission electron microscope (TEM). 2 % w/v uranyl acetate or ammonium molybdate solution is used as a negative stain for TEM (*see* **Note 2**) and a flexible plastic membrane (Parafilm®) can be used for transferring the nanoparticles onto carbon-coated grids.

2.2.3 Materials for Zeta Potential

Disposable folded capillary cells (Malvern® Instruments, Westborough, MA, USA) are required for measuring zeta potential (*see* **Note 3**). Zetasizer Nano ZS (Malvern® Instruments, Westborough, MA, USA) can be used for measuring the zeta potential.

2.2.4 Materials for Drug Loading

Organic solvents like DCM or chloroform and aqueous solvents like distilled and de-ionized water or Tris-EDTA buffer (TE buffer) or 70:30 acetonitrile–water mixture are required.

2.2.5 Materials for In Vitro Drug Release

Phosphate-buffered saline (PBS) pH 7.4, a dialysis membrane (Spectra/Por® 1-7 regenerated cellulose membranes, Spectrum Laboratories, Inc, CA) with a molecular weight cut off in the range of 6,000–50,000 Da (*see* **Note 4**) and sodium azide.

2.2.6 Materials for Syringeability and Injectability

1 ml syringe and 30 or 32G needles.

2.2.7 Materials for Physical Stability

5 ml glass vials, rubber stoppers, and aluminum caps.

3 Methods

3.1 Preparation of Nanoparticles

Various materials and methods can be employed to prepare nanoparticles of diverse sizes, morphologies, and compositions. Nanoparticles can be broadly classified as reservoir and matrix type delivery systems [10]. Reservoir systems consist of a drug core, which is surrounded by a polymer layer that controls drug release [11, 12]. Matrix type of systems have the drug distributed throughout a polymeric carrier [10]. Although there are some reports on the preparation of reservoir type systems of a nanoscale [13], matrix type systems are more commonly prepared, due to the ease of their preparation. While aseptic manufacturing of nanoparticles using sterile raw materials is ideal, depending on the drug stability in response to radiation, gamma irradiation may be used for end-stage sterilization of nanoparticles discussed in this chapter. With end-stage sterilization, the stability of the drug as well as particles has to be ascertained.

3.1.1 Selection of Carrier Material

PLA and PLGA polymers belong to the class of synthetic biodegradable polymers. Being synthetic in nature, as mentioned above, they are available in various molecular weights, lipophilicities, and rates of degradation. Thus, the duration of drug release can be modulated based on the polymer choice. PLA and PLGA polymers are degraded to lactic and glycolic acids in the presence of water due to hydrolytic cleavage of the ester bonds in the polymer matrix. The acids that are formed further catalyze the degradation of the parent polymer, through a process known as autocatalysis and increase the degradation rate with time [14, 15]. As a result, these polymers are degraded at the site of administration and can be easily eliminated from the body. Owing to these properties, they are a preferred choice for preparing nanoparticles intended for sustained delivery. This chapter focuses on preparation of nanoparticles using the PLA and PLGA family of polymers.

3.1.2 Emulsion Solvent Evaporation Method

PLA and PLGA nanoparticles can be prepared by various methods including emulsion solvent evaporation, emulsion solvent diffusion, nanoprecipitation, and supercritical fluid technology, among others. Of these, emulsion solvent evaporation technique is the most commonly used and described in greater detail below.

Emulsion solvent evaporation involves two major steps, namely emulsification followed by solvent evaporation. Emulsion formation is accomplished by providing energy in the form of sonication or homogenization and solvent evaporation is achieved either by stirring at room temperature or by increasing the temperature and reducing pressure. Based on the nature of the drug, the emulsion solvent evaporation method can be further divided into single emulsion method or double emulsion method. Hydrophobic drugs are typically formulated using a single oil-in-water (o/w) emulsion since the drug is soluble in the inner organic phase along with the polymer. Hydrophilic drugs are generally formulated using (water-in-oil)-in-water (w/o/w) double emulsion method since the drug is insoluble in the organic phase but soluble in the aqueous phase. Peptides, proteins, and nucleic acids including plasmids can be entrapped into nanoparticles by the double emulsion method. To reduce the degradation of peptides/proteins (solid-in-oil)-in-water (s/o/w) methods may be employed. Figure 1 presents the general methodology for preparing o/w and w/o/w emulsions. These two methods are further described below.

Single Emulsion Method for Hydrophobic Drugs

Single o/w emulsion method is used for loading hydrophobic drugs in PLA/PLGA nanoparticles and is comprised of two principal steps. In the first step, polymer solution is prepared in a volatile

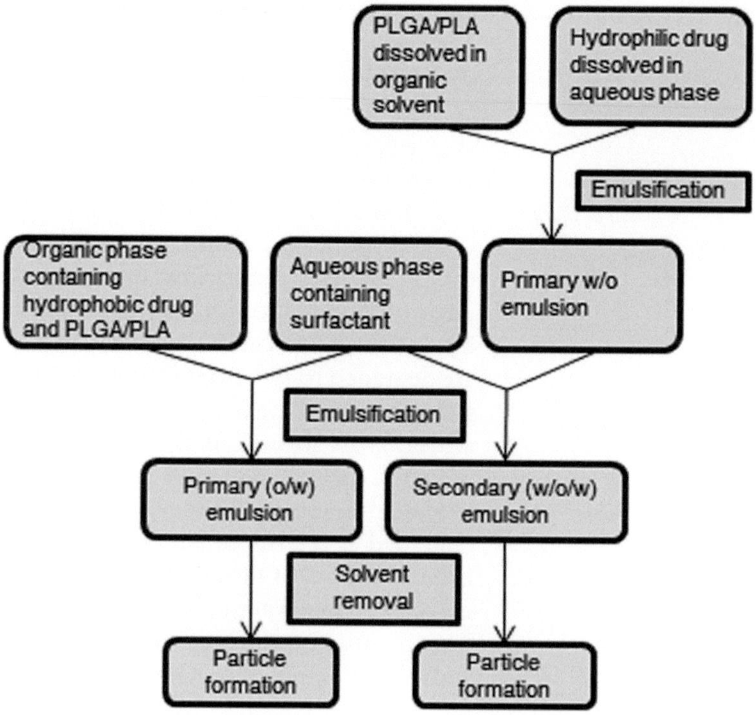

Fig. 1 Schematic representation of o/w single emulsion and w/o/w double emulsion methods

organic solvent and the hydrophobic active substance is also dissolved in the internal organic phase. This polymer solution is emulsified in water, which is the continuous phase immiscible with the internal organic phase. Formation of an o/w emulsion requires a surfactant with a hydrophilic–lipophilic balance (HLB) value in the range of 10–20. PVA has an HLB value of 18 and hence it is useful for forming an o/w emulsion. Thus, emulsifiers like PVA are added to the aqueous phase to stabilize the oil droplets and prevent them from coalescing. In the second step, the emulsion is converted into a nanoparticle suspension by evaporating the volatile solvent and inducing precipitation of the polymer as nanoparticles. The solidified nanoparticles are then collected by centrifugation and washed with distilled and de-ionized water to remove free drug and partly additives such as surfactants. The washed nanoparticles are typically freeze dried for storage because freeze drying increases the on shelf long-term stability of these products. Kompella et al. have prepared budesonide PLA nanoparticles for transscleral delivery of the drug to the retina for inhibiting VEGF expression [16]. Kadam et al. have prepared PLA nanoparticles for studying the effect of choroidal neovascularization on transscleral delivery of triamcinolone acetonide [17]. Yang et al. prepared PLGA nanoparticles of brimonidine and timolol maleate for achieving sustained anti-glaucoma effect following topical administration [18]. The step-by-step procedure for preparing nanoparticles entrapping hydrophobic drugs is outlined below:

1. 100 mg of PLGA-Resomer RG 503H [18] or 200 mg of L-PLA [17] is dissolved in 1 or 5 ml DCM taken in 5 and 10 ml glass vials (*see* **Notes 5–7**).
2. Drug (e.g., brimonidine 20 mg, timolol maleate 40 mg, triamcinolone acetonide 100 mg) is dissolved or dispersed in the polymer solution.
3. The polymer-drug dispersion is added under sonication to ~10–30 ml of a prechilled 2 % w/v aqueous solution of PVA taken in a 50 ml glass beaker. PVA functions as the emulsifier (*see* **Notes 8–10**).
4. Sonication in step 3 is done using a probe sonicator (Misonix Sonicator® 3000, Farmingdale, NY) for 1 min at a power of 10 W and is done on ice (*see* **Notes 11–15**).
5. The primary o/w emulsion obtained after sonication is added to 100 ml [17] or 50 ml [18] chilled 2 % w/v PVA solution under probe sonication. Sonication is done for 3 min at 30 W power (*see* **Note 16**).
6. The emulsion thus obtained is kept under stirring at room temperature for 3 h to evaporate the organic solvent. Residual solvent, if any, is further evaporated by using a rotary evaporator (Buchi Rotavapor R-200, Buchi Corporation, New Castle, DE, USA) for 2 h at 40 °C (*see* **Notes 17–20**).
7. The nanoparticles thus formed are centrifuged using a Sorvall RC 6 plus centrifuge (Thermo Scientific, Asheville, NC, USA) at ~25,000–30,000 × *g* for 15–20 min at 4 °C to obtain a pellet of the nanoparticles (*see* **Notes 21** and **22**).
8. The supernatant is removed and the pellet is redispersed in 25 ml distilled, de-ionized water and centrifuged again. This washing step ensures further removal of free drug and additives like surfactants (*see* **Note 23**).
9. Another round of washing followed by centrifugation is repeated.
10. The pellet is redispersed in 10 ml distilled, de-ionized water and frozen by storing at −80 °C for 30 min.
11. After the primary freezing step, the nanoparticles are lyophilized in a Labconco freeze dryer (Labconco Corporation, Kansas City, MO) at −80 °C and at a pressure of 0.1 mBar for 24 h (*see* **Notes 24–26**).

Double Emulsion Method for Hydrophilic Drugs

A (w/o/w) double emulsion is formed for entrapping hydrophilic drugs in PLA/PLGA nanoparticles. In the emulsification step, the aqueous drug solution is emulsified with organic polymer solution by means of sonication with or without the use of a surfactant

(HLB value in the range of 3–6). The resulting w/o droplets are dispersed in an external aqueous phase containing PVA, allowing the formation of secondary emulsion (w/o/w). Singh et al. reported the preparation of Flt23k PLGA nanoparticles and their functionalization with RGD peptide and transferrin to treat laser-induced CNV by intravenous delivery [7]. Luo et al. [19] and Cho et al. [20] also described the use of PLGA nanoparticles entrapping Flt23k plasmid, for controlling angiogenesis and fibrosis associated with CNV. The step-by-step procedure for preparing nanoparticles entrapping hydrophilic drugs like plasmids is described below:

1. 100 mg polymer (PLGA-Resomer RG 503H) is dissolved in 2 ml DCM in a 5 ml glass vial (*see* **Note 27**).
2. Drug (e.g., Flt23k plasmid 4 mg in buffer) is dissolved in about 500 μl distilled, de-ionized water.
3. The drug solution is added to the polymer solution in a glass vial under probe sonication (Misonix Sonicator® 3000, Farmingdale, NY) for 1 min at a power of 6–10 W (*see* **Notes 11–15**).
4. The primary w/o emulsion obtained in step 3 is added under probe sonication to 10 ml of prechilled 2 % w/v PVA solution taken in a 50 ml glass beaker and sonicated for 3 min at 24–30 W power to obtain the (w/o/w) emulsion (*see* **Note 28**).
5. The secondary emulsion thus obtained is kept under stirring at room temperature for 3 h to evaporate the organic solvent. Residual solvent, if any, is further evaporated by using a rotary evaporator (Buchi Rotavapor R-200, Buchi Corporation, New Castle, DE, USA) for 2 h at 40 °C (*see* **Notes 17–20**).
6. The nanoparticles thus formed are centrifuged using a Sorvall RC 6 plus centrifuge (Thermo Scientific, Asheville, NC, USA) at ~25,000–30,000 × *g* for 15–20 min to obtain a pellet of the nanoparticles (*see* **Notes 21** and **22**).
7. The supernatant is removed and the pellet is redispersed in 25 ml distilled, de-ionized water and centrifuged again. This washing step ensures further removal of the free drug and additives like emulsifiers (*see* **Note 23**).
8. Another round of washing followed by centrifugation is repeated.
9. The pellet is redispersed in 10 ml distilled, de-ionized water and frozen by storing at −80 °C for 30 min.
10. After the primary freezing step, the nanoparticles are lyophilized in a Labconco freeze dryer (Labconco Corporation, Kansas city, MO) at −80 °C and at a pressure of 0.1 mBar for 24 h (*see* **Notes 24–26**).

3.2 Characterization of Nanoparticles

3.2.1 Particle Size

Particle size is an important parameter that not only affects the degradation of the polymer matrix but also influences the disposition of the particles once they have been injected into the eye [21, 22]. There is no single standard technique for measuring the particle size of nanoparticles. A variety of methods like dynamic light scattering (DLS), scanning electron microscopy (SEM), transmission electron microscopy (TEM), and nanoparticle tracking analysis (NTA) can be employed for determining the particle size [7, 16, 17, 23, 24]. DLS, which is one of the most commonly used methods for measuring particle size is discussed here. DLS is a characterization technique that reports the particle size in terms of the hydrodynamic diameter of the particles [25]. It is advantageous because it is non-destructive, making sample recovery possible, uses a small amount of sample and is quick and easy to perform [26]. Step-by-step procedure for measuring particles size by DLS is as follows:

1. 1 mg of PLA/PLGA nanoparticles are weighed in an eppendorf tube.
2. 1 ml filtered, de-ionized water is added to the particles (*see* **Notes 29** and **30**).
3. The particles are suspended in water by gently shaking the eppendorf tube (*see* **Note 31**).
4. The dispersion prepared in step 3 can be analyzed using the Zetasizer Nano ZS (Malvern® Instruments) (*see* **Note 32**).

3.2.2 Morphology

Particle geometry and surface features of the nanoparticles can be studied using SEM and TEM. The detailed procedure for the two methods is as follows.

Scanning Electron Microscopy (SEM)

1. The particles are mounted on aluminum stubs.
2. Following mounting, the particles are coated with a layer of gold using a sputter coater (Anatech, CA, USA).
3. After coating, the particles are examined under an electron microscope set at 5–10 kV [16, 17] (*see* **Note 33**).

Transmission Electron Microscopy (TEM)

1. A droplet of the nanoparticle suspension is placed on a flexible plastic film (Parafilm®) (*see* **Note 34**).
2. Carbon-coated grid is floated on the droplet of nanoparticle suspension to permit the adsorption of the nanoparticles onto the grid.
3. The grid is blotted with a filter paper and air dried for 5 min (*see* **Note 35**).
4. After drying, the grid is transferred onto a drop of uranyl acetate or ammonium molybdate.

5. Following staining in step 4, the grid is blotted with a filter paper and air dried for 5 min.
6. The sample is examined under an electron microscope set at 60–100 kV (*see* **Note 36**).

3.2.3 Zeta Potential

Essentially, the same sample preparation used for particle size determination can be used for zeta measurements. If the sample is at the right dilution for size measurements, but is too concentrated or dilute for zeta potential measurements, a fresh dispersion suitable for zeta potential measurements should be prepared in such cases. Because zeta potential measures the potential difference between the dispersion medium and the stationary layer of liquid attached to the dispersed particle, the dispersion medium in which the sample is prepared can affect the zeta potential measurement. Different media that are commonly employed are de-ionized water, PBS, and saline. Selection of the medium would depend on the conditions in which the zeta potential is desired. If the actual zeta potential of the particles is desired without any influence of the dispersion medium on the particle charge, de-ionized water would be the ideal choice. However, if the zeta potential of a particle in a physiological medium such as serum is desired, then the measurement should be done in PBS. Zeta potential measurements can be done using the Zetasizer Nano ZS (Malvern® Instruments) and are based on the principle of laser doppler micro-electrophoresis. Zeta potential measurements require the disposable folded capillary cells, which are specially designed for measuring zeta potential (*see* **Note 37**). PLGA nanoparticles prepared by the methods described are reported to have a negative zeta potential in water [7, 19].

3.2.4 Drug Loading

Drug loading is an estimate of the amount of drug entrapped in the nanoparticles and can be used for calculating the entrapment efficiency of the particles.

$$\text{Percent drug loading} = \frac{\text{Mass of the drug in nanoparticles}}{\text{Mass of nanoparticles weighed}} \times 100$$

$$\text{Percent entrapment efficiency} = \frac{\text{Experimental drug loading}}{\text{Theoretical drug loading}} \times 100$$

Drug loading can be quantified by following the steps described below:

1. 2 mg of the lyophilized nanoparticles are weighed (*see* **Note 38**).
2. The weighed nanoparticles are dissolved in 2 ml DCM (or chloroform) and vortexed for about 1 h at room temperature (*see* **Note 39**).

3. The organic solvent is evaporated under nitrogen and the drug in residue is reconstituted using a suitable solvent. For instance, for the budesonide loaded PLA nanoparticles, 1 ml acetonitrile--water (70:30) mixture was used for extraction. For Flt23k plasmid loaded, RGD and transferrin-functionalized PLGA nanoparticles, TE buffer was employed for plasmid extraction from the residue [7] and for Flt23k loaded RGD-functionalized PLGA nanoparticles, 1 ml water was used [20] (*see* **Note 40**).
4. The dispersion in step 3 is vortexed for about 1–2 h (*see* **Note 41**).
5. The extract is used for drug quantification. Quantification can be done by a suitable method like absorbance [7, 20] or fluorescence spectroscopy, HPLC [16] or LC-MS (*see* **Note 42**).

3.2.5 In Vitro Drug Release Studies

These studies are performed in a buffer, which acts as the release medium and dissolves the drug. In vitro release studies are typically carried out at 37 °C and employ a dialysis membrane for small molecule drugs, peptides, and small nucleic acids. For large molecules such as proteins and plasmids, a membrane free method such as ultracentrifugation for collection of full amount of dispersion medium at various time points is more appropriate. For the small molecule drugs, the drug-loaded nanoparticles are added to a dialysis bag, sealed, placed in a release medium. The drug released from the particles penetrates across the dialysis membrane into the release medium. Aliquots are withdrawn from the bulk medium at specific pre-determined time points. The drug released into the dissolution medium is then quantified using a suitable technique like absorbance, fluorescence, or mass spectroscopy. PBS at pH 7.4 is generally chosen as the buffer because it simulates physiological conditions.

Detailed procedure to be followed while performing release study by the dialysis method for small molecule drugs is as follows:

1. 1–2 mg of drug-loaded PLA/PLGA particles are weighed in 1.5 ml eppendorf tubes (*see* **Note 43**).
2. 1 ml water is added to the particles in the eppendorf tubes.
3. PBS (pH 7.4) containing 0.05 % w/v sodium azide as preservative is prepared (*see* **Note 44**).
4. 50 ml buffer from step 3 is added to centrifuge tubes (*see* **Note 45**).
5. Dialysis membrane with a suitable molecular weight cut off in the range of 6,000–50,000 Da is chosen based on the difference between the molecular weights of the drug and the polymer used to prepare nanoparticles (*see* **Note 46**). The membrane is sealed at one end to form a bag.

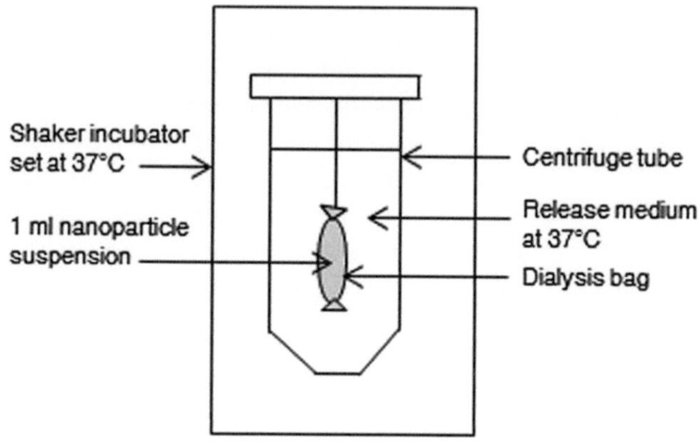

Fig. 2 Set up for performing in vitro drug release study by dialysis method

6. 1 ml of the nanoparticle suspension from step 2 is added to this dialysis bag.
7. The other end of the dialysis bag containing the nanoparticle suspension is now sealed and the bag is immersed in centrifuge tubes from step 4.
8. The centrifuge tubes are capped and placed in a shaker incubator at 37 °C with gentle shaking.
9. 1–2 ml aliquots are withdrawn at pre-determined time points (*see* **Notes 47** and **48**).
10. The volume withdrawn at each withdrawal time point is replaced by an equal volume of fresh buffer containing sodium azide, pre-equilibrated to 37 °C (*see* **Note 49**).
11. Samples collected in step 8 can be stored at −20 °C till analysis and can be analyzed using a suitable technique.

Figure 2 represents the set up for performing in vitro release study by the dialysis method.

3.2.6 Syringeability and Injectability

The PLA/PLGA nanoparticles prepared by one of the above methods are administered in the eye as intravitreal, subretinal, suprachoroidal, periocular, or intravenous injections. For the successful delivery of these particles, they should be injectable. In order to be injectable they should be easily withdrawn into a syringe by means of a needle. Details of the method used for assessing the syringeability and injectability of these particles are outlined below. We previously reported this method for microparticles [27].

1. A stock of nanoparticle dispersion at a concentration to be used for in vivo injections is prepared in PBS at pH 7.4.
2. 50 μl of the nanoparticle dispersion from step 1 is withdrawn into a 1 ml syringe using a 30 or 32G needle (*see* **Note 50**).

3. 50 μl of the suspension from step 2 is added to pre-weighed eppendorf tubes.
4. Additionally, using a micropipette, 50 μl of the nanoparticle suspension from step 1 is added to another set of pre-weighed eppendorf tubes.
5. The weight of the suspension in the two sets of eppendorf tubes is noted. The two sets represent the two withdrawal methods as described in step 2 and step 4, respectively.
6. Drug present in the eppendorf tubes is extracted and analyzed by methods similar to those described in Section 3.2.4.
7. Weight of the nanoparticle suspension and percent drug transferred to the eppendorf tubes by both withdrawal methods is compared. If the results obtained indicate 95 % or greater amount of dose delivery, it can be concluded that the nanoparticles are syringeable, and can be withdrawn into a syringe and injected without substantial loss of the entrapped drug. Based on the percent delivery, volume withdrawn can be adjusted as needed for dosing.

3.2.7 Physical Stability

The physical stability studies can be carried out on both the lyophilized nanoparticle formulation and the reconstituted product intended for delivery. Since the nanoparticles are reconstituted with PBS before ocular delivery and are dispersed in the physiological fluids after injection, monitoring the stability of the reconstituted product in PBS can prove to be useful. A study assessing the physical stability of the reconstituted particles can throw light on the aggregation tendency of the particles when dispersed in a medium simulating physiological conditions. Physical stability of the nanoparticles can be assessed by measuring the particle size, zeta potential, and the amount of drug retained in the particles, in addition to visually examining the appearance of the nanoparticles at pre-determined time points. Stability studies can be performed according to the ICH guidelines on stability testing of new drug substances and drug products [28]. The following stability study design can be adopted:

For lyophilized nanoparticles:

1. 4 mg of nanoparticles are weighed in clear glass vials (one set of vials per analysis time point for each condition).
2. The vials are closed with rubber stoppers and sealed with aluminum caps.
3. Samples are stored at different conditions of temperature and relative humidity (RH) in stability chambers that have controlled temperatures and RHs. Temperature and RH conditions are described in Table 2.

Table 2
Stability study design for assessing the stability of PLA/PLGA nanoparticles

Study	Storage condition	Duration	Time points for analysis
Long term	5 ± 3 °C	12 months	At the end of 0.5, 1, 2, 3, 6 and 12 months
Accelerated	25 ± 2 °C/60 ± 5 % RH	6 months	At the end of 0.5, 1, 2, 3, and 6 months

4. Samples are withdrawn at time points as depicted in Table 2.
5. 1 mg sample is used for measurement of particle size and zeta potential as described in Sections 3.2.1 and 3.2.3. 2 mg sample is used for determining the drug loading by the method described in Section 3.2.4.

For reconstituted nanoparticles:

1. 10 mg of nanoparticles are weighed and reconstituted with 10 ml PBS pH 7.4 and are stored at 37 °C.
2. Samples are withdrawn at 0, 24, and 48 h and analyzed for particle size and zeta potential as described in Sections 3.2.1 and 3.2.3, respectively.

4 Notes

1. L-PLA (Lactel®) should be stored at ≤ −10 °C and DL-PLGA (50:50) (Resomer® RG 503H) should be stored at 2–8 °C.
2. Negative stain solution should be stored at 4 °C. Each time before using the solution, it should be centrifuged to remove the undissolved uranyl acetate or ammonium molybdate that may have precipitated during storage.
3. For the disposable folded capillary cell (Malvern® Instruments, Westborough, MA, USA) to measure zeta potential, the manufacturer recommends single use and proper wetting of the container with ethanol or methanol followed by flushing of the container five times with de-ionized water or the vehicle. The cell is not compatible with organic solvents.
4. Spectra/Por® regenerated cellulose (RC) dialysis membranes (Spectrum Laboratories, Inc.) are superior to cellulose ester membranes in terms of tolerated pH and temperature range and the tolerance of exposure to acids, basis, and organic solvents. Therefore, RC membranes are recommended for dialysis. Supplier recommends that the RC dialysis membranes should be stored at 4 °C. The supplier provides the RC membranes

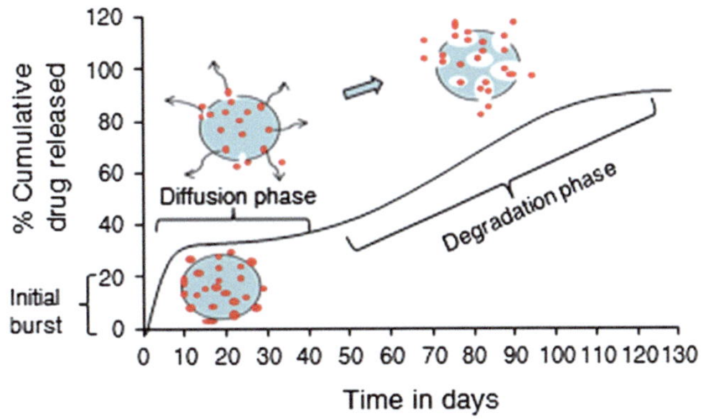

Fig. 3 Typical in vitro drug release profile for drug-loaded PLA/PLGA nanoparticles. Initial burst release is characterized by dissolution of drug molecules (in *red*) present on or near the nanoparticle (in *blue*) surface, diffusion phase is characterized primarily by drug molecules diffusing from the polymer matrix, and degradation phase is characterized by drug molecules primarily being released following bulk degradation of the polymer matrix

packaged in the dry form with glycerine as the preservative or in the wet form with 0.05 % w/v sodium azide as the preservative. It is recommended that the wet membranes must not be allowed to dry out as drying can lead to an irreversible collapse of the pore structure; hence, they should be kept wetted in 0.05 % w/v sodium azide during storage. Before using the dialysis membrane for the in vitro release study, the membrane should be soaked in distilled and de-ionized water for 15–30 min to remove the preservative. Soaking should be followed by thorough rinsing in running distilled and de-ionized water.

5. Volume of DCM for dissolving the polymer is based on the amount of polymer weighed, the type of polymer, and the molecular weight of the polymer. In general, PLA polymers have a lower solubility than PLGA polymers in most solvents. Further, as the intrinsic viscosity of the polymer increases, the molecular weight increases and the solubility decreases [29, 30]. In the methods described, while 100 mg PLGA of 0.32–0.44 dl/g intrinsic viscosity was dissolved in 1 ml DCM, 200 mg L-PLA which had a higher intrinsic viscosity of 0.95–1.2 dl/g was dissolved in 5 ml of DCM. About 5 min of vortexing can help dissolve the polymers in DCM.

6. PLA/PLGA particles designed for sustained release are characterized by a triphasic drug release profile as depicted in Fig. 3 [31]. The initial burst release is due to dissolution of the drug present on or near the particle surface. The burst release is followed by a slow release phase that is controlled by diffusion of the drug from the polymer matrix [14, 15, 32]. The diffusion phase is followed by a more rapid drug release due to bulk degradation of the polymer matrix [14, 15]. It has been

reported that while drug release occurs mainly through diffusion from the polymer matrix in the early phases, in the later phases, drug release is mediated through both diffusion of the drug and degradation of the polymer matrix [21]. Polymer degradation is influenced by the polymer composition (lactide:glycolide ratio), intrinsic viscosity and molecular weight, and crystallinity [27, 33]. Hence, selection of a suitable polymer from a wide variety of PLA/PLGA polymers available becomes critical.

Polymer composition: The more hydrophilic the polymer, more rapid is its degradation [34, 35]. The hydrophilicity is determined by copolymer composition. Glycolic acid, being more hydrophilic than lactic acid, PLGA copolymers with higher glycolide content are more hydrophilic and have a faster degradation rate due to higher water uptake [34–37]. Generally, if drug release up to 4–6 weeks is desired, PLGA 50:50 with low to medium molecular weight (e.g., Resomer® RG 502 or 503) can be used and if a slower release is required, PLGA with a higher lactide/glycolide ratio (e.g., PLGA 65:35, PLGA 75:25, or PLGA 85:15) or PLA can be used [33, 38].

Polymer molecular weight: In general, for a particular lactide/glycolide composition of PLA/PLGA polymer, employing high molecular weight polymers has been found to decrease their degradation rate, thereby sustaining drug release [27, 32, 36, 37, 39].

Polymer crystallinity: L-PLA and PGA are crystalline while D, L-PLA is amorphous [40]. In general, crystalline polymers are able to sustain drug release for longer periods of time because they are degraded at a slower rate compared to semi-crystalline and amorphous polymers [27, 41].

Polymer concentration: Increasing the polymer concentration increases the viscosity of the polymer giving rise to a dense and compact internal structure that prevents drug diffusion to external phase during the evaporation step [42]. Generally, higher drug loading can be achieved by increasing the polymer concentration.

Polymer end group: The nature of the end group of the polymer chain affects the degradation rate of the polymer by controlling the water uptake by the polymer. Hydrophilic end groups such as free carboxyl groups exhibit faster degradation rates than hydrophobic end groups such as ester or alkyl ester groups [43, 44]. For instance, Resomer® RG 503H which is acid terminated degrades faster than Resomer® RG 503 which is ester terminated.

It should be noted that apart from the polymer properties discussed above, nanoparticle size, pH, ionic strength, and temperature of release medium also affect the polymer degradation [45, 46].

Table 3
List of commonly used organic solvents for dissolving the polymers

Solvents	Solvent class	Concentration limit in pharmaceutical formulations (ppm[a,b])	Boiling point (°C)	Miscibility with water
Dichloromethane	2	600	40	Immiscible
Chloroform	2	60	61	Immiscible
Ethyl acetate	3	5,000	77	Immiscible

As per ICH guidelines for residual solvents Q3C (R4) and United States Pharmacopeia, class 2 solvents are solvents to be limited in pharmaceutical products and class 3 solvents are solvents with low toxic potential
[a]United States Pharmacopeia
[b]Values according to ICH guidelines Q3C (R4)

7. The solvent choice for the emulsion solvent evaporation method should be based on the following criteria:
   (a) Polymer should be soluble in the solvent
   (b) Solvent should be immiscible with the aqueous phase
   (c) Solvent should be completely and easily removed

   Solvents that can be employed apart from DCM are ethyl acetate and chloroform [9]. Table 3 lists the solvents that can be employed for dissolving the polymers and their physical properties.
8. Surfactants function as emulsifiers by adsorbing on the surface of the oil globules and preventing them from aggregating [47]. PVA has been reported to aid in nanoparticle formation at concentrations as low as 0.1 % w/v [48]. However, the higher the PVA concentration used, the smaller is the size of the nanoparticles obtained [49, 50]. At higher PVA concentration, more number of surfactant molecules would be adsorbed on the particle surface, thereby preventing the oil droplets from coalescing. PVA at 2 % w/v has been found to give rise to stable nanoparticles with particle size in the range of ~200–500 nm by the methods described.
9. The PVA solution should be stored at 4 °C.
10. The phase ratio (organic to aqueous solvent ratio) may influence the size of the nanoparticles [48]. In general, a ratio of 1:10 of organic/aqueous phase produced nanoparticles of ~350 nm size when prepared by the method described [16].
11. Strong agitation force is required to reduce the droplet size for forming a stable emulsion. The emulsification step is a key aspect of the emulsion solvent evaporation method because the emulsion droplet size is directly related to the final nanoparticle size [9]. The higher the sonication power input and longer the sonication time, the smaller the particle size achieved [47, 49].

12. The glass beaker used for sonication should be of a suitable size to achieve satisfactory size reduction. If a large beaker is used, particles near the walls might not experience enough sonication and will remain as larger-sized particles, increasing the polydispersity.
13. It has been observed that when the probe touches the glass walls, it gives rise to particle impurities in the final product. Hence it is advisable to use a wide mouthed container for sonication and care should be taken that the probe does not touch the glass walls during sonication.
14. The Tg for L-PLA is around 55–60 °C and Tg for DL-PLGA (Resomer® RG 503H) is in the range of 44–48 °C. Therefore, the heat generated during probe sonication can degrade these polymers. Hence sonication is done on ice using prechilled preparations to prevent heat generation and thermal degradation of thermolabile actives and the polymer.
15. The quality of the probe controls the quality of the nanoparticles formed. A new good quality probe with a high power input yields monodisperse small-sized particles as compared to an old probe.
16. Sonication of the primary emulsion after it has been added to 2 % w/v PVA ensures a further reduction in the droplet size of the emulsion.
17. Organic solvent removal method would largely depend on the type of the solvent employed. The most common approach for removing the solvent is a rotary evaporator placed in a hood, which uses heat to force the liquid solvent into a gaseous state and simultaneously applies vacuum to remove the solvent gases. Rotary evaporator can be used for removal of most of the solvents. Stirring at room temperature in a hood to remove the organic solvent can be a good alternative method for drugs that are sensitive to temperature or vacuum pressure. However, stirring at room temperature mandates the use of a low boiling point solvent like DCM (B.P. 40 °C).
18. The temperature of the water bath in the rotary evaporator should not exceed glass transition temperature (Tg) of the polymer being used. Temperature of the bath is generally set at 40 °C (Buchi Heat Bath B490) if DCM is used as the solvent.
19. Organic solvent removal is a critical step in particle preparation because the rate of solvent removal influences the particle size and drug entrapment efficiency [51]. Fast rate of solvent removal has been reported to decrease the particle size and increase the drug loading [51]. Faster removal decreases the aggregation of nanoparticles, thereby promoting formation of smaller-sized particles. The rate of polymer precipitation during solvent evaporation step influences drug partitioning into the external phase and subsequently affects the amount of drug entrapped. Slow rate of solvent removal can lead to polymer

precipitating slowly, giving the drug more time to diffuse into the external phase from the internal phase, resulting in low entrapment efficiencies [51].

20. The solvents typically employed are organic and traces of these solvents in the final product, at concentrations above the permissible limits can lead to toxicity issues in humans. There are strict guidelines in place for residual organic solvents in pharmaceutical formulations [52]. Table 3 lists the permissible limits for the commonly used solvents in pharmaceutical formulations. The limit for DCM in pharmaceutical formulations as specified in the United States Pharmacopeia is 600 ppm (parts per million). Residual DCM in TG-0054-loaded PLA microparticles (L-PLA of intrinsic viscosity 0.9–1.2 dl/g, Lactel®) prepared by a similar method has been reported to be ~1 ppb (parts per billion) as determined by EPA Method 8260 using gas chromatography-mass spectrometry (GC-MS) [27]. For microparticle preparation, evaporation was done for 3 h by magnetic stirring at room temperature, followed by rotary evaporation for 2 h. Although it is essential that the solvent be completely removed, care should be taken to minimize the removal of drug from the internal phase into the external phase while doing so.

21. Centrifugation speed should be selected such that all the particles get settled. If centrifugation is done at low speeds, lighter particles may be left in the supernatant and will not get pelleted and will be lost during the washing step resulting in a lower yield of nanoparticles. Shorter centrifugation times can also have a similar effect. Centrifugation can be typically done at 27,000 × *g* for 20 min using the Sorvall RC 6 plus centrifuge for settling particles in the range of 250–500 nm.

22. Tubes used for centrifugation should be sturdy, inert and should not interact with the solvent and the nanoparticles. The tubes should be strong enough to sustain the high centrifugal force and should not crack during centrifugation. Moreover, they should not leach any material into the nanoparticle suspension. The Nalgene oak ridge centrifuge tubes and Nalgene centrifuge bottles are made of polypropylene copolymer and have excellent mechanical strength and chemical resistance and are leak proof. These tubes can be used for centrifugation using the Sorvall RC 6 Plus centrifuge.

23. Washing step is important for the removal of unentrapped drug and free emulsifiers like surfactants.

24. The temperature at which freeze drying is conducted should be below the Tg of the polymer. Variations in the vacuum pressure (0.1–0.5 mBar) can affect the lyophilization time. High pressure would increase the lyophilization time. For particles prepared by the method described and lyophilized using the

Labconco freeze dryer (Labconco Corporation, Kansas City, MO), a pressure of 0.1 mBar applied for 24 h yielded nanoparticles in the form of a dry powder.

25. PLGA and PLA polymers are degraded to lactic and glycolic acids in the presence of water and the degradation is further catalyzed through autocatalysis; thereby increasing the parent polymer degradation rate with time [14, 15]. If freeze drying has not gone to completion, then the sample will have high water content, which can decrease the shelf life of the nanoparticles by degrading the polymers. Residual water can also give rise to higher-than-usual burst release due to the drug being carried to the surface of the particles along with water. Residual water in the freeze-dried particles can be determined by using techniques like Karl Fisher method or thermal gravimetric analysis.
26. Lyoprotectants like trehalose, sucrose, mannitol, and glucose can be added to the product before freeze drying to help maintain the integrity of product during and after lyophilization and to aid in easy redispersibility of the lyophilized product after reconstitution [50, 53].
27. The low entrapment efficiencies of hydrophilic drugs observed with the double emulsion method, owing to diffusion of drug from the internal phase to the external phase, can be overcome by employing high polymer concentration or by choosing a polymer with high molecular weight, leading to an increase in the viscosity of the internal phase and preventing drug leakage [9]. Alternatively, the pH and salt concentration in the external phase can be controlled to minimize drug solubility, and hence, diffusion into the external phase [54].
28. Application of high shear stress helps in droplet size reduction and in achieving small-sized nanoparticles by the double emulsion method. However, the second sonication step should be controlled to minimize the diffusion of hydrophilic drug to the external aqueous phase, leading to low drug loading.
29. DLS is sensitive to contamination and cannot differentiate between particle types such as the analyte particles (nanoparticles) and contaminant particles like dust or air bubbles [25, 26]. Hence, any extraneous contaminants other than the analyte can affect the measurement and give an erroneous result. Therefore, water filtered through a 0.2 μm filter is used for obtaining accurate readings.
30. DLS technique is highly dependent on sample concentration [25]. The instrument cannot accurately estimate the size of the particles if the solution is too concentrated or too dilute.

31. Gentle shaking generally helps in dispersing the particles. If the particles are not easily dispersed, vortexing or mild sonication in a bath sonicator can be helpful in dispersing the particles.
32. Follow instrument manufacturer's instructions for operating the instrument.
33. 5–10 kV setting generally works for PLA/PLGA nanoparticles. However, if the particles are observed to change shape at the high voltage, then the voltage can be set to a lower value.
34. Concentration of the nanoparticle suspension depends on the characteristics of particles and the image desired. If the particles have a tendency to stick together, a dilute suspension is preferred so that the individual particles can be imaged. Furthermore, if one desires to capture more number of particles in a field, then the suspension should be sufficiently concentrated.
35. Drying can cause the nanoparticles to clump together giving rise to black blotches in the image. The sample concentration needs to be decreased in this case.
36. Depending on the quality of the image obtained, the concentration of the negative staining solution, and staining time should be adjusted. If there are black blotches in the image, the concentration of the staining solution can be reduced (from 2 to 1 % w/v and lower) or the staining time can be decreased.
37. The sample should be introduced into the cell in the inverted position in order to not introduce bubbles. Any bubbles present in the cell should be removed before use by gentle tapping.
38. The lyophilized particles weighed should be dry and should not be in the form of a wet cake. If there is excess water in the formulation, then the amount weighed will be inaccurate and this will affect the estimation of drug loading, which is expressed as mg drug per mg particles. Storing in a desiccator is recommended for hygroscopic particles.
39. The organic solvent employed should be able to dissolve PLA/PLGA. Vortexing ensures that the drug is completely extracted from the PLA/PLGA matrix. In cases where the drug is soluble in the organic solvent, the drug content can be directly quantified in this solvent. For example, drug loading of triamcinolone acetonide in PLGA nanoparticles was determined by measuring the absorbance of the drug in chloroform at 238 nm [17].
40. Hydrophilic drugs and genes are not soluble in the organic solvent, and hence require an additional step of extraction in a second aqueous solvent. The aqueous solvent used should be capable of selectively dissolving the drug. Moreover, the choice of this solvent is also governed by the method used for

quantification. For example, extraction solvent can be kept similar to the solvent used in HPLC quantification.

41. Drug extraction into a separate phase, typically involves vortexing for 1–2 h to allow the drug to completely move into the new phase. Extraction efficiency must be calculated to ensure that the entire drug is being extracted with the method. Extraction efficiency can be determined by adding a known amount of drug to PLA/PLGA and dissolving in organic solvent and then evaporating the solvent to form a film. Films with different drug quantities in the range of interest are prepared. The drug in the film is extracted and analyzed by the same method that is used for extracting the drug from the nanoparticles. The extraction recovery should be near 100 %. If not, then the method needs to be revised either by increasing the time of vortexing for extraction or by using a different solvent for extraction. Alternatively, the drug quantities measured can be corrected for extraction efficiency, in order to estimate the actual drug loading.
42. The analytical technique selected should be sensitive and selective for the drug being analyzed.
43. Amount of particles to be weighed for analysis depends on the drug loading and solubility of the drugs. Lesser amounts can be weighed for drugs with good solubility and higher drug loading.
44. Since PLA and PLGA nanoparticles are used for sustained drug delivery, duration of release studies with these particles tends to be anywhere between 15 days and 6 months. Hence, a preservative is needed in the buffer to prevent microbial growth in the medium during the length of the study.
45. Volume of release medium chosen for the study depends on the drug solubility in the medium. The volume of medium should be at least three times that required to dissolve the total amount of drug present in the nanoparticles weighed for the study in order to maintain sink conditions.
46. The membrane should allow only the drug molecules to pass through while nanoparticles with a larger dimension should be retained in the dialysis bag. To achieve efficient separation by means of dialysis with Spectra/Por® membranes, the ratio of the molecular weights of the two species to be separated should be at least 25. Moreover, the supplier recommends selecting a membrane with a molecular weight cutoff that is about 50 % of the molecular weight of the species to be retained for achieving a minimum of 90 % retention and is 50–100 times larger than the molecular weight of the species to be eliminated for optimal separation.

47. The volume of aliquot withdrawn depends on the drug solubility and the analytical technique being used for quantification.
48. The time points selected should be such that they are able to provide information about both initial burst release and complete release of the drug from the nanoparticles.
49. To ensure there is no change in the overall volume of the release medium in the centrifuge tubes over the length of the study, aliquot withdrawn at any point of time must be replaced with an equal volume of the same buffer. Moreover, the buffer should be previously equilibrated to 37 °C to maintain physiological conditions. In cumulative drug release analysis, the volumes removed should be corrected for.
50. If the nanoparticles do not pass through a 32G needle, 30G needle can be used.

Acknowledgments

This work was supported in part by the NIH grant EY018940. The authors are thankful to lab members including Puneet Tyagi, Shelley Durazo, Ruchit Trivedi, and Dr. Jiban Jyoti Panda and past lab member Dr. Sarath Yandrapu for helpful discussions during the preparation of this chapter.

References

1. Akpek EK, Smith RA (2013) Overview of age-related ocular conditions. Am J Manag Care 19 (5 Suppl):s67–s75
2. Clark AF, Yorio T (2003) Ophthalmic drug discovery. Nat Rev Drug Discov 2 (6):448–459. doi:10.1038/nrd1106
3. Shah SS, Denham LV, Elison JR, Bhattacharjee PS, Clement C, Huq T, Hill JM (2010) Drug delivery to the posterior segment of the eye for pharmacologic therapy. Exp Rev Ophthalmol 5 (1):75–93. doi:10.1586/eop.09.70
4. Amrite AC, Ayalasomayajula SP, Cheruvu NP, Kompella UB (2006) Single periocular injection of celecoxib-PLGA microparticles inhibits diabetes-induced elevations in retinal PGE2, VEGF, and vascular leakage. Invest Ophthalmol Vis Sci 47(3):1149–1160. doi:10.1167/iovs.05-0531
5. Kompella UB, Amrite AC, Pacha Ravi R, Durazo SA (2013) Nanomedicines for back of the eye drug delivery, gene delivery, and imaging. Prog Retin Eye Res. doi:10.1016/j.preteyeres.2013.04.001
6. D'Souza SS, DeLuca PP (2006) Methods to assess in vitro drug release from injectable polymeric particulate systems. Pharm Res 23 (3):460–474. doi:10.1007/s11095-005-9397-8
7. Singh SR, Grossniklaus HE, Kang SJ, Edelhauser HF, Ambati BK, Kompella UB (2009) Intravenous transferrin, RGD peptide and dual-targeted nanoparticles enhance anti-VEGF intraceptor gene delivery to laser-induced CNV. Gene Ther 16(5):645–659. doi:10.1038/gt.2008.185
8. Mitra M, Misra R, Harilal A, Sahoo SK, Krishnakumar S (2011) Enhanced in vitro antiproliferative effects of EpCAM antibody-functionalized paclitaxel-loaded PLGA nanoparticles in retinoblastoma cells. Mol Vis 17:2724–2737
9. Astete CE, Sabliov CM (2006) Synthesis and characterization of PLGA nanoparticles. J Biomater Sci Polym Ed 17(3):247–289
10. Peyman GA, Yang D, Khoobehi B, Rahimy MH, Chin SY (1996) In vitro evaluation of

polymeric matrix and porous biodegradable reservoir devices for slow-release drug delivery. Ophthalmic Surg Lasers 27(5):384–391

11. Thombre AG, Himmelstein KJ (1984) Modelling of drug release kinetics from a laminated device having an erodible drug reservoir. Biomaterials 5(5):250–254
12. Richards Grayson AC, Cima MJ, Langer R (2004) Molecular release from a polymeric microreservoir device: Influence of chemistry, polymer swelling, and loading on device performance. J Biomed Mater Res A 69 (3):502–512. doi:10.1002/jbm.a.30019
13. Kawashima Y, Yamamoto H, Takeuchi H, Hino T, Niwa T (1998) Properties of a peptide containing DL-lactide/glycolide copolymer nanospheres prepared by novel emulsion solvent diffusion methods. Eur J Pharm Biopharm 45(1):41–48. doi:10.1016/S0939-6411(97) 00121-5
14. Gopferich A (1996) Mechanisms of polymer degradation and erosion. Biomaterials 17 (2):103–114
15. Siepmann J, Elkharraz K, Siepmann F, Klose D (2005) How autocatalysis accelerates drug release from PLGA-based microparticles: a quantitative treatment. Biomacromolecules 6 (4):2312–2319. doi:10.1021/bm050228k
16. Kompella UB, Bandi N, Ayalasomayajula SP (2003) Subconjunctival nano- and microparticles sustain retinal delivery of budesonide, a corticosteroid capable of inhibiting VEGF expression. Invest Ophthalmol Vis Sci 44 (3):1192–1201
17. Kadam RS, Tyagi P, Edelhauser HF, Kompella UB (2012) Influence of choroidal neovascularization and biodegradable polymeric particle size on transscleral sustained delivery of triamcinolone acetonide. Int J Pharm 434 (1–2):140–147. doi:10.1016/j.ijpharm.2012.05.025
18. Yang H, Tyagi P, Kadam RS, Holden CA, Kompella UB (2012) Hybrid dendrimer hydrogel/PLGA nanoparticle platform sustains drug delivery for one week and antiglaucoma effects for four days following one-time topical administration. ACS Nano 6 (9):7595–7606. doi:10.1021/nn301873v
19. Luo L, Zhang X, Hirano Y, Tyagi P, Barabas P, Uehara H, Miya TR, Singh N, Archer B, Qazi Y, Jackman K, Das SK, Olsen T, Chennamaneni SR, Stagg BC, Ahmed F, Emerson L, Zygmunt K, Whitaker R, Mamalis C, Huang W, Gao G, Srinivas SP, Krizaj D, Baffi J, Ambati J, Kompella UB, Ambati BK (2013) Targeted intraceptor nanoparticle therapy reduces angiogenesis and fibrosis in primate and murine macular degeneration. ACS Nano 7 (4):3264–3275. doi:10.1021/nn305958y
20. Cho YK, Uehara H, Young JR, Tyagi P, Kompella UB, Zhang X, Luo L, Singh N, Archer B, Ambati BK (2012) Flt23k nanoparticles offer additive benefit in graft survival and anti-angiogenic effects when combined with triamcinolone. Invest Ophthalmol Vis Sci 53 (4):2328–2336. doi:10.1167/iovs.11-8393
21. Panyam J, Dali MM, Sahoo SK, Ma W, Chakravarthi SS, Amidon GL, Levy RJ, Labhasetwar V (2003) Polymer degradation and in vitro release of a model protein from poly(D, L-lactide-co-glycolide) nano- and microparticles. J Control Release 92(1–2):173–187
22. Amrite AC, Kompella UB (2006) Nanoparticles for ocular drug delivery. In: Gupta RB, Kompella UB (eds) Nanoparticle technology for drug delivery, vol 159. Taylor and Francis Group, New York, pp 319–360
23. Shmueli RB, Bhise NS, Green JJ (2013) Evaluation of polymeric gene delivery nanoparticles by nanoparticle tracking analysis and high-throughput flow cytometry. J Vis Exp (73): e50176. doi:10.3791/50176
24. Wright M (2012) Nanoparticle tracking analysis for the multiparameter characterization and counting of nanoparticle suspensions. Methods Mol Biol 906:511–524. doi:10.1007/978-1-61779-953-2_41
25. Zolls S, Tantipolphan R, Wiggenhorn M, Winter G, Jiskoot W, Friess W, Hawe A (2012) Particles in therapeutic protein formulations, Part 1: overview of analytical methods. J Pharm Sci 101(3):914–935. doi:10.1002/jps.23001
26. den Engelsman J, Garidel P, Smulders R, Koll H, Smith B, Bassarab S, Seidl A, Hainzl O, Jiskoot W (2011) Strategies for the assessment of protein aggregates in pharmaceutical biotech product development. Pharm Res 28 (4):920–933. doi:10.1007/s11095-010-0297-1
27. Shelke NB, Kadam R, Tyagi P, Rao VR, Kompella UB (2011) Intravitreal poly(L-lactide) microparticles sustain retinal and choroidal delivery of TG-0054, a hydrophilic drug intended for neovascular diseases. Drug Deliv Transl Res 1(1):76–90. doi:10.1007/s13346-010-0009-8
28. ICH Q1A (R2) (2003) Guidance (International Conference on Harmonisation). Stability testing of new drug substances and products

29. McCrackin FL (1987) Relationship of intrinsic viscosity of polymer solutions to molecular weight. Polymer 28(11):1847–1850
30. Wang N, Wu XS, Lujan-Upton H, Donahue E, Siddiqui A (1997) Synthesis, characterization, biodegradation, and drug delivery application of biodegradable lactic/glycolic acid oligomers: I synthesis and characterization. J Biomater Sci Polym Ed 8(12):905–917
31. Dawes GJ, Fratila-Apachitei LE, Necula BS, Apachitei I, Witkamp GJ, Duszczyk J (2010) Release of PLGA-encapsulated dexamethasone from microsphere loaded porous surfaces. J Mater Sci Mater Med 21(1):215–221. doi:10.1007/s10856-009-3846-6
32. Mittal G, Sahana DK, Bhardwaj V, Ravi Kumar MN (2007) Estradiol loaded PLGA nanoparticles for oral administration: effect of polymer molecular weight and copolymer composition on release behavior in vitro and in vivo. J Control Release 119(1):77–85. doi:10.1016/j.jconrel.2007.01.016
33. Wischke C, Schwendeman SP (2008) Principles of encapsulating hydrophobic drugs in PLA/PLGA microparticles. Int J Pharm 364(2):298–327. doi:10.1016/j.ijpharm.2008.04.042
34. Kenley RA, Maryann Ott Lee T, Randolph Mahoney II, Sanders LM (1987) Poly(lactide-co-glycolide) decomposition kinetics in vivo and in vitro. Macromolecules 20(10):2398–2403
35. Wang N, Wu XS (1997) Synthesis, characterization, biodegradation, and drug delivery application of biodegradable lactic/glycolic acid oligomers: Part II Biodegradation and drug delivery application. J Biomater Sci Polym Ed 9(1):75–87
36. Park TG (1995) Degradation of poly(lactic-co-glycolic acid) microspheres: effect of copolymer composition. Biomaterials 16(15):1123–1130
37. Jalil R, Nixon JR (1990) Microencapsulation using poly (L-lactic acid) III: effect of polymer molecular weight on the microcapsule properties. J Microencapsul 7(1):41–52. doi:10.3109/02652049009028422
38. Beck LR, Pope VZ, Flowers CE Jr, Cowsar DR, Tice TR, Lewis DH, Dunn RL, Moore AB, Gilley RM (1983) Poly(DL-lactide-co-glycolide)/norethisterone microcapsules: an injectable biodegradable contraceptive. Biol Reprod 28(1):186–195
39. Braunecker J, Baba M, Milroy GE, Cameron RE (2004) The effects of molecular weight and porosity on the degradation and drug release from polyglycolide. Int J Pharm 282(1–2):19–34. doi:10.1016/j.ijpharm.2003.08.020
40. Makadia HK, Siegel SJ (2011) Poly Lactic-co-Glycolic Acid (PLGA) as Biodegradable Controlled Drug Delivery Carrier. Polymers 3(3):1377–1397. doi:10.3390/polym3031377
41. Vert M, Mauduit J, Li S (1994) Biodegradation of PLA/GA polymers: increasing complexity. Biomaterials 15(15):1209–1213
42. Yandrapu S, Kompella UB (2013) Development of sustained-release microspheres for the delivery of SAR 1118, an LFA-1 antagonist intended for the treatment of vascular complications of the eye. J Ocul Pharmacol Ther 29(2):236–248. doi:10.1089/jop.2012.0210
43. Tracy MA, Ward KL, Firouzabadian L, Wang Y, Dong N, Qian R, Zhang Y (1999) Factors affecting the degradation rate of poly(lactide-co-glycolide) microspheres in vivo and in vitro. Biomaterials 20(11):1057–1062
44. Houchin ML, Topp EM (2008) Chemical degradation of peptides and proteins in PLGA: a review of reactions and mechanisms. J Pharm Sci 97(7):2395–2404. doi:10.1002/jps.21176
45. Chu CC (1981) The in-vitro degradation of poly(glycolic acid) sutures—effect of pH. J Biomed Mater Res 15(6):795–804. doi:10.1002/jbm.820150604
46. Dunne M, Corrigan I, Ramtoola Z (2000) Influence of particle size and dissolution conditions on the degradation properties of polylactide-co-glycolide particles. Biomaterials 21(16):1659–1668
47. Jain A, Jain SK (2013) Formulation and optimization of temozolomide nanoparticles by 3 factor 2 level factorial design. Biomatter 3(2)
48. Julienne MC, Alonso MJ, Gomez Amoza JL, Benoit JP (1992) Preparation of poly(DL lactide/glycolide) nanoparticles of controlled particle size distribution: application of experimental designs. Drug Dev Ind Pharm 18(10):1063–1077. doi:10.3109/03639049209069315
49. Gomez-Gaete C, Bustos GL, Godoy RR, Saez CK, Novoa GP, Fernandez EM, Tsapis N, Fattal E (2013) Successful factorial design for the optimization of methylprednisolone encapsulation in biodegradable nanoparticles. Drug Dev Ind Pharm 39(2):310–320. doi:10.3109/03639045.2012.676049
50. Lalani J, Rathi M, Lalan M, Misra A (2013) Protein functionalized tramadol-loaded PLGA nanoparticles: preparation, optimization, stability and pharmacodynamic studies. Drug Dev Ind Pharm 39(6):854–864. doi:10.3109/03639045.2012.684390

51. Zhou YZ, Alany RG, Chuang V, Wen J (2013) Optimization of PLGA nanoparticles formulation containing L-DOPA by applying the central composite design. Drug Dev Ind Pharm 39 (2):321–330. doi:10.3109/03639045.2012.681054
52. ICH Q3C (R4) (2003) Guidance (International Conference on Harmonisation). Impurities: Guideline for Residual Solvents
53. Abdelwahed W, Degobert G, Stainmesse S, Fessi H (2006) Freeze-drying of nanoparticles: formulation, process and storage considerations. Adv Drug Deliv Rev 58 (15):1688–1713. doi:10.1016/j.addr.2006.09.017
54. Luan X, Skupin M, Siepmann J, Bodmeier R (2006) Key parameters affecting the initial release (burst) and encapsulation efficiency of peptide-containing poly(lactide-co-glycolide) microparticles. Int J Pharm 324(2):168–175. doi:10.1016/j.ijpharm.2006.06.004

Methods in Pharmacology and Toxicology (2014): 317–316
DOI 10.1007/978-1-62703-745-7

INDEX

E

F

G

H

I

M

N

O

MIX
Papier aus verantwortungsvollen Quellen
Paper from responsible sources
FSC® C105338

If you have any concerns about our products,
you can contact us on
ProductSafety@springernature.com

In case Publisher is established outside the EU,
the EU authorized representative is:
Springer Nature Customer Service Center GmbH
Europaplatz 3, 69115 Heidelberg, Germany

Printed by Libri Plureos GmbH
in Hamburg, Germany